T0259607

Bovine Theriogenology

Editor

ROBERT L. LARSON

VETERINARY CLINICS OF NORTH AMERICA: FOOD ANIMAL PRACTICE

www.vetfood.theclinics.com

Consulting Editor
ROBERT A. SMITH

July 2016 • Volume 32 • Number 2

ELSEVIER

1600 John F. Kennedy Boulevard • Suite 1800 • Philadelphia, Pennsylvania, 19103-2899

http://www.vetfood.theclinics.com

VETERINARY CLINICS OF NORTH AMERICA: FOOD ANIMAL PRACTICE Volume 32, Number 2
July 2016 ISSN 0749-0720, ISBN-13: 978-0-323-44858-1

Editor: Patrick Manley
Developmental Editor: Meredith Clinton

Veterinary Clinics of North America: Food Animal Practice (ISSN 0749-0720) is published in March, July, and November by Elsevier Inc., 360 Park Avenue South, New York, NY 10010-1710. Subscription prices are $240.00 per year (domestic individuals), $361.00 per year (domestic institutions), $100.00 per year (domestic students/residents), $265.00 per year (Canadian individuals), $476.00 per year (Canadian institutions), $335.00 per year (international individuals), $476.00 per year (international institutions), and $165.00 per year (international and Canadian students/ residents). To receive student/resident rate, orders must be accompanied by name of affiliated institution, date of term, and the signature of program/residency coordinator on institution letterhead. *Clinics* subscription prices. All prices are subject to change without notice. **POSTMASTER:** Send address changes to *Veterinary Clinics of North America*: *Food Animal Practice*, Elsevier Health Sciences Division, Subscription Customer Service, 3251 Riverport Lane, Maryland Heights, MO 63043. Customer Service (orders, claims, online, change of address): Elsevier Health Sciences Division, Subscription **Customer Service, 3251 Riverport Lane, Maryland Heights, MO 63043. Tel: 1-800-654-2452 (U.S. and Canada); 314-447-8871 (ouside U.S. and Canada). Fax: 314-447-8029. E-mail: journalscustomerservice-usa@elsevier.com (for print support); journalsonlinesupport-usa@elsevier.com (for online support).**

Reprints. For copies of 100 or more, of articles in this publication, please contact the Commercial Reprints Department, Elsevier Inc., 360 Park Avenue South, New York, NY 10010-1710. Tel.: 212-633-3874; Fax: 212-633-3820; E-mail: reprints@elsevier.com.

Veterinary Clinics of North America: Food Animal Practice is covered in *Current Contents/Agriculture, Biology and Environmental Sciences, MEDLINE/PubMed (Index Medicus), and Excerpta Medica.*

Contributors

CONSULTING EDITOR

ROBERT A. SMITH, DVM, MS
Diplomate, American Board of Veterinary Practitioners; Veterinary Research and
Consulting Services, LLC, Greeley, Colorado

EDITOR

ROBERT L. LARSON, DVM, PhD, ACT, ACAN, ACVPM-Epi
Coleman Chair, Food Animal Production Medicine, Department of Clinical Sciences,
College of Veterinary Medicine, Kansas State University, Manhattan, Kansas

AUTHORS

MATTHEW S. AKINS, PhD Dairy Science
Assistant Scientist and Extension Dairy Specialist, Department of Dairy Science,
University of Wisconsin-Madison, Madison, Wisconsin

RICARDO C. CHEBEL, DVM, MPVM
Associate Professor, Departments of Large Animal Clinical Sciences and Animal
Sciences, University of Florida, Gainesville, Florida

BETHANY J. FUNNELL, DVM
Clinical Assistant Professor, College of Veterinary Medicine, Purdue University, West
Lafayette, Indiana

ROBERT O. GILBERT, BVSc, MMedVet, MRCVS
Diplomate, American College of Theriogenologists; Professor of Reproductive Medicine,
Department of Clinical Sciences, College of Veterinary Medicine, Cornell University,
Ithaca, New York

DANIEL GIVENS, DVM, PhD
Professor of Pathobiology, Office of Academic Affairs, College of Veterinary Medicine,
Auburn University, Auburn, Alabama

W. MARK HILTON, DVM
Diplomate, American Board of Veterinary Practitioners; Clinical Professor, College of
Veterinary Medicine, Purdue University, West Lafayette, Indiana; Elanco Animal Health,
Greenfield, Indiana

RICHARD M. HOPPER, DVM
Diplomate, American College of Theriogenologists; Professor and Section Head,
Theriogenology, Food Animal Medicine and Ambulatory, Department of Pathobiology and
Population Medicine, College of Veterinary Medicine, Mississippi State University,
Starkville, Mississippi

MARIANNA M. JAHNKE, MS
Lecturer/Embryologist, Veterinary Diagnostic and Production Animal Medicine, Iowa State University College of Veterinary Medicine, Ames, Iowa

SHELIE LAFLIN, DVM
Laflin Angus Ranch, Olsburg, Kansas

GRAHAM CLIFFORD LAMB, PhD
North Florida Research and Education Center, Assistant Director and Professor, University of Florida, Marianna, Florida

ROBERT L. LARSON, DVM, PhD, ACT, ACAN, ACVPM-Epi
Coleman Chair, Food Animal Production Medicine, Department of Clinical Sciences, College of Veterinary Medicine, Kansas State University, Manhattan, Kansas

MILTON M. McALLISTER, DVM, PhD
Diplomate, American College of Veterinary Pathologists; School of Animal and Veterinary Sciences, University of Adelaide, Roseworthy, South Australia, Australia

VITOR R.G. MERCADANTE, PhD
Assistant Professor, Department of Animal and Poultry Sciences, Virginia Tech, Blacksburg, Virginia

BENJAMIN W. NEWCOMER, DVM, PhD
Assistant Professor, Department of Pathobiology, College of Veterinary Medicine, Auburn University, Auburn, Alabama

JEFF D. ONDRAK, DVM, MS
Assistant Professor, Great Plains Veterinary Educational Center, University of Nebraska-Lincoln, Clay Center, Nebraska

COLIN W. PALMER, DVM, MVSc
Diplomate, American College of Theriogenologists; Associate Professor of Theriogenology, Department of Large Animal Clinical Sciences, Western College of Veterinary Medicine, University of Saskatchewan, Saskatoon, Saskatchewan, Canada

PATRICK E. PHILLIPS, DVM
Diplomate, American College of Theriogenologist; Senior Clinician, Veterinary Diagnostic and Production Animal Medicine, Iowa State University College of Veterinary Medicine, Ames, Iowa

EDUARDO S. RIBEIRO, DVM, MSc, PhD
Assistant Professor, Department of Animal and Biosciences, University of Guelph, Guelph, Ontario, Canada

NORA SCHRAG, DVM
Assistant Clinical Professor, Field Service, Department of Clinical Sciences, Kansas State College of Veterinary Medicine, Manhattan, Kansas

JEFFREY S. STEVENSON, MS, PhD
Department of Animal Sciences and Industry, Kansas State University, Manhattan, Kansas

BRAD J. WHITE, DVM, MS
Interim Director, Beef Cattle Institute, Department of Clinical Sciences, College of Veterinary Medicine, Kansas State University, Manhattan, Kansas

Contents

A systems approach to beef cattle reproduction facilitates evaluating the flow of cattle through the herd population based on temporal changes in reproductive and production state. The previous years' timing of calving has either a positive or negative effect on the present year's reproductive success. In order to create and maintain high reproductive success, one must focus on: developing heifers to become pregnant early in the breeding season, ensuring bull breeding soundness, aligning the calving period with optimal resource availability, managing forage and supplementation to ensure good cow body condition going into calving, and minimizing reproductive losses due to disease.

Reproductive inefficiency compromises the profitability of dairy herds and the health and longevity of individual cows. In the average dairy herd, the combination of estrus detection and ovulation synchronization protocols yields the best economic return. Genomic selection of animals is particularly profitable in situations in which little is known about their genetic potential. Biosensor systems in milking parlors may allow for the design of reproductive strategies tailored for cows according to their physiologic needs while optimizing economic return.

Replacement heifer management has a large influence on the reproductive success of beef herds. Overall herd productivity increases when a high percentage of heifers become pregnant early in the first breeding season and a high percentage of first-calf heifers conceive early in the breeding season for a second pregnancy. In order to become pregnant early in the breeding season as a heifer (nulliparous), deliver a live calf, and become pregnant early in the breeding season as a first-calf cow, management of heifer development must optimize nutrition, heifer maturity at the onset of breeding, bull fertility, and overall reproductive success.

Commercial embryo transfer has evolved as an art and as a science since the early 1970s. Today's multiple ovulation embryo transfer is a widely used reproductive tool on many farms and is performed by veterinarians throughout the world. Propagation of the female genomes of select donors, through embryo transfer, has allowed a rapid progression of genetic gain in many breeds, much like what happened with artificial insemination since the 1940s. Advancement of this technology is migrating to in vitro fertilization technology today, allowing a higher volume of offspring to be produced with sex selection in the laboratory.

Postpartum diseases are common in dairy cows, and their incidence contributes to reduced fertility and increased risk of culling, making their prevention and management extremely important. Reproductive efficiency has a major impact on economic success of any dairy production unit. Optimizing reproductive efficiency contributes to overall efficiency of production units, minimizing environmental impacts and contributing to sustainability of food production. Additionally, control of reproductive diseases is important for maintenance of health and welfare of dairy cows; for minimizing use of antibiotics; and ensuring a wholesome, safe, and nutritious product.

Bovine trichomoniasis has been recognized as a pathogen of the bovine reproductive tract for nearly 100 years. Although characteristics of the causative organism, *Tritrichomonas foetus* lend to control and there are examples of disease eradication, cattle producers are still faced with this disease. This article highlights the clinical presentation, magnitude of effect, risk factors, epidemiology, and sample collection and suggests applications in developing herd-level control measures for beef cattle producers including testing strategies for control, testing strategies for surveillance, strategies to eliminate trichomoniasis from infected herds, and strategies for prevention in uninfected herds.

Both bovine viral diarrhea virus and bovine herpesvirus 1 can have significant negative reproductive impacts on cattle health. Vaccination is the primary control method for the viral pathogens in US cattle herds. Polyvalent, modified-live vaccines are recommended to provide optimal protection against various viral field strains. Of particular importance to bovine viral diarrhea control is the limitation of contact of pregnant cattle with potential viral reservoirs during the critical first 125 days of gestation.

Neosporosis is one of the most common and widespread causes of bovine abortion. The causative parasite is transmitted in at least two ways, horizontally from canids, and by endogenous transmission within maternal lines of infected cattle. The prevalence of neosporosis is higher in the dairy industry than in the beef industry because of risk factors associated with intensive feeding. There are no vaccines, but logical management options are discussed that can lower the risk of abortion outbreaks and gradually reduce the prevalence of infection within herds. Steps should be taken to prevent total mixed rations from becoming contaminated by canine feces. If a herd has a high rate of infection that is associated with abortions in heifers, then the rate of reduction of infection prevalence can be speeded by only selecting seronegative replacement heifers to enter the breeding herd. Elimination of all infected cattle is not a recommended goal.

Accurate assessment of yearling bulls is important for the bottom line of all interested parties: the buyer, the seller, and the veterinarian performing the BSE. Special considerations and current research are highlighted and their application to the evaluation of yearling bulls is discussed.

Mature bulls must be fed a balanced ration, vaccinated appropriately, and undergo a breeding soundness evaluation to ensure they meet what is required of a short, but intense breeding season. To be classified as a satisfactory potential breeder, minimum standards for physical soundness, scrotal circumference, sperm motility, and sperm morphology must be achieved using an accepted bull-breeding soundness evaluation format. Sperm production requires approximately 70 days. Heat and stress are the most common insults to spermatogenesis, causing an increase in morphologic abnormalities with obesity-associated scrotal fat accumulation being the most frequent cause of elevated testicular temperature in mature bulls.

Medical and surgical management can be used to restore a bull that has suffered a reproductive tract malady. The economic cost of treatment weighed against the bull's replacement value as well as prognosis for recovery is of prime consideration. In turn, early recognition of a treatable condition and immediate initiation of action are factors that impact both treatment cost and prognosis in many cases. Common problems are penile hair rings, fibropapillomas, vesicular adenitis, penile hematoma, and traumatic injury to the prepuce. Less frequent problems are injuries that lead to denervation of the penis, penile shunts, and penile deviation.

Video content accompanies this article at http://www.vetfood.
theclinics.com

Dystocia is an inevitable challenge in the livestock industries, particularly
with primiparous female animals. Prevention and appropriate management will decrease cow and calf morbidity and mortality, which will
improve the economic status of the beef or dairy operation. Early identification and proper intervention improves outcomes, and the use of selection tools to decrease the potential for dystocia will have positive returns.
Assisted reproductive technologies present a unique set of challenges to
the calving process that both the producer and practitioner should be prepared to address.

VETERINARY CLINICS OF NORTH AMERICA: FOOD ANIMAL PRACTICE

THE CLINICS ARE NOW AVAILABLE ONLINE!
Access your subscription at:
www.theclinics.com

Preface

Bovine Theriogenology

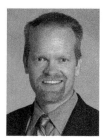

Robert L. Larson, DVM, PhD, ACT, ACAN, ACVPM-Epi
Editor

Ensuring that a high percentage of bovine females exposed to breeding by natural service and/or artificial insemination give birth to a healthy calf is critical for high efficiency of beef and milk production. High reproductive efficiency requires that heifers reach puberty at an appropriate age, that cows are fertile and able to conceive at an appropriate time postparturition, that fertile semen is delivered to the female reproductive tract via natural service by bulls or by artificial insemination at a time that is optimal for conception, that gestational pregnancy wastage is minimized, and that parturition results in the birth of a vigorous calf delivered by a healthy dam. Successful bovine reproduction is the culmination of many complex biologic processes that can each be influenced by management decisions. The purpose of this issue of *Veterinary Clinics of North America: Food Animal Practice* is to provide an overview of the current knowledge of some of the most important aspects of successful bovine reproduction for veterinary practitioners, animal scientists, students, and researchers.

I would like to thank each of the contributing authors for agreeing to allocate time from their busy schedules to organize and communicate their wealth of knowledge and experience related to the multifaceted topics addressed by each article. Each author provides practical applications to enhance the efficiency of bovine reproduction and improve animal health and well-being based on a rigorous review of the available literature that combines a commitment to the scientific method with the need for effective action steps that can be taken at the herd and individual animal levels.

I would also like to extend my thanks to Meredith Clinton and the staff at Elsevier for their support during production. I believe that the contributing authors and Elsevier editors who have devoted so much time to create a valuable resource should be very proud of the final product. Last, I would like to thank my wife and family for their love

Vet Clin Food Anim 32 (2016) xi–xii
http://dx.doi.org/10.1016/j.cvfa.2016.05.001
0749-0720/16/$ – see front matter © 2016 Published by Elsevier Inc.

vetfood.theclinics.com

and support as they make going to work each morning and coming home at the end of the day truly a blessing.

Robert L. Larson, DVM, PhD, ACT, ACAN, ACVPM-Epi
Department of Clinical Sciences
College of Veterinary Medicine
Kansas State University
1800 Denison Avenue
Manhattan, KS 66506-5606, USA

E-mail address:
RLarson@vet.k-state.edu

Reproductive Systems for North American Beef Cattle Herds

Robert L. Larson, DVM, PhD, ACT, ACVPM-Epi*, Brad J. White, DVM, MS

KEYWORDS

- Beef cattle • Reproductive momentum • Postpartum anestrous
- Heifer development • Breeding soundness examination of bulls • Veterinary services

KEY POINTS

- A systems approach to beef cattle reproduction recognizes the diversity of interacting components that affect herd-level reproductive efficiency and that the whole system is more than the sum of its parts.
- The systems approach facilitates evaluating the flow of cattle through the herd population based on temporal changes in reproductive and production state.
- The previous year's timing of calving has either a positive or negative effect on the present year's reproductive success.
- The ability of cow herds to maintain a 365-day calving interval requires active management of the impact that age and body condition have on the length of postpartum infertility.

INTRODUCTION

A systems approach to beef cattle reproduction recognizes the diversity of interacting components that affect the number of calves weaned per cow present in the herd at the start of the breeding season, and the need to recognize that the whole system is more than the sum of its parts.[1,2] The systems approach facilitates an evaluation of the dynamic reproductive system in beef cow-calf herds by evaluating flow of cattle through the production unit based on temporal changes in reproductive and production state. An important concept within a systems approach to beef herd reproduction is the realization that the previous year's timing of calving has either a positive or

Disclosure: The authors have received grants, or research contracts, from the National Cattlemen's Beef Association, the United States Department of Agriculture, Zoetis Animal Health, Merck & Company, CEVA Biomune, Boehringer Ingelheim Vetmedica, and Merial Animal Health.
Department of Clinical Sciences, College of Veterinary Medicine, Kansas State University, 1800 Denison Avenue, Manhattan, KS 66506, USA
* Corresponding author.
E-mail address: RLarson@vet.ksu.edu

Vet Clin Food Anim 32 (2016) 249–266
http://dx.doi.org/10.1016/j.cvfa.2016.01.001
0749-0720/16/$ – see front matter © 2016 Elsevier Inc. All rights reserved.

negative effect on this year's reproductive success. This article defines herd momentum as the impact of historical reproductive outcomes on the subsequent herd reproductive performance.

CONSTRAINING BIOLOGICAL REALITIES AFFECTING BEEF REPRODUCTION

A few key facts regarding biological constraints of beef cow-calf production systems must be known to accurately model the flow of cows through several stages of reproduction:

- A reproductive system that optimizes beef cow-calf production requires that nutritional demands (primarily energy and protein) for mature (multiparous) cows that vary throughout the production year based on pregnancy and lactation status can be met by available grazed forage and body reserves with limited need for supplementation. This system requires that herd managers consider the timing of calving and peak lactation as well as mature cow size and lactation level relative to the nutrient levels present in available grazed forage.[3,4]
- In order to match the cow production cycle with the forage production cycle, it is necessary for beef cows to calve at about the same time each year (ie, at 365-day intervals).
  - Nutritional requirements vary throughout the production cycle with highest energy and protein requirements occurring during early lactation and the lowest requirements occurring during midgestation when the cows are not lactating.[5–7]
  - Nutrients available per acre of grazed forage vary throughout the year with highest levels coinciding with vegetative growth and lower levels occurring when plants are dormant.[8,9] The timing of highest forage productivity is influenced by the mixture of species and time of year.
  - Plotting lactation curves for cows with peak lactations of 4.5, 9.1, or 13.6 kg (10, 20, and 30 pounds) of milk production per day shows that high nutritional demands of lactation coincide with the breeding season when targeting a calving interval of 365 days (**Fig. 1**).

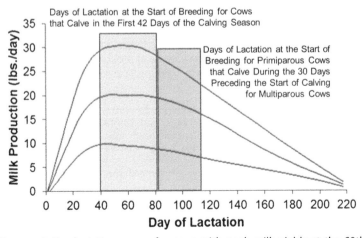

Fig. 1. Representative lactation curves for cows with peak milk yields at the 60th day of lactation of 4.5, 9.1, or 13.6 kg (10, 20, or 30 lb).

- Overall cow costs (eg, depreciation, land, feed, labor) are reduced if heifers calve by 24 months of age rather than delaying breeding to result in calving at 36 to 48 months of age.[10]
- In order for beef heifers to reach puberty at an age consistent with breeding to calve at 23 months of age, average daily weight gain from weaning to breeding must be sufficient to reach expected body weight at puberty (typically 55%–65% of mature body weight). This rate of weight gain is difficult to achieve on forage alone; therefore, growing heifers usually require supplementation with feeds that exceed the energy density of moderate-quality forage.
- Recognizing that there are 283 days of gestation means that there are 82 days from the time a cow calves to the time it needs to become pregnant again to maintain a 365-day calving interval.
- Although cattle are able to become pregnant anytime throughout the year (nonseasonal reproduction), cattle managers prefer that beef herds give birth during short (2-month to 3-month) predetermined times of the year that optimize the forage production of a region or to meet some other management or marketing goal (eg, uniformity of calf crop and ability to manage calves as a more homogenous unit).
- Female cattle have 21-day estrous cycles such that, approximately every 21 days, a nonpregnant, fertile heifer or cow expresses behavior that initiates mating and ovulates an oocyte (egg).
- The likelihood of a fertile mating resulting in pregnancy that can be detected 50 days later is 60% to 70%.[11]
  ○ Following approximately 30% of matings between a fertile female and a fertile bull either fertilization fails to take place or fertilization occurs and an early embryo is formed but, because of the complexity of mammalian reproduction, the embryo is imperfect and dies within the first 14 days.
  ○ When fertilization fails or an embryo is lost before day 14 of gestation, the cow expresses estrus and ovulates a fertile oocyte about 21 days after her last estrus and has another 60% to 70% probability of conceiving and maintaining a pregnancy.
- Beef cows have a period of time after calving, called postpartum anestrus, when they do not display the behavioral aspects of estrus necessary to initiate mating and they do not ovulate fertile eggs.
  ○ Postpartum anestrus in mature (multiparous) cows lasts an average of about 50 to 80 days if the cows are in good body condition and is prolonged if cows are thin[12–16] (**Table 1**).
  ○ Although reporting the average length of time from calving to the resumption of fertile estrous cycles for mature cows is informative, it is important to recognize that approximately one-half of cows in groups described by these averages do not resume fertile cycles during that length of time.
  ○ A more important length of time to know is how long it takes for 90% of cows in a herd to resume fertile cycles. An estimate of 70 to 100 days from calving to the resumption of fertile cycles for 90% of the cows is reasonable for many herds if the average length of postpartum anestrus is 50 to 80 days (**Fig. 2**).
  ○ Important assumption: cows that calve in good body condition during the first 42 to 52 days of calving are likely to resume fertile cycles before the start of breeding or during the first 21 days of breeding, meaning that this group of cows are the only cows that are likely to become pregnant in the first 21 days of the breeding season. In contrast, cows that calve later than the

Table 1
Mean length of postpartum anestrous in beef cows

Cow Description	Treatment Groups	Mean Length of Postpartum Anestrous (d)
Brangus females: cows and heifers Rutter and Randel,[12] 1984	BCS 7 at calving 90% NRC postpartum	57.5
	BCS 7 at calving 100% NRC postpartum	40.3
	BCS 7 at calving 110% NRC postpartum	34.7
Charolais × Angus cows Houghton et al,[13] 1990	Low energy prepartum (7.4 Mcal/d) + low energy postpartum (10.1 Mcal/d)	72.6 33.3% in estrus w/n 60
	Low energy prepartum (7.4 Mcal/d) + high energy postpartum (16.9 Mcal/d)	54.3 56.3% in estrus w/n 60
	Maintenance energy prepartum (10.6.4 Mcal/d) + low energy postpartum (10.1 Mcal/d)	65.7 52.9% in estrus w/n 60
	Maintenance energy prepartum (10.6.4 Mcal/d) + high energy postpartum (16.9 Mcal/d)	68.4 54.3% in estrus w/n 60
4-year-old cows Perry et al,[14] 1991	70% NRC energy prepartum + 70% NRC energy postpartum	0% ovulated by 150
	70% NRC energy prepartum + 150% NRC energy postpartum	96 (of those that ovulated) (83% ovulated by 150)
	150% NRC energy prepartum + 70% NRC energy postpartum	74 (of those that ovulated) (29% ovulated by 150)
	150% NRC energy prepartum + 150% NRC energy postpartum	74 (100% ovulated by 150)
Mature cows Cushman et al,[15] 2007	Simmental-sired cows (BCS 6)	55.5
	Gelbvieh-sired cows (BCS 6)	57.5
	Red Angus–sired cows (BCS 6)	60.8
	Hereford-sired cows (BCS 6)	61.2
	Charolais-sired cows (BCS 6)	62.6
	Angus-sired cows (BCS 6)	62.9
	Limousin-sired cows (BCS 6)	66.7
Multiparous cows Lents et al,[16] 2008	<5 BCS at calving	93.1
	≥5 BCS at calving	63.5
First-calf heifers Ciccioli et al,[17] 2003	BCS 4–5 at calving Fed to gain 450 g (1 lb)/d postpartum	120
	BCS 4–5 at calving Fed to gain 900 g (2 lb)/d postpartum	100
First-calf heifers Berardinelli and Joshi,[18] 2005	Not exposed to bulls	84–88
	Exposed to bulls	68–71

Abbreviations: BCS, body condition score; NRC, national research council; w/n, within.

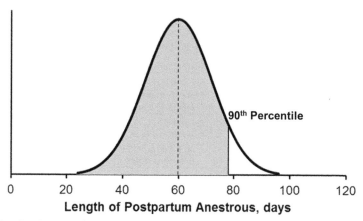

Fig. 2. The distribution of postpartum anestrous length for a cow herd if the distribution is nearly normal with a mean of 60 days and a standard deviation of 12 days.

52nd day of calving are not likely to resume fertile cycles until the second 21 days of the breeding season or later (**Table 2**).

- The timing of calving in the current calving season affects the timing of breeding in the subsequent breeding season; therefore, cow-calf herds have inherent momentum from year to year. This momentum can be positive (most cows calve early in the calving season and breed early in the following breeding season) or negative (most cows calve late in the calving season and breed late in the following breeding season).
- Herd reproductive momentum is important to consider when implementing changes to improve reproductive performance.
  - The average length of time for the postpartum anestrous period is longer following the first (primiparous) pregnancy (80–100 days)[17,18] compared with later (multiparous) pregnancies (50–80 days).
    - In order to schedule the start of calving for the mature herd at the same date each year, first-calf heifers (primiparous cows) need to calve at least 100 days ahead of breeding, which means that heifers must calve in good body condition at least 20 days ahead of the mature cows to ensure that they have resumed fertile cycles by the start of breeding for their second pregnancies.
    - Many primiparous cows require 100 days or more to resume fertile estrous cycles. Evaluating primiparous cows to determine the percentage that have resumed fertile cycles by observing behavioral estrus, detecting the presence of corpus luteum (CL) via palpation or ultrasonography, or measuring blood progesterone levels that exceed a predetermined cutoff such as 1 ng/mL allows veterinarians to determine herd-specific estimates for the length of postpartum anestrus in this important cohort of breeding females.
- Cows with 3 opportunities to be mated to a fertile bull (each with a 65% probability of a successful pregnancy) during a breeding season have a 96% probability of giving birth to a calf at the end of gestation (**Table 3**). Animals in the herd expected to have completed the postpartum anestrous period and to be having fertile estrous cycles by the start of the subsequent breeding season include:
  - Nearly all mature (multiparous) cows that calve in good body condition during the first 21 days of calving

Table 2
Effect of timing of calving on the likelihood of having 90% of mature cows to resume fertile cycles by the start of breeding and every 21 days thereafter based on a target of 70 to 100 days

Cows that Calve During the First 21 d of Calving Season

Days between calving and start of breeding	62–82 d More than one-half are likely to have resumed fertile cycles
Days between calving and end of first 21 d of breeding	83–103 d Even if thin at the time of calving, 90% are likely to be having fertile cycles by end of first 21 d of breeding if grazing high-quality forage

Cows that Calve During the Second 21 d of Calving Season

Days between calving and start of breeding	41–61 d Up to one-half will have resumed fertile cycles if calve in good body condition (particularly those calving in the first half of the second 21 d)
Days between calving and end of first 21 d of breeding	62–82 At least one-half are likely to have resumed fertile cycles if calved in good body condition and have access to diet that maintains body weight
Days between calving and end of second 21 d of breeding	83–103 d Even if thin at the time of calving, 90% are likely to be having fertile cycles by end of second 21 d of breeding if grazing high-quality forage

Cows that Calve During the Third 21 d of Calving Season

Days between calving and start of breeding	20–40 d Not expected to be having fertile cycles at the start of the breeding season
Days between calving and end of first 21 d of breeding	41–61 d Up to one-half will have resumed fertile cycles if calve in good body condition (particularly those calving in the first half of the third 21 d)
Days between calving and end of second 21 d of breeding	62–82 d At least one-half are likely to have resumed fertile cycles if calved in good body condition and have access to diet that maintains body weight
Days between calving and end of third 21 d of breeding	83–103 d Even if thin at the time of calving, 90% are likely to be having fertile cycles by end of third 21 d of breeding if grazing high-quality forage

Cows that Calve During the Fourth 21 d of Calving Season

Days between calving and start of breeding	0–19 d Almost impossible to be having fertile cycles at the start of the breeding
Days between calving and end of first 21 d of breeding	20–40 d Not expected to be having fertile cycles at the end of the first 21 d of the breeding season
Days between calving and end of second 21 d of breeding	41–61 d Up to one-half will have resumed fertile cycles if calve in good body condition (particularly those calving in the first half of the third 21 d)

(continued on next page)

Table 2 (continued)	
Days between calving and end of third 21 d of breeding	62–82 d At least one-half are likely to have resumed fertile cycles if calved in good body condition and have access to diet that maintains body weight
Days between calving and end of fourth 21 d of breeding	83–103 d Even if thin at the time of calving, 90% are likely to be having fertile cycles by end of fourth 21 d of breeding if grazing high-quality forage

- ○ At least one-half of multiparous cows that calve in good body condition in the second 21 days
- ○ First-calf heifers (primiparous cows) that calve before the start of the multiparous cow calving season
- Cows with 2 opportunities to be mated to a fertile bull during a breeding season have about an 84% to 91% probability of becoming pregnant and maintaining a pregnancy to the end of gestation (see **Table 3**). Cows with only 2 or fewer opportunities for mating include:
  - ○ Mature (multiparous) cows that give birth to a calf more than 42 days after the start of the calving season
  - ○ First-calf heifers (primiparous cows) that calve after the start of the mature (multiparous) cow calving season
  - ○ Primiparous or multiparous cattle that are thin and have a prolonged period of postpartum anestrus[19]

REPRODUCTIVE GOALS FOR BEEF CATTLE HERDS

- Two key measures of reproductive success in beef cow herds are:
  - ○ The percentage of cows that become pregnant in the first 21 days of the breeding season
  - ○ The percentage of cows that become pregnant in the first 60 to 65 days of the breeding season
- A herd with a very good reproductive profile (depicted by the percentage of the herd that becomes pregnant in each 21-day interval) can achieve 95% pregnancy success in a breeding season approximately 63 days long (**Fig. 3**).

Table 3 Expected percentages of bovine females present in a beef cow-calf herd at the start of a breeding season that become pregnant and maintain a pregnancy based on the pregnancy success per mating and the number of mating opportunities in the breeding season			
	Mating Opportunities (%)		
Pregnancy Success Per Mating (%)	**1**	**2**	**3**
55	55	80	91
60	60	84	94
65	65	88	96
70	70	91	97

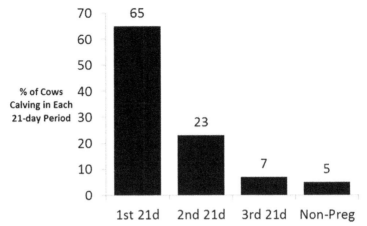

Fig. 3. A front-end loaded reproductive profile with 65% of the herd becoming pregnant (or calving) in the first 21 days of the breeding (calving) season and 65% of remaining cows becoming pregnant (calving) in each of the subsequent 21-day periods. Non-Preg, nonpregnant.

- First 21 days: ideally 60% to 65% of the herd becomes pregnant in the first 21 days. To achieve this goal, nearly every cow needs to be cycling by the end of the first 21 days of the breeding season and the bulls must be fertile and pregnancies maintained once they are established.
- Second 21 days: fertile cows that failed to conceive or maintain a pregnancy from the first mating have another normal estrus cycle and have another 60% to 70% probability to become pregnant at the next estrus approximately 21 days later, resulting in another 23% of the herd becoming pregnant in the second 21 days of the breeding season.
- Third 21 days: if fertile cows have not established a pregnancy after 2 matings, 60% to 70% of the remaining cows in the third 21 days of the breeding season will become pregnant, leaving the herd with about 5% nonpregnant cows after a 63-day breeding season.
- Herds should be managed so that most cows have 3 opportunities to be mated by fertile bulls in a short (eg, 60–75 days) breeding season.
  - If all cows are cycling and bulls are fertile, 3 opportunities for breeding should allow 95% (or a herd-specific goal selected to optimize economic return) of cows to conceive and maintain a pregnancy.
- Herds should be front-end loaded, in that 60% or more of the cows should establish a viable pregnancy in the first 21 days and 85% of the cows in the herd become pregnant in the first 2 cycles.
- Maintain high pregnancy success and front-end loading every year (positive reproductive momentum) regardless of forage production variation and risk of injury, disease, and other vagaries of beef cattle production.
  - In order to create and maintain herd positive reproductive momentum, it is necessary to focus on developing heifers to become pregnant early in the breeding season, ensuring bull breeding soundness, aligning the calving period with optimal resource availability, managing forage and supplementation to ensure good cow body condition going into calving, and minimizing reproductive losses caused by disease.

PRODUCTION AND REPRODUCTION BENEFITS OF FRONT-END LOADING

- Front-end loaded herds produce weaned calves that have greater average age and body weight compared with non–front-end loaded herds that have the same breeding season and weaning dates, but that do not have a high percentage of the calves born in the first 21 days of the calving season (**Fig. 4**, Document S1).
- Overall percentage of exposed cows that become pregnant and the percentage of cows that become pregnant in the first 21 days of the breeding season have significant impact on the weight weaned per cow exposed. Numerous studies have indicated that there are substantial profitability differences between cow-calf producers; although cost-control is of primary importance in this profitability spread, differences in calving percentage and weight weaned per cow exposed between ranches also has a significant impact on profitability.[4,20–22]
- A front-end loaded herd is likely to have the same calving distribution in subsequent years because of the effect of momentum in beef herd reproduction:
  - Cows that calve early in the calving season can complete the postpartum anestrus period before the start of the breeding season and be eligible for breeding early in the season.
  - Calving early in the season leads to increased lifetime weight of calves weaned as well as increased longevity in the herd.[23]
  - Increased herd longevity decreases cow depreciation costs, which is one of the major expenses associated with long-term cow ownership.
- Land, labor, feed, and breeding costs for the mature (multiparous) cows do not need to be increased to obtain a front-end loaded herd if the calving season and mature cow size are appropriately matched to available resources.

IDENTIFICATION OF THE OPTIMUM BREEDING SEASONS (MULTIPAROUS AND NULLIPAROUS COWS)

- Reproductive momentum in beef herds is created when nulliparous (replacement) heifers are selected and developed so that the entire cohort of replacement heifers calves early enough to have a sufficient (80–100 days or more) period of time between calving and the start of the breeding season to resume fertile estrous cycles before the start of the breeding season for the second pregnancy.
  - This system results in the first-calf heifers (primiparous cows) having 3 potential estrous cycles to establish a viable pregnancy for their second calf if exposed to a 65-day breeding season.
  - Cows that calve early in their second calving season have ample time to resume fertile estrous cycles before the start of their third breeding season and have 3 opportunities to establish a viable pregnancy.
  - Increasing the front-end loading of the heifers and mature cows establishes positive momentum because a greater percentage of the herd is fertile and cycling at the start of the subsequent breeding season.
- Timing of calving of replacements that are pregnant with their first calves relative to the onset of the mature cow herd calving season has an important impact on herd reproductive momentum.
  - The breeding period for replacement (nulliparous) heifers should begin and end before the breeding period for mature (multiparous) cows.
  - Because the period of postpartum anestrous is prolonged following the birth of the first calf, few first-calf heifers (primiparous cows) are expected to have

A

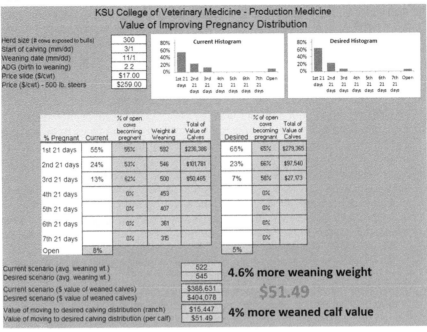

B

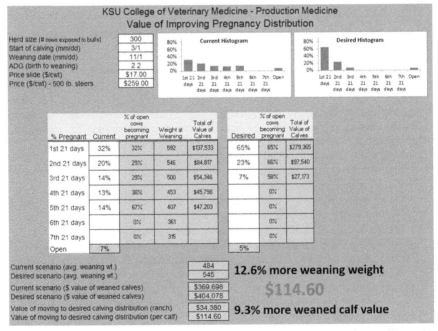

Fig. 4. Comparison of the weaning weight and gross income advantage from selling calves from a herd with an ideal pregnancy distribution to a herd with (*A*) a good, but not ideal, pregnancy distribution; and (*B*) a herd with only 50% of cows cycling at the start of a prolonged breeding season.

resumed fertile cycles by 62 to 82 days after calving and it takes 100 or more days until all or nearly all have fertile estrous cycles.

- ○ Replacement heifers that have their first calves late enough that they have not resumed fertile estrous cycles by the end of the first 21 days of the breeding only have 1 or 2 opportunities to become pregnant in a 65-day breeding season; consequently, about 12% to 35% are expected to be nonpregnant at the end of the breeding season.
  - These heifers likely have normal reproductive potential, but are limited in the number of days eligible for breeding following the period of postpartum anestrus.
- ○ Extending the breeding season longer than 65 days allows more cows to become pregnant, but cows that conceive more than 52 days after the start of breeding are unlikely to begin fertile estrous cycles until the second or later 21-day period of the breeding season, and cows that conceive more than 82 days after the start of breeding do not calve until after the start of the following breeding season. This scenario is described as negative reproductive momentum.
- The desired timing of the onset and length of the breeding season for nulliparous heifers is influenced by:
  - ○ The desire to optimize calving timing of the mature cows in the herd based on forage availability, marketing, or labor constraints.
  - ○ The length of the period of postpartum anestrous of first-calf (primiparous) cows.
- Once the first day of the breeding season necessary to obtain the optimum multiparous cow calving season is identified by a herd manager, the expected length of the postpartum anestrous period needed to ensure that a high percentage of first-calf heifers (primiparous cows) have resumed fertile estrous cycles can be subtracted to identify the last day of the calving season for the replacement heifers.
- The length of the replacement heifer breeding season (and subsequent calving season) should be long enough to allow 1 or more matings based on management goals.
- Use of estrous synchronization protocols to cause a high percentage of the replacement cohort to express a fertile estrus or ovulate a fertile oocyte at the start of the identified breeding season results in the most breeding opportunities for the cohort for any selected breeding season length.
  - ○ For example, most fertile heifers (heifers showing estrus and ovulating a fertile oocyte) in a cohort exposed to a 42-day breeding season are expected to have 2 opportunities to be mated, with a few heifers (those expressing estrus on the first or second day of the breeding season) having 3 opportunities.
  - ○ If estrous synchronization is implemented, most cycling heifers in the cohort have 3 opportunities to be mated in the same 42-day breeding season.
  - ○ Studies have indicated that about 60% to 70% of bovine matings result in a viable pregnancy at midgestation.[11] Using this range of pregnancy success, an expected percentage of cycling replacement heifers that should become pregnant in a controlled breeding season can be calculated based on the length of the breeding season and the subsequent expected number of mating opportunities (see **Table 3**).

BULL CONSIDERATIONS FOR OBTAINING AND MAINTAINING FRONT-END LOADING (POSITIVE MOMENTUM FROM ONE YEAR TO THE NEXT)

- Bulls represent a significant monetary investment associated with purchase price, housing costs, feed, and veterinary care.

- Bulls also serve as a source of risk to the ranch, with poor reproductive performance having a great impact on the percentage of heifers and cows that become pregnant and the average calf age at weaning.
- Careful attention to selection based on predictions of genetic contribution to desirable traits, management to protect health, breeding soundness examination to remove bulls with questionable breeding ability, and appropriate bull/cow breeding ratios are required to optimize the investments that ranchers make in their bulls.
- A breeding soundness examination of bulls (BSEB) is a comprehensive examination of the bull to estimate his ability to successfully initiate pregnancy.
  - Breeding soundness examinations of bulls before each breeding season are done to reduce the risk that breeding failure is caused by inadequate semen volume, sperm cell fertilizing ability, and semen delivery.
  - Although individual situations vary, 10% to 20% or more of bulls perform poorly in the breeding pasture.[24–27]
  - The overall effect of BSEB is to eliminate many infertile bulls and to improve the genetic base for fertility within the herd and breed.
- Carefully monitor bulls during the breeding season.
  - Semen quality can deteriorate after a bull passes a BSEB, but in most situations in which the quality and quantity of sperm production decline significantly in a previously fertile bull, the bull shows at least moderate signs of illness or injury.
  - Bulls should be evaluated frequently to detect any early signs of injury, excessive weight loss, or illness; if problems are detected, affected bulls should be replaced by fertile bulls.
  - Although many matings occur at times that are not convenient for observation, witnessing successful matings ensures that a bull is able to mount and breed effectively, which justifies the time and effort to watch for matings.
- An adequate number of bulls that are fertile and able to inseminate cows must be present throughout the breeding season.
  - In a front-end loaded herd, the greatest demand is at the beginning of the breeding season, and the number of fertile bulls required declines rapidly as a high percentage of the herd becomes pregnant during the first 21 days.
  - In a herd that is not front-end loaded, the number of fertile bulls required to breed cows in estrus may not peak until midway through the breeding season. Because bulls are likely to be the healthiest, most injury free, and most fertile at the beginning of the breeding season, the likelihood of adequate numbers of fertile bulls per cow in estrus is higher in front-end loaded herds than in herds that fail to have high numbers of cycling cows until later in the breeding season.

DISEASE CONTROL CONSIDERATIONS FOR OBTAINING AND MAINTAINING FRONT-END LOADING (POSITIVE MOMENTUM FROM ONE YEAR TO THE NEXT)

- Biosecurity is the attempt to keep infectious agents (eg, bacteria, virus, fungi, parasites) away from a herd. One aspect of biosecurity is a vaccination program that improves the immunity of cattle against the infectious agents that they may encounter.
- For most North American beef herds, the potential list of antigens in a vaccination program includes brucellosis, infectious bovine rhinotracheitis (IBR), bovine viral diarrhea (BVD), vibriosis (campylobacteriosis), and leptospirosis.

○ Some herds at high risk of exposure to trichomoniasis benefit from use of the vaccine to decrease the magnitude of pregnancy loss. However, the vaccine is not expected to prevent an exposed herd from becoming infected or to replace testing and culling strategies to prevent or eradicate herd infections.
- Herd additions (replacement females and bulls) should only be purchased from herds with a known and effective vaccination and disease prevention program.
  ○ Avoid purchasing animals from unknown sources or that have been mixed with other cattle before sale.
  ○ Herd additions should be isolated from the resident herd for at least 1 month before introduction to the herd. Isolated cattle should not share feeders, waterers, or airspace (distance depends on wind velocity and direction). During the isolation period the additions should be tested for and vaccinated against transmissible diseases.

OPTIONS TO MOVE A POOR REPRODUCTIVE PROFILE TO A FRONT-END LOADED PROFILE

- Determine what caused the profile to become poor and correct; considerations include:
  ○ Heifers are bred to calve at a time that does not allow many in the cohort to become pregnant early in the breeding season for their second pregnancy
  ○ Bull failure (eg, subfertility, insufficient number of bulls) that delayed the establishment of pregnancy even though cows were having fertile cycles
  ○ Pregnancy wasting disease that delayed or ended pregnancy
  ○ Cows (particularly primiparous cows) that calve in thin body condition and have a prolonged period of postpartum anestrus so that many cows in the herd have not resumed having fertile cycles when expected based on days since calving
- Postpartum anestrous in lactating cows is difficult to appreciably shorten by moderately increasing the energy density of the diet.[17,28,29]
  ○ An appropriate level of energy to maintain body condition is necessary for cows to express expected length of postpartum anestrous (ie, not prolonged). However, increased energy density of the diet (eg, provision of high-quality forage or supplementation of moderate-quality forage with an energy-dense concentrate) is not expected to transition a herd with a poor reproductive profile to a herd with a front-end loaded distribution.
- Estrous synchronization protocols that include progestogens or gonadotropin-releasing hormone can shorten the period of postpartum anestrus in cows with sufficient time since calving. However, this intervention, applied 7 to 30 days ahead of breeding, will affects few cows that calve later than the first 40 to 50 days of the calving season (ie, at least 30–40 days postpartum by start of breeding), and herds with a poor reproductive profile are not likely to have enough cows that calve in the first 40 to 50 days to improve the pregnancy distribution appreciably.
- Short-term (48-hour) weaning of calves can shorten the period of postpartum anestrus by several days in cows with sufficient time since calving. However, this intervention applied 2 days ahead of breeding (80 days after the first multiparous cow calves) is only expected to affect cows that calve in the first 40 to 50 days of the calving season.
- Because it is difficult to change the pregnancy profile of the primiparous and multiparous cows in the herd, making the herd profile more front-end loaded

requires that replacement (nulliparous) heifers are developed so that they can calve ahead of the mature herd with sufficient time before the start of the breeding season for their second pregnancies so that nearly all of the cohort has resumed fertile cycles and can be mated during the first 21 days.

- ○ Replacements that become pregnant at a time that does not allow a reasonable expectation for resumption of fertile cycles by the end of the first 21 days of the breeding season for their second pregnancies must not be added to the herd if the profile is to be improved.
- ○ Herds that have a poor reproductive profile have a low number of heifers born early in the calving season, and must either obtain heifers from outside sources that meet the genetic, structural, and behavioral standards for the herd or keep a high percentage of the herd's heifers, develop them postweaning to meet a conservative target weight (60%–65% of expected mature weight) by the start of breeding, and only keep as replacements those that will calve ahead of the mature cows.
- Replacing 15% of the herd each year for 4 years with heifers that calve ahead of the cows and that are likely to become pregnant during the first 21 days of their second breeding season results in nearly 60% of the cows that comprised the original pregnancy distribution being replaced by animals that have the potential to maintain front-end loading. Four years into a management effort focused on front-end loading, a herd with a previously poor pregnancy distribution will only consist of cows from the original distribution that calved early and herd additions selected to calve early.

VETERINARY SERVICES ASSOCIATED WITH NORTH AMERICAN BEEF HERD REPRODUCTIVE SYSTEMS

- Veterinarians provide 3 types of service that help ranchers meet their economic goals (**Table 4**):
  - ○ First, to increase herd income by enhancing reproductive and growth efficiency as well as improving the market value of all cattle sold
  - ○ Second, to help control costs through nutritional and input cost counseling
  - ○ Third, to protect the herd from biological and economic losses caused by disease and injury
- The income side of cow-calf ranches is driven by reproductive efficiency and market value of cattle sold.
  - ○ Reproductive efficiency is often measured by calculating the weight (or value) of calves sold divided by the number of cows exposed for breeding.
  - ○ Calf weight at weaning is greatly influenced by age at weaning. Calves born early in the calving season weigh more and therefore are worth more dollars than calves that are born later in the calving season. To ensure older calves, strategies must be used that result in cows becoming pregnant early in the breeding season.
  - ○ In order to achieve high reproductive success, nearly all the replacement heifers and cows need to be cycling by the start of the breeding season. In order for mature cows to be cycling at the start of the breeding season, they need to have calved in the first 42 to 52 days of the calving season in good body condition.
  - ○ Because cycling cows can only become pregnant if they are mated to fertile bulls, doing breeding soundness examinations in the weeks leading up to the breeding season ensures that infertile bulls are not counted on to get cows pregnant in the breeding pastures.

Table 4
Veterinary services associated with establishing and maintaining an optimum reproductive profile

	Interventions	Timing
Cow and Heifer Considerations		
Body condition	BCS at appropriate times, forage management, and supplement formulation	Midgestation and 60 d before calving
Heifer selection and development	Select heifers born early	Weaning
	Select crossbred heifers and heifers from sires with EPD for scrotal circumference and heifer pregnancy that ensures adequately young age at puberty	Weaning
	Plan ration to meet goal of 55%–65% of mature weight before start of breeding	Weaning to breeding
	Breeding soundness examination 1–45 d before start of breeding (reproductive tract score, weight, pelvic area)	Yearling
Herd-specific age at puberty	Reproductive tract evaluation before breeding allows estimation of the age when 90% (or an appropriate target percentage based on overall herd goals) of a herd's heifers will reach puberty	Yearling
Heifer breeding	Estrous synchronization and AI to calving ease bull	Breeding
	Limit breeding season to 45 d or less	
Primiparous cows (first-calf heifers)	Estrous detection or palpation of CL to estimate when 90% of primiparous cows resume fertile cycles after calving	Breeding
Bull Considerations		
BSEB yearlings	Complete physical examination: feet, legs, walking, lungs, skin, eyes, and so forth (and visually recheck during breeding season)	1–30 d before breeding season
	Examine penis (yearlings): warts, persistent frenulum, hair rings	
	Palpate testicles (soft, fibrotic, scrotal hematoma, scrotal frostbite)	
	Examination of accessory sex glands: seminal vesicles	
	Evaluate semen: motility, sperm morphology	
BSEB mature	Complete physical examination: feet, legs, walking, lungs, skin, eyes, and so forth (and visually recheck during breeding season)	1–30 d before breeding season
	Examine penis (mature): deviations of penis, failure to extend, hematoma	
	Palpate epididymis (spermatocele, sperm granuloma, epididymitis)	
	Examination of accessory sex glands: seminal vesicles	
	Evaluate semen: motility, sperm morphology	

(continued on next page)

Table 4
(continued)

	Interventions	Timing
Diseases Considerations		
Trichomonas	Test at-risk bulls (preputial scrapings: 3×)	Before breeding
Neospora	Limited	—
IBR	Vaccinate annually	Before breeding
BVD	Biosecurity to prevent contact with persistently infected cattle and vaccinated annually	Before breeding
Leptospirosis	Vaccinate (and sanitation to lesser extent)	Midgestation
Fungal/toxins	Feed quality and access	Gestation

Abbreviations: AI, artificial insemination; EPD, expected progeny differences.

- ○ Veterinarians can also provide advice and services to monitor heifer selection and development from weaning through breeding by monitoring body weight, body condition, skeletal size, and reproductive tract maturity.
- The cost side of the cow-calf business ledger is controlled by optimizing grazing forage use, supplementation plans, and input purchases.
  - ○ Although other expertise is often necessary to optimize grazing management, veterinarians can use data collected throughout the year to evaluate the appropriateness of the herd's stocking density and cow maintenance requirements as determined by genetic selection for mature size, growth, and milking ability.
  - ○ Veterinarians can assist producers to attain high reproductive productivity by monitoring mature cow body condition at several key times in the year, particularly in midgestation to late gestation and from a few weeks before the start of the calving season to the next breeding season.
  - ○ Veterinary data that provide information about the appropriateness of the current genetic selection and grazing management strategies include body condition scores, percentage of pregnant cows exposed to bulls, and the amount of supplemental feed needed to maintain current body condition scores.
- An additional area of veterinary advice and services that affects a rancher's bottom line is the need to provide reasonable protection against health risks.
  - ○ Abortion-causing diseases and diseases or injuries that affect bull health and the bulls' ability to get a high percentage of the herd pregnant in a controlled breeding season can be damaging to the reproductive efficiency and economic health of a cow-calf operation.
  - ○ Veterinarians can help to optimize the use of vaccines, testing, and quarantine of herd additions, and management strategies to limit breeding herd exposure to infectious disease, toxins, parasites, and physical dangers.

SUPPLEMENTARY DATA

Supplementary data related to this article can be found at http://dx.doi.org/10.1016/j.cvfa.2016.01.001.

REFERENCES

1. Ebersohn JP. A commentary on systems studies in agriculture. Agric Syst 1976;3: 173–84.

2. Rountree JH. Systems thinking – some fundamental aspects. Agric Syst 1977;4: 247–54.
3. Mulliniks JT, Rius AG, Edwards MA, et al. Improving efficiency of production in pasture- and range-based beef and dairy systems. J Anim Sci 2015;93:2609–15.
4. Ramsey R, Doye D, Ward C, et al. Factors affecting beef cow-herd costs, production, and profits. J Ag Appl Econ 2005;37:91–9.
5. Buskirk DD, Lemenager RP, Horstman LA. Estimation of net energy requirements (NEm and NEΔ) of lactating beef cows. J Anim Sci 1992;70:3867–76.
6. National Research Council. Nutrient requirements of beef cattle. 7th edition. Washington, DC: National Academy Press; 1996.
7. Larson RL. Heifer development – reproduction and nutrition. In: Olson KC, editor. Veterinary clinics of North America: food animal practice bovine nutrition, vol. 23. Philadelphia: WB Saunders; 2007. p. 53–68.
8. Varel VH, Kreikemeier KK. Low- and high-quality forage utilization by heifers and mature beef cows. J Anim Sci 1999;77:2774–80.
9. Brink GE, Jackson RD, Alber NB. Residual sward height effects on growth and nutritive value of grazed temperate perennial grasses. Crop Sci 2013;53: 2264–74.
10. Núñez-Dominquez R, Cundiff LV, Dickerson GE, et al. Lifetime production of beef heifers calving first at two vs three years of age. J Anim Sci 1991;69:3467–79.
11. BonDurant RH. Selected diseases and conditions associated with bovine conceptus loss in the first trimester. Theriogenology 2007;68:461–73.
12. Rutter LM, Randel RD. Postpartum nutrient intake and body condition: effect on pituitary function and onset of estrus in beef cattle. J Anim Sci 1984;58:265–74.
13. Houghton PL, Lemenager RP, Horstman LA, et al. Effects of body composition, pre- and postpartum energy level and early weaning on reproductive performance of beef cows and preweaning calf gain. J Anim Sci 1990;68:1438–46.
14. Perry RC, Corah LR, Cochran RC, et al. Influence of dietary energy on follicular development, serum gonadotropins, and first postpartum ovulation in suckled beef cows. J Anim Sci 1991;69:3762–73.
15. Cushman RA, Allan MF, Thallman RM, et al. Characterization of biological types of cattle (Cycle VII): influence of postpartum interval and estrous cycle length on fertility. J Anim Sci 2007;85:2156–62.
16. Lents CA, White FJ, Ciccioli NH, et al. Effects of body condition score at parturition and postpartum protein supplementation on estrous behavior and size of the dominant follicle in beef cows. J Anim Sci 2008;86:2549–56.
17. Ciccioli NH, Wettemann RP, Spicer LJ, et al. Influence of body condition at calving and postpartum nutrition on endocrine function and reproductive performance of primiparous beef cows. J Anim Sci 2003;81:3107–20.
18. Berardinelli JG, Joshi PS. Introduction of bulls at different days postpartum on resumption of ovarian cycling activity in primiparous beef cows. J Anim Sci 2006;83:2106–10.
19. Waldner CL, Guerra AG. Cow attributes, herd management, and reproductive history events associated with the risk of nonpregnancy in cow-calf herds in Western Canada. Theriogenology 2013;79:1083–94.
20. Bruce LB, Torrell RC, Hussein HS. Profit predictions in cow-calf operations: part 2, influence of major management practices. J Prod Agri 1999;12:647–9.
21. Miller AJ, Faulkner DB, Knipe RK, et al. Critical control points for profitability in the cow-calf enterprise. Prof Anim Sci 2001;17:295–302.
22. Dhuyvetter KC. Differences between high, medium, and low profit producers: an analysis of 2006-2010 Kansas Farm Management Association cow-calf

enterprise. 2011. Am-KCD-2011.2. Available at: http://www.agmanager.info/livestock/budgets/production/beef/Cow-calf_EnterpriseAnalysis(Jun2011).pdf.

23. Cushman RA, Kill LK, Funston RN, et al. Heifer calving date positively influences calf weaning weights through six parturitions. J Anim Sci 2013;91:4486–91.

24. Carson RL, Wenzel JGW. Observations using the new bull-breeding soundness evaluation forms in adult and young bulls. Vet Clin North Am Food Anim Pract 1997;13:305–11.

25. Parkinson TJ. Evaluation of fertility and infertility in natural service bulls. Vet J 2004;168:215–29.

26. Kastelic JP, Thundathil JC. Breeding soundness evaluation and semen analysis for predicting bull fertility. Reprod Domest Anim 2008;43:368–73.

27. Van Eenennaam AL, Weber KL, Drake DJ. Evaluation of pull prolificacy on commercial beef cattle ranches using DNA paternity analysis. J Anim Sci 2014;92:2693–701.

28. Marston TT, Lusby KS, Wettemann RP, et al. Effects of feeding energy or protein supplements before or after calving on performance of spring-calving cows grazing native range. J Anim Sci 1995;73:657–64.

29. Lalman DL, Williams JE, Hess BW, et al. Effect of dietary energy on milk production and metabolic hormones in thin, primiparous beef heifers. J Anim Sci 2000;78:530–8.

Reproductive Systems for North American Dairy Cattle Herds

Ricardo C. Chebel, DVM, MPVM[a,b,*], Eduardo S. Ribeiro, DVM, MSc, PhD[c]

KEYWORDS

- Dairy cattle • Reproductive efficiency • Reproductive management • Economics

KEY POINTS

- Reproductive inefficiency compromises the health and longevity of individual cows and the profitability of herds.
- In the average dairy herd, the combination of estrous detection and ovulation synchronization protocols yields the best economic return.
- Genomic selection of animals is particularly profitable in situations in which little is known about their genetic background.
- Biosensor systems in milking parlors may allow for the design of reproductive strategies tailored for cows according to their physiologic needs while optimizing economic return.

INTRODUCTION

Reproductive management of dairy animals has been marked by extensive progress in the past 50 years, from the creation of prostaglandin drugs (prostaglandin F2 alpha [PGF$_{2\alpha}$]) that allow the synchronization of estrus in the 1970s to the implementation of on-farm *in vitro* embryo production programs and the use of genomic selection to aid in breeding strategies. Such progress has been realized because reproductive efficiency has long been identified as critical for the profitability of dairy herds. Herds with efficient reproductive programs benefit from having a large proportion of cows in the most productive phase of lactation,[1] greater availability of replacement animals, greater genetic progress,[2,3] reduced proportion of reproduction culls,[4,5] reduced

Disclosure: The authors have nothing to disclose.
[a] Department of Large Animal Clinical Sciences, University of Florida, 2030 Shealy Drive, Gainesville, FL 32608, USA; [b] Department of Animal Sciences, University of Florida, 2030 Shealy Drive, Gainesville, FL 32608, USA; [c] Department of Animal Biosciences, University of Guelph, 50 Stone Road East, Guelph, Ontario N1G 2W1, Canada
* Corresponding author. Department of Large Animal Clinical Sciences, University of Florida, 2030 Shealy Drive, Gainesville, FL 32608.
E-mail address: rcchebel@ufl.edu

Vet Clin Food Anim 32 (2016) 267–284
http://dx.doi.org/10.1016/j.cvfa.2016.01.002
0749-0720/16/$ – see front matter © 2016 Elsevier Inc. All rights reserved.
vetfood.theclinics.com

cost of reproductive programs,[2,4] and improved health. Furthermore, improved reproductive performance might reduce emission of greenhouse gases because of the reduced number of animals per unit of production and the reduced retention of replacement animals.[6,7]

For years, fertility in dairy cows has declined in multiple regions of the world and diverse production systems.[8–11] Changes in cow physiology associated with greater milk production, nutritional management, housing, increased herd size, reduced expression of estrus, and genetic makeup of the dairy cattle population have been identified as reasons for the decrease in reproductive efficiency.[8,12,13] Nonetheless, the downward trend in reproductive efficiency has been virtually halted because of the extensive progress in the knowledge of reproductive biology, physiology, and management.[14] For example, calving interval (CI) has declined significantly in the past 10 years (**Fig. 1**A), most likely because of reduced calving to first artificial insemination (AI) interval (**Fig. 1**B, C).[14] The positive trend in daughter pregnancy rate (DPR) observed in the past 10 years (**Fig. 1**D)[14] may be a result of more controlled voluntary waiting periods (VWPs) and shorter calving to first AI intervals. However, the importance of modern genetic selection programs that have focused on milk yield, productive life, reproduction, and health should not be disregarded.[3,6,13]

REPRODUCTIVE EFFICIENCY AND DAIRY HERD PROFITABILITY

The income of dairy herds is mainly originated from sales of milk (88% of gross income), cows for dairy purposes, cull animals, and calves (12% of gross income),[15] whereas the largest expenses are associated with feeding the herd (60% of total operating costs) and rearing replacement animals (25% of total operating costs).[15] Reproductive efficiency affects the profitability of dairies in several ways that are not always easy to account for. Improved reproductive performance has many beneficial effects: increased efficiency of milk production by shifting the milking herd to a more productive phase of the lactation[1]; improved income over feed cost (IOFC) and milk yield per day of CI[16]; reduced reproductive culls,[5] reduced need for replacement animals and increased percentage of the lactating herd that is multiparous[4,15]; improved genetic gain because of more selective culling of lactating cows and more stringent selection of replacement animals[13,15]; and, reduced cost of reproductive interventions.[2,4] However, significant improvement in reproductive performance results in a greater proportion of the adult herd dry,[4] demanding proper planning to accommodate dry cows and maternity needs.

The lactation curve and the dry matter intake (DMI) of mature cows determine that the efficiency of milk production is significantly greater during early versus late lactation (**Fig. 2**).[16] Consequently, the highest efficiency of milk production is achieved when most of the cows in a herd conceive within the first 100 days in milk (DIM). For example, consider 2 herds that have a VWP of 50 days, an average DIM at first AI of 60 days, and cows that are eligible to become pregnant for 13 consecutive cycles (from 50 to 312 DIM). In the herd with average milk yield of 12,500 kg per 305 days of lactation, improving 21-day pregnancy rates (PR; i.e., the percentage of eligible cows that become pregnant every 21 days) from 12% to 33% would reduce the average CI by 63 days (from 440 to 377 days) and result in an increase of 7% in the IOFC and 1.51 kg of milk per cow per day of CI (551 kg of milk per cow per year; **Fig. 3**A).[16] If the same improvements in 21-day PR are achieved in the herd with average milk yield of 9000 kg per 305 days of lactation, IOFC would increase 8% and milk yield would increase by 1.11 kg per cow per day of CI (405 kg of milk per cow per year;

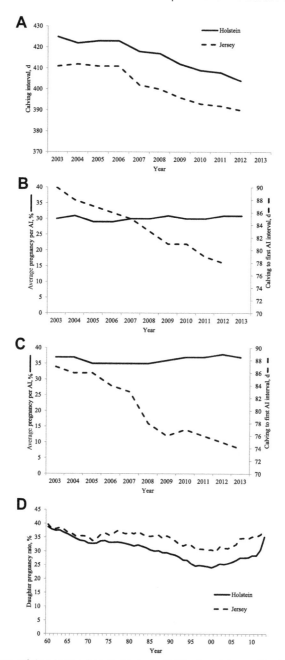

Fig. 1. (*A*) Average calving interval in Holstein (*solid line*) and Jersey (*dashed line*) cows in dairy herd improvement programs in the United States. (*B*) Average pregnancy per AI (*solid line*) and interval from calving to first postpartum AI (*dashed line*) among Holstein cows enrolled in dairy herd improvement programs in United States. (*C*) Average pregnancy per AI (*solid line*) and interval from calving to first postpartum AI (*dashed line*) among Jersey cows enrolled in dairy herd improvement programs in United States. (*D*) Average DPR of Holstein (*solid line*) and Jersey (*dashed line*) sires. (*Data from* Norman HD, Walton LM, Durr J. Reproductive status of cows in dairy herd improvement programs and bred using artificial insemination. Council on Dairy Cattle Breeding; 2013. Available at: https://www. cdcb.us/publish/dhi/current/reproall.html.)

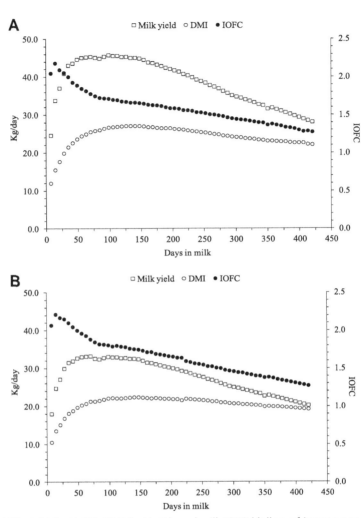

Fig. 2. Milk yield (kg/d; □), DMI (kg/d; ○), and milk IOFC (dollars of income per dollars of feed consumed; •) according to days in milk. Milk price was set at $0.35/kg in all scenarios. (*A*) High-producing herd (12,500 kg per 305 days of lactation) with feed price at $0.35/kg of dry matter. (*B*) A moderate-producing herd (9000 kg per 305 days of lactation) and feed price at $0.29/kg of dry matter. (*From* Ribeiro ES, Galvão KN, Thatcher WW, et al. Economic aspects of applying reproductive technologies to dairy herds. Anim Reprod 2012;9:370–87.)

Fig. 3B).[16] The economic gains of improving reproductive performance in herds with higher productivity and more persistent lactation curve may not be as dramatic.[17]

The economic value of improved reproductive performance is not easily determined, is particular for given production systems, and is affected by several factors. Several researchers have created models to estimate the value of increasing 21-day PR or reducing the calving to pregnancy interval (days open) according to different scenarios. De Vries[17] suggested that the cost of a day open varies from $0 to $6.00 depending on DIM, milk production and price, feeding costs, persistency of lactation curve, lactation number, culling policies, and availability of replacement heifers. Groenendaal and colleagues[18] estimated the cost of a day open to be $1.25, $2.10, and

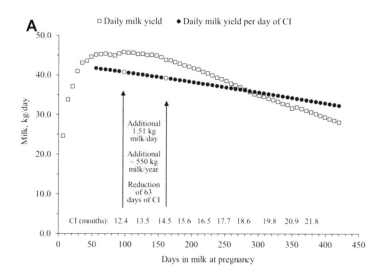

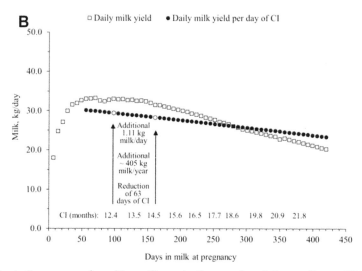

Fig. 3. Lactation curve and resulting milk production per day of CI according to DIM at pregnancy in a high-producing herd (12,500 kg in 305 days of lactation [A]) and in a moderate-producing herd (9000 kg of milk in 305 days of lactation [B]). (*From* Ribeiro ES, Galvão KN, Thatcher WW, et al. Economic aspects of applying reproductive technologies to dairy herds. Anim Reprod 2012;9:370–87.)

$2.75 up to 90, 150, and 210 DIM, respectively. Researchers have also created models to estimate the value of newly established pregnancies and the cost of pregnancy losses. De Vries[17] proposed that the difference in retention pay off (RPO; the economic benefit of keeping a cow in the herd vs. culling and replacing it with a replacement heifer) of pregnant and nonpregnant cows provides an estimate of the value of a new pregnancy (assuming equal milk yield, DIM, lactation curve persistency, and lactation number).[19] According to this theory, the value of a pregnancy is less early postpartum because there is little difference in RPO between pregnant and nonpregnant cows. The value of a pregnancy increases dramatically in later stages of lactation. For example, when evaluating 2 cows in later stages of lactation with equal milk yield, lactation curve persistency, and lactation number, it is more profitable to replace the nonpregnant cow for a replacement heifer, whereas it is profitable to keep the pregnant cow.[19] According to De Vries,[17] establishing a new pregnancy in the early stages of lactation is highly valuable for low-producing cows and cows with low persistency of the lactation curve but establishing a new pregnancy too early postpartum in high-producing cows and cows with high persistency of the lactation curve may result in economic losses.[19] The value of a new pregnancy has been estimated to range from −$100 to $500[19] and from $128 to $232.[20] In contrast, the cost of a pregnancy loss ($0 to $1373[19]; $128 to $897[20]) increases as stage of lactation, stage of gestation, and milk yield increase.[19]

The aforementioned research may lead to the suggestion that reproductive management should be tailored to the individual to optimize economic return. Although this may be possible in small herds, and in the future in large herds, the present reality of large herds demands reproductive management systems that are robust and meet the needs of most cows in a group. With that in mind, many herds adopt robust reproductive strategies for first postpartum AI and reinsemination of all cows,[21] and some herds adopt different VWP according to parity. The average VWP is approximately 55 days in US dairy herds, with nearly 75% of dairies having a VWP of 41 to 60 DIM (**Fig. 4**),[22] and the average interval from calving to first AI is 78 ± 0 and 74 ± 0.1 days for Holstein and Jersey cows, respectively.[14] The VWP should be established based on the anticipated optimum time for establishment of pregnancy and on the reproductive efficiency of the herd. In most herds it is not possible to precisely control when a cow becomes pregnant and it is necessary to adopt a short VWP. **Fig. 5** shows the estimated VWP for herds according to the desired interval from calving to pregnancy and 21-day PR, maintaining a maximum of 13 reproductive cycles. To achieve an average days open of 110 days, herds with 21-day PR less than 25% need to have VWPs less than 50 DIM, which is often associated with reduced

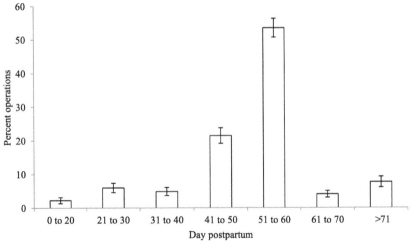

Fig. 4. Observed VWP in dairy farms in the United States according to a recent survey. (*Data from* Norman HD, Walton LM, Durr J. Reproductive status of cows in dairy herd improvement programs and bred using artificial insemination. Council on Dairy Cattle Breeding; 2013. Available at: https://www.cdcb.us/publish/dhi/current/reproall.html.)

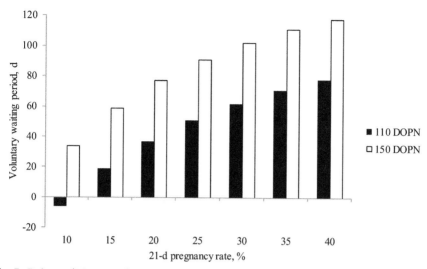

Fig. 5. Estimated VWP to achieve median days open (DOPN) of 110 or 150 days according to the 21-day pregnancy rate (breeding cycles kept constant = 13). Negative VWP values are the result of calculations and are not possible to achieve.

fertility. In contrast, herds that need to achieve 150 days open and have 21-day PR greater than 25% may have VWPs greater than 80 DIM. De Vries[17] suggested that the ideal interval from calving to pregnancy is, on average, 133 days for first-lactation cows and 112 days for second-lactation cows, but could be reduced to 63 and 51 days for cows with low production and low lactation persistency. In summary, herds with reduced milk yield, poor lactation curve persistency, and low 21-day PR must have short VWP and aggressive reproductive management. In contrast, herds with persistent lactation curves, high milk yield, and increased 21-day PR may benefit from extending the VWP.

Greater reproductive efficiency reduces the number of reproductive culls, which affects replacement policies because dairy managers may make culling decisions based on economic aspects rather than biological considerations.[18] In most scenarios, reduced reproductive efficiency forces managers to either reduce selection pressure, otherwise number of lactating cows may be reduced, affecting cash flow, or purchase replacement heifers to replace cows culled for reproduction failure, jeopardizing genetic improvement and the biosecurity of the herd. Dairies that have efficient reproductive management often have a surplus of replacement heifers.[4] Rearing replacement heifers accounts for approximately 25% of the total cost of dairy operations,[15] but herds with good reproductive performance may be more selective in replacement selection and may profit from the sale of heifers for dairy purposes.

REPRODUCTIVE EFFICIENCY AND BREEDING STRATEGIES

Development of $PGF_{2\alpha}$ in the 1970s produced significant advancements in reproductive management of dairy cattle. Although $PGF_{2\alpha}$ treatment causes luteolysis and induces estrus in a large proportion of cyclic animals, accuracy and efficiency of estrous detection are variable and depend on animal, environmental, and management factors.[23–25] In the late 1990s, ovulation synchronization protocols (OVSPs; eg, Ovsynch[26]) were developed, allowing the fixed-time AI of cows while producing acceptable pregnancy per AI (P/AI; number of cows pregnant divided by the number of cows inseminated). Implementation of OVSP for timed AI increases yearly profit per cow by $30 compared with AI on detected estrus (DE) alone[27] and reduces the cost per pregnancy by 80 to $148 compared with AI on DE alone.[17]

The use of OVSP for timed AI of lactating dairy cows has become popular to the point of some producers using it exclusively to manage their herds. However, questions arise concerning what is the most profitable reproductive management strategy (eg, 100% OVSP, 100% AI on DE, combination of OVSP and AI on DE). To answer this question, it is important to consider a few facts. One of the most important is that identification of nonpregnant cows following AI may be done by observed return to estrus or by nonpregnancy diagnosis. In most herds that adopt estrous detection, 40% to 60% of nonpregnant cows are observed in estrus and reinseminated between 3 and 28 days after a previous AI (average 22 days). In contrast, nonpregnancy diagnosis by transrectal ultrasonography may be done as early as 26 days after AI with proper accuracy and efficiency and, if an aggressive OVSP for timed AI is adopted, cows could be reinseminated as early as 29 days after previous AI. Thus, the interval to reinsemination in herds that adopt estrous detection may be reduced by 4 or more days when compared with herds that do not reinseminate cows based on signs of estrus. Although this may lead to the suggestion that adopting estrous detection is advisable, this is not always the case. In herds in which efficiency of estrous detection is high but accuracy is low, it may be deleterious to increase the number of cows inseminated in estrus. Giordano and colleagues[28] indicated that when P/AI of cows inseminated in estrus is 25%, increasing the percentage of cows inseminated in estrus from 30% to 80% decreases net return per cow per year from −$7.91 to −$14.84 per cow per year compared with 100% OVSP and timed AI. Tenhagen and colleagues[29] showed that when P/AI of cows inseminated in estrus is adequate (35%–40%) and the estrous detection rate is approximately 55%, herds may rely more heavily on AI on DE but when estrous detection rate is extremely low (<30%) it may be more advantageous to implement aggressive OVSP for timed AI. Galvão and colleagues[4] simulated in a herd of 1000 cows the best economic outcomes of reproductive programs that used 100% OVSP and timed AI with differing levels of compliance (85% and 95%), 100% AI on DE with differing levels of efficiency (40% and 60%) and accuracy (85% and 95%), and a combination of OVSP and timed AI and AI on DE. Pregnancies per AI of the different protocols were estimated from the literature. According to this simulation, the reproductive programs that resulted in the best return per cow per year, the greatest 21-day PR, and the shortest average DIM were programs that combined OVSP for timed AI and AI on DE.[4] As expected, poor compliance with OVSP and poor estrous detection efficiency and accuracy had important detrimental effects on the profitability of the herds (**Fig. 6**).[4] According to Kalantari and Cabrera[30] the best economic return was obtained when 80% of cows were inseminated on DE, P/AI of cows inseminated on DE was 35%, and P/AI of cows inseminated at fixed time following OVSP were 30% and 28% for first AI and reinseminations, respectively. This finding raises an important topic that is often overlooked when discussing reproductive management of lactating dairy cows and heifers: labor force. Proper training and education of the labor involved in all aspects of reproductive management is fundamental for the success of such programs. Veterinarians and consultants have a prime opportunity to make themselves indispensable to dairy producers when they become involved in training, educating, and monitoring the performance of the labor involved in these tasks. In conclusion, no single reproductive management strategy fits all dairy herds in North America. Before a reproductive management strategy is recommended, it is important to evaluate facilities (eg, freestall, open lots, tie stalls) and management (eg, severe overstocking), personnel (eg, training, education),

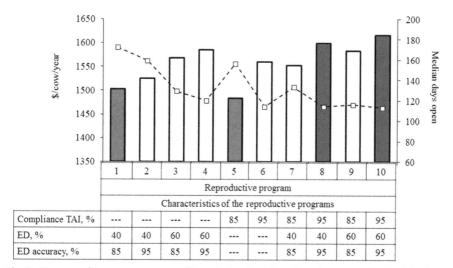

Characteristics of the reproductive programs									
Compliance TAI, %	---	---	---	---	85	95	85	95	85	95
ED, %	40	40	60	60	---	---	40	40	60	60
ED accuracy, %	85	95	85	95	---	---	85	95	85	95

Fig. 6. Mean profit per cow per year ($/cow/y; bars) and median days open (dashed line) according to 10 breeding programs. Milk price set at $0.44/kg. Red bars represent the breeding programs with the lowest profit per cow per year and the green bars represent the breeding programs with the highest profit per cow per year. ED, estrous detection; TAI, timed artificial insemination. (*Data from* Galvão KN, Federico P, De Vries A, et al. Economic comparison of reproductive programs for dairy herds using estrous detection, timed artificial insemination, or a combination. J Dairy Sci 2013;96:2681–93.)

herd composition (eg, breed, percentage of first lactation cows), adoption of new technologies, record keeping, and cow health.

Automated estrous detection systems (eg, pedometers or activity monitors) have had greater penetration in the US dairy industry in the past 10 years. These systems predict estrus with 70% to 80% accuracy based on changes in behavioral patterns[31] and their performance is comparable with that of mount detection devices.[32] Although it has often been suggested that the adoption of automated estrous detection systems in the management of dairy herds may eliminate the need for OVSP for timed AI and reduce hormone use in dairy herds, this is not necessarily true. Unquestionably, herds with poor estrous detection efficiency and accuracy may benefit significantly from the use of automated estrous detection systems. However, the automated estrous detection systems do not detect in estrus cows that do not display estrus (eg, anovular cows). In recent experiments, 7% to 44% of cows were not detected in estrus by such systems.[32–34] Therefore, most herds that adopt automated estrous detection systems still need to implement OVSP for timed AI of cows that do not display estrus. The cost of the automated estrous detection systems may easily be compensated for by significant improvements in estrous detection efficiency and accuracy, which lead to improved 21-day PR. Thus, it may be assumed that herds with low estrous detection efficiency and poor P/AI of cows inseminated on DE would realize economic gains when adopting automated estrous detection systems, particularly when such systems have long durability. Furthermore, automated estrous detection systems may help to optimize the timing of insemination of heifers and lactating cows with sex-sorted semen and improve their P/AI,[35,36] which may be an attractive strategy for herds that desire a larger pool of replacement heifers.

According to the NAHMS (2009)[22], 25% of the dairy calves born in the United States are from cows sired by natural service.[22] Although many producers defend the use of natural service with the belief that reproductive performance may be improved compared with AI systems, epidemiologic studies have shown that reproductive performance is not altered[37] or worsened[38] for natural service compared with AI based on DE or OVSP systems. Lima and colleagues[39,40] compared reproductive performance and economic return of reproductive management based on 100% OVSP for timed AI versus 100% natural service. The OVSP for timed AI was aggressive to ensure timely reinsemination of cows that failed to conceive to a previous AI. Similarly, sires were aggressively managed and underwent a breeding soundness examination every 3 months (including trichomoniasis screening), the bull to open cow ratio was 1:20, exposure period to rest period pattern was 14:14 days, and bulls were evaluated weekly for health problems and replaced if necessary. The median interval to pregnancy was slightly shorter for the natural service (111 vs 116 days) but, because of the cost of feeding sires and gains in genetic merit by using semen for timed AI, the economic return was approximately $32.47 per cow per year greater for the 100% OVSP for timed AI versus the 100% natural service.[39,40] In summary, natural service may be a reproductive strategy for managers who do not have the ability to manage the activities necessary for AI (estrous detection or OVSP, labor, semen inventory, inventory of AI consumables); however, natural service is not a strategy to improve the reproductive performance or genetic composition of the herd, and it is more costly than AI programs.

REPRODUCTIVE EFFICIENCY AND HEALTH

Although constantly overlooked, reproductive efficiency also is associated with overall health of dairy herds and individual cow health. As mentioned earlier, improved reproductive efficiency reduces both the number of reproductive culls[5] and the need for replacement heifers,[4] whereas the availability of replacement heifers increases.[4] Therefore, herds with efficient reproductive management that are not expanding do not need to purchase replacement heifers to maintain a constant number of lactating cows in the herd, reducing the risk of a breach in biosecurity and introduction of contagious and infectious diseases.

Improved reproductive performance is also expected to improve the health of individual cows. Success of the reproductive program and gestation length determine the CI. In most herds the dry period is constant (45–60 days in most US dairy herds)[22] and extending the CI results in cows spending a larger amount of time in the less efficient stages of lactation.[1] Therefore, cows that do not conceive promptly after the VWP tend to gain a significant amount of body fat reserves during the final stages of lactation, even when herds adjust rations according to milk yield. According to a large data set (8989 lactations from 2 CA herds), body condition score (BCS) at dry-off was mainly explained by 305-day mature equivalent milk yield, interval from calving to establishment of pregnancy, and number of lactations (**Fig. 7**; Chebel and Mendonça, unpublished data, 2012). In general, there was a positive correlation between interval from calving to conception and BCS at dry-off and a negative correlation between 305-day mature equivalent milk yield and BCS at dry-off.

Excessive accumulation of fat poses a significant risk for the health of periparturient dairy cows because obese cows have more dramatic immunosuppression during this period than thinner cows.[41,42] Predisposing factors for reduced innate immune function during the prepartum period are hormonal alterations associated with parturition,[43] reduced DMI,[44] increased concentrations of nonesterified fat acids and beta-hydroxy butyrate,[44–47] and decreased concentration of insulin-like growth factor-1.[48,49] Consequently, conditions that limit DMI and exacerbate negative energy balance during the periparturient period increase the risk of infectious diseases.[50]

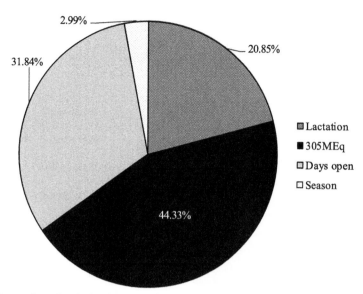

Fig. 7. Proportion of variation in BCS at dry-off accounted for by 305-day mature equivalent milk yield, interval from calving to pregnancy (days open), lactation, and season (winter vs summer). R^2 of multivariate model = 0.184 (Chebel and Mendonça, unpublished data, 2012).

Obese cows (BCS ~ 4.0) had reduced DMI during the last 21 days of gestation and had a more dramatic decrease in DMI from 21 to 1 day before calving.[51] Furthermore, BCS 21 days before calving explained 9.7% of the variability in DMI from 21 to 1 day before calving.[51] Consequently, obese cows are more likely to lose BCS and body weight during the periparturient period than thinner cows.[52,53] In a model that explained 38.7% of the variability in BCS change during the dry period, BCS at dry-off explained 90.6% of its variability (**Fig. 8**; Chebel and Mendonça, unpublished data, 2012). The association between BCS loss during the dry period and incidence of postpartum diseases also was investigated. Loss of BCS during the prepartum period increased the likelihood of diseases such as retained fetal membranes, metritis, and digestive disorders and increased the likelihood of cows being removed from the herd within 30 and 60 DIM (**Table 1**; Chebel and Mendonça, unpublished data, 2012).

In summary, excessive BCS at dry-off reflects poor milk yield and/or poor reproductive efficiency. Obese cows have compromised immune and metabolic functions in the prepartum period and are more likely to present postpartum health disorders. Because the occurrence of metabolic and infectious diseases early postpartum has a negative impact on reproductive performance,[25,54] a so-called revolving-door scenario is established, jeopardizing the lifetime production of cows.

THE ROLE OF GENOMIC SELECTION IN REPRODUCTIVE MANAGEMENT OF DAIRY HERDS

Genetic selection of the Holstein breed was focused mainly on milk yield until approximately 10 years ago. However, a negative correlation exists between genetic traits for milk yield and other traits, including reproductive efficiency.[55,56] Consequently, compared with genetically inferior cows for milk yield, a population of genetically superior cows for milk yield presents important physiologic and behavioral alterations that may, at least in part, be the cause of the reduced reproductive efficiency observed

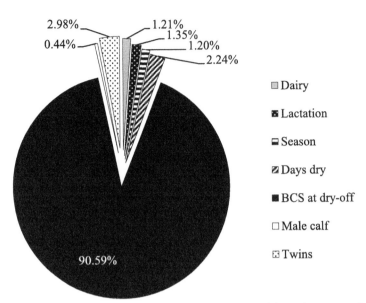

Fig. 8. Proportion of variation in BCS loss accounted for by herd, lactation, season (winter vs summer), length of the dry period, BCS at dry-off, calf sex, and number of calves (singleton vs twins). R^2 of multivariate model = 0.387 (Chebel and Mendonça, unpublished data, 2012).

from the 1950s to the beginning of the current century. A breeding project that started in 1964 at the University of Minnesota provides evidence that genetic selection for high milk yield is associated with physiologic alterations of dairy cows that affect fertility. Cows bred continuously with semen of sires and sons of sires with predicted

Table 1
Association between BCS change during the dry period and incidence of postpartum health disorders, removal from the herd within 30 and 60 DIM, and rate of removal from the herd up to 305 days postpartum (Chebel and Mendonça, unpublished data, 2012)

Items	≥+0.25	0	−0.25 to −0.5	≤−0.75	P Value
		BCS Change During the Dry Period			
Cows, n (%)	1384 (15)	3852 (43)	3551 (40)	202 (2)	—
RFM (%)	3.0[a,B]	3.4[a,B]	5.5[b]	7.4[B]	<.01
Metritis (%)	10.0[a]	12.3[a]	15.7[b,A]	20.8[b,B]	<.01
GI disorders, %	2.6[a]	2.4[a]	4.8[b]	9.9[c]	<.01
At least 1 disease (%)	15.0[a,c,A]	17.4[a]	24.7[b,B]	34.2[c]	<.01
Removal by 30 DIM (%)	3.0[a]	2.8[a]	5.1[b]	12.9[c]	<.01
Removal by 60 DIM (%)	5.1[a]	4.5[a]	7.6[b]	15.4[c]	<.01
Culling rate (AHR and 95% confidence interval)	0.88[a] (0.77, 1.01)	Reference[a]	1.14[b] (1.04, 1.25)	1.73[c] (1.36, 2.19)	<.01

Abbreviations: AHR, adjusted hazard ratio; GI, gastrointestinal; RFM, retention of fetal membranes.
[a,b,c] Within a row, values with different superscripts differ ($P < 0.05$).
[A,B] Within a row, values with different superscripts differ ($0.05 < P < 0.10$).

transmitting ability (PTA) milk average for the 1960s (unselected = 6890 ± 403 kg per 305-day lactation) have milk yield ~4000 kg per 305-day lactation less than cows bred continuously to sires with the highest PTA milk from each year (selected = 11,078 ± 329 kg per 305-day lactation).[57,58] Unselected and selected cows had similar body weight, degree of fat depot mobilization during the peripartum period, and energy balance during the postpartum period.[59,60] However, unselected cows had lower growth hormone concentration during lactation and higher insulin like growth factor-1 concentration until 12 weeks of lactation.[59–61] These differences in somatotropic axis are critical for resumption of ovarian cycles following parturition.[62] Consequently, unselected cows resumed ovarian cycles ~10 days sooner and had greater progesterone concentration during the first 3 estrous cycles postpartum compared with selected cows.[60,63] These experiments show that genetic selection for high milk yield alters reproductive physiology of lactating dairy cows directly or indirectly (as suggested by Sangsritavong and colleagues[64]).

Conventional methods of genetic selection (parental average [PA] and PTA) are limited in their ability to improve the genetic progress of traditional fertility traits (eg, DPR, CI) because such traits have low heritability.[3,65–67] Heritability of productive traits ranges from 0.30 (mature equivalent milk, fat, and protein yield) to 0.58 (fat percentage), whereas heritability of reproductive traits ranges from 0.04 (interval from calving to first insemination) to 0.23 (interval from calving to first ovulation). The low heritability of traditional reproductive traits may reflect a dependence on a multitude of cow and managerial factors. For example, DPR is the speed at which animals become pregnant, assuming a 60-day VWP. Consequently, this variable is highly affected by the actual VWP adopted on-farm, use of fixed-time AI, and use of natural service. Similarly, CI depends on the interval from calving to resumption of ovarian cycles, estrous expression, estrous detection efficiency, establishment and maintenance of pregnancies, and length of gestation.[68] Despite the low heritability of traditional reproductive traits, the implementation of genetic evaluation for DPR starting in 2003 is thought to have contributed to increases in reproductive performance of Holstein and Jersey breeds.[3] Physiologic characteristics of cows that depend less on management and affect reproductive performance (eg, postpartum resumption of ovarian cycles and pregnancy loss) may present higher heritability and may be better candidates for genetic selection.[12,69,70]

The generation of PA and PTA data demands large investments of time and resources, which still do not guarantee 100% accurate information because of inherent confounding of some phenotypes (eg, DPR and CI).[71] In recent years, cattle breeders and producers have gained access to more affordable genomic evaluation. Initially (late 2007), only young males and elite females were tested using the 50,000 (50K) bovine single-nucleotide polymorphism probes because cost limited its broader use in the cattle population. Since 2010 a more affordable array (3K probes) has been available to the dairy industry. The low-density array (3K) may be used effectively for imputation of the 50K probes and produces results (genomic PTA [GPTA]) that are almost as accurate as the results produced with the 50K probes.[72,73] The use of GPTA for selection of future sires presents economic advantages because of its higher reliability compared with PA or PTA, because it expedites genetic gains through shortening of generation intervals, and because it allows the elimination of lower GPTA animals soon after birth.[74] In recent years, 90% of young Holstein and Jersey sires have been selected using GPTA.[75] However, questions remain on how commercial producers may use GPTA information in their reproductive programs. The cost of genomic testing is ~$40 per animal, demanding that a clear strategy to use the GPTA information generated be designed to result in profits. Weigel and colleagues[76] simulated lifetime net merit (LNM$) gains that dairy herds may realize by using GPTA for selection of females, taking into consideration reliability of the test and selection strategy. According to this simulation, reliability of selection would be smallest when heifer calves of unknown pedigree are selected based on phenotype alone, and reliability of selection would be maximum when sixth-lactation cows with complete pedigree are selected based on GPTA. According to the investigators, genomic testing is more valuable when less is known about an animal's genetic potential (heifer calves or animals with no pedigree).[76] Use of GPTA for selection of heifer calves with no pedigree resulted in an increase in LNM$ of $66 to $259 per animal, whereas use of GPTA for selection of heifer calves with full pedigree resulted in increase in LNM$ of $19 to $87 per animal.[76] Claus and colleagues[77] also estimated the benefits of using GPTA to select replacement heifers according to different scenarios. In general, an economic advantage was observed when using GPTA to select replacement heifers, particularly when little was known about their genetic potential, replacement heifers were abundant, cost of testing was low, accuracy of GPTA was significantly higher than PTA, and benefits of genetic improvement were higher.[77] In summary, genomic testing may result in significant economic gains when a clear strategy exists to make use of the GPTA data. Increased use of GPTA for selection of replacement heifers will improve the quality of genetic information of herds, increasing the reliability of PTA selection and, possibly, reducing the economic advantage of using GPTA, unless niche markets are explored (stock farms) or the cost of genomic testing is reduced significantly.

FUTURE CONSIDERATIONS

Biosensor systems within the milking parlor (eg, AfiLab system and Herd Navigator) are currently available in Israel, Europe, Canada, and a few select markets of the United States. Such systems allow the daily monitoring of dairy cows for several metabolites and biological markers that are used to estimate energy balance, identify occurrence of metabolic (eg, ketosis) and infectious (eg, mastitis) diseases, and to predict stage of the estrous cycle and pregnancy status (eg, in-line determination of progesterone and pregnancy-associated glycoprotein concentrations). Such systems coupled with technologies currently available (eg, GPTA, activity monitors/pedometers, rumination monitors, ultrasonography, OVSP for timed AI, sex-sorted semen) will facilitate the design of reproductive strategies for specific groups of cows according to their physiologic needs while maximizing profitability.

REFERENCES

1. Ferguson JD, Galligan DT. Veterinary reproductive programs. In: Proceedings of 32nd Annual Convention of the American Association of Bovine Practitioners (AABP). Nashville (TN): American Association of Bovine Practitioners; 1999. p. 133–7.
2. Giordano JO, Kalantari AS, Fricke PM, et al. A daily herd Markov-chain model to study the reproductive and economic impact of reproductive programs combining timed artificial insemination and estrus detection. J Dairy Sci 2012; 95(9):5442–60.
3. Norman HD, Wright JR, Hubbard SM, et al. Reproductive status of Holstein and Jersey cows in the United States. J Dairy Sci 2009;92:3517–28.
4. Galvão KN, Federico P, De Vries A, et al. Economic comparison of reproductive programs for dairy herds using estrus detection, timed artificial insemination, or a combination. J Dairy Sci 2013;96:2681–93.

5. Pinedo PJ, de Vries A, Webb DW. Dynamics of culling risk with disposal codes reported by Dairy Herd Improvement dairy herds. J Dairy Sci 2010;93:2250–61.
6. Bell MJ, Wall E, Russell G, et al. The effect of improving cow productivity, fertility, and longevity on the global warming potential of dairy systems. J Dairy Sci 2011; 94:3662–78.
7. Garnsworthy PC. The environmental impact of fertility in dairy cows: a modeling approach to predict methane and ammonia emissions. Anim Feed Sci Tech 2004; 112:211–23.
8. Lucy MC. Reproductive loss in high-producing dairy cattle: where will it end? J Dairy Sci 2001;84:1277–93.
9. VanRaden PM, Sanders AH, Tooker ME, et al. Development of a national genetic evaluation for cow fertility. J Dairy Sci 2004;87:2285–92.
10. Hare E, Norman HD, Wright JR. Trends in calving ages and calving intervals for dairy cattle breeds in the United States. J Dairy Sci 2006;89:365–70.
11. Walsh SW, Williams EJ, Evans ACO. A review of the causes of poor fertility in high milk producing dairy cows. Anim Reprod Sci 2011;123:127–38.
12. Royal MD, Flint AP, Woolliams JA. Genetic and phenotypic relationships among endocrine and traditional fertility traits and production traits in Holstein-Friesian dairy cows. J Dairy Sci 2002;85:958–67.
13. Weigel KA. Prospects for improving reproductive performance through genetic selection. Anim Reprod Sci 2006;96:323–30.
14. Norman HD, Walton LM, Durr J. Reproductive status of cows in dairy herd improvement programs and bred using artificial insemination. 2013. Available at: https://www.cdcb.us/publish/dhi/current/reproall.html.
15. Santos JEP, Bisinotto RS, Ribeiro ES, et al. Applying nutrition and physiology to improve reproduction in dairy cattle. Soc Reprod Fertil Suppl 2010;67:387–403.
16. Ribeiro ES, Galvão KN, Thatcher WW, et al. Economic aspects of applying reproductive technologies to dairy herds. Anim Reprod 2012;9:370–87.
17. De Vries A. Economics of reproductive performance. In: Risco CA, Melendez P, editors. Dairy production medicine. Hoboken (NJ): Wiley-Blackwell; 2011. p. 139–51.
18. Groenendaal H, Galligan DT, Mulder HA. An economic spreadsheet model to determine optimal breeding and replacement decisions for dairy cattle. J Dairy Sci 2004;87:2146–57.
19. De Vries A. Economic value of pregnancy in dairy cattle. J Dairy Sci 2006;89: 3876–85.
20. Cabrera VE. Economics of fertility in high-yielding dairy cows on confined TMR systems. Animal 2014;8(Suppl 1):211–21.
21. Caraviello DZ, Weigel KA, Fricke PM, et al. Survey of management practices on reproductive performance of dairy cattle on large US commercial farms. J Dairy Sci 2006;89:4723–35.
22. National Animal Health Monitoring System (NAHMS). Dairy 2007. Part IV: reference of dairy cattle health and management practices in the United States, 2007. #N494.0209. Fort Collins (CO): Centers for Epidemiology and Animal Health/USDA/APHIS/VS; 2009.
23. Vailes LD, Britt JH. Influence of footing surface on mounting and other sexual behaviors of estrual Holstein cows. J Anim Sci 1990;68:2333–9.
24. Wiltbank M, Lopez H, Sartori R, et al. Changes in reproductive physiology of lactating dairy cows due to elevated steroid metabolism. Theriogenology 2006; 65:17–29.

25. Santos JE, Rutigliano HM, Sá Filho MF. Risk factors for resumption of postpartum estrous cycles and embryonic survival in lactating dairy cows. Anim Reprod Sci 2009;110:207–21.

26. Pursley JR, Mee MO, Wiltbank MC. Synchronization of ovulation in dairy cows using PGF2alpha and GnRH. Theriogenology 1995;44:915–23.

27. LeBlanc S. Economics of improving reproductive performance in dairy herds. WCDS Adv Dairy Technol 2007;19:201–14.

28. Giordano JO, Fricke PM, Wiltbank MC, et al. An economic decision-making support system for selection of reproductive management programs on dairy farms. J Dairy Sci 2011;94:6216–32.

29. Tenhagen BA, Drillich M, Surholt R, et al. Comparison of timed AI after synchronized ovulation to AI at estrus: reproductive and economic considerations. J Dairy Sci 2004;87:85–94.

30. Kalantari AS, Cabrera VE. The effect of reproductive performance on the dairy cattle herd value assessed by integrating a daily dynamic programming model with a daily Markov chain model. J Dairy Sci 2012;95:6160–70.

31. Roelofs J, López-Gatius F, Hunter RH, et al. When is a cow in estrus? Clinical and practical aspects. Theriogenology 2010;74:327–44.

32. Valenza A, Giordano JO, Lopes G Jr, et al. Assessment of an accelerometer system for detection of estrus and treatment with gonadotropin-releasing hormone at the time of insemination in lactating dairy cows. J Dairy Sci 2012;95:7115–27.

33. Fricke PM, Giordano JO, Valenza A, et al. Reproductive performance of lactating dairy cows managed for first service using timed artificial insemination with or without detection of estrus using an activity-monitoring system. J Dairy Sci 2014;97:2771–81.

34. Stevenson JS, Hill SL, Nebel RL, et al. Ovulation timing and conception risk after automated activity monitoring in lactating dairy cows. J Dairy Sci 2014;97:4296–308.

35. Bombardelli GD, Soares HF, Chebel RC. Time of insemination relative to reaching activity threshold is associated with pregnancy risk when using sex-sorted semen for lactating Jersey cows. Theriogenology 2016;85(3):533–9.

36. Sá Filho MF, Mendanha MF, Sala RV, et al. Use of sex-sorted sperm in lactating dairy cows upon estrus detection or following timed artificial insemination. Anim Reprod Sci 2013;143:19–23.

37. De Vries A, Steenholdt C, Risco CA. Pregnancy rates and milk production in natural service and artificially inseminated dairy herds in Florida and Georgia. J Dairy Sci 2005;88:948–56.

38. Overton MW, Sischo WM. Comparison of reproductive performance by artificial insemination versus natural service sires in California dairies. Theriogenology 2005;64:603–13.

39. Lima FS, Risco CA, Thatcher MJ, et al. Comparison of reproductive performance in lactating dairy cows bred by natural service or timed artificial insemination. J Dairy Sci 2009;92:5456–66.

40. Lima FS, De Vries A, Risco CA, et al. Economic comparison of natural service and timed artificial insemination breeding programs in dairy cattle. J Dairy Sci 2010;93:4404–13.

41. Samartín S, Chandra RK. Obesity, overnutrition and the immune system. Nutr Res 2001;21:243–62.

42. Sauerwein H, Bendixen E, Restelli L, et al. The adipose tissue in farm animals: a proteomic approach. Curr Protein Pept Sci 2014;15:146–55.

43. Kimura K, Goff JP, Kehrli ME Jr. Effects of the presence of the mammary gland on expression of neutrophil adhesion molecules and myeloperoxidase activity in periparturient dairy cows. J Dairy Sci 1999;82:2385–92.

44. Hammon DS, Evjen IM, Dhiman TR, et al. Neutrophil function and energy status in Holstein cows with uterine health disorders. Vet Immunol Immunopathol 2006; 113:21–9.

45. Hill AW, Reid IM, Collins RA. Influence of liver fat on experimental *Escherichia coli* mastitis in periparturient cows. Vet Rec 1985;117:549–51.

46. Kaneene JB, Miller R, Herdt TH, et al. The association of serum nonesterified fatty acids and cholesterol, management and feeding practices with peripartum disease in dairy cows. Prev Vet Med 1997;31:59–72.

47. Rukkwamsuk T, Kruip TA, Wensing T. Relationship between overfeeding and over conditioning in the dry period and the problems of high producing dairy cows during the postparturient period. Vet Q 1999;21:71–7.

48. Heemskerk VH, Daemen MARC, Buurman WA. Insulin-like growth factor-1 (IGF-1) and growth hormone (GH) in immunity and inflammation. Cytokine Growth Factor Rev 1999;10:5–14.

49. Kasimanickam RK, Kasimanickam VR, Olsen JR, et al. Associations among serum pro- and anti-inflammatory cytokines, metabolic mediators, body condition, and uterine disease in postpartum dairy cows. Reprod Biol Endocrinol 2013;11:103.

50. Huzzey JM, Veira DM, Weary DM, et al. Prepartum behavior and dry matter intake identify dairy cows at risk for metritis. J Dairy Sci 2007;90:3220–33.

51. Hayirli A, Grummer RR, Nordheim EV, et al. Animal and dietary factors affecting feed intake during the prefresh transition period in Holsteins. J Dairy Sci 2002;85: 3430–43.

52. Fronk TJ, Schultz LH, Hardie AR. Effect of dry period overconditioning on subsequent metabolic disorders and performance of dairy cows. J Dairy Sci 1980;63:1080.

53. Treacher RJ, Reid IM, Roberts CJ. Effect of body condition at calving on the health and performance of dairy cows. Anim Prod 1986;43:1–6.

54. Ribeiro ES, Lima FS, Greco LF, et al. Prevalence of periparturient diseases and effects on fertility of seasonally calving grazing dairy cows supplemented with concentrates. J Dairy Sci 2013;96:5682–97.

55. Hansen LB, Freeman AE, Berger PJ. Yield and fertility relationships in dairy cattle. J Dairy Sci 1983;66:293–305.

56. Rauw WM, Kanis E, Noordhuizen-Stassen EN, et al. Undesirable side effects of selection for high production efficiency in farm animals: a review. Livest Prod Sci 1998;56:15–33.

57. Hansen LB. Consequences of selection for milk yield from a geneticist's viewpoint. J Dairy Sci 2000;83:1145–50.

58. Jones WP, Hansen LB, Chester-Jones H. Response of health care to selection for milk yield of dairy cattle. J Dairy Sci 1994;77:3137–52.

59. Crooker BA, Weber WJ, Ma LS, et al. Effect of energy balance and selection for milk yield on the somatotropic axis of the lactating Holstein cow: endocrine profiles and hepatic gene expression. In: Energy metabolism of animals (15th Symposium). EAAP Energy Symposium. Snekkersten (Denmark): 2001. p. 345–8. EAAP Publ. No. 103.

60. Lucy MC, Crooker BA. Physiological and genetic differences between low and high index dairy cows. In: Fertility in the high producing dairy cow, vol. 1. Galway (Ireland): British Society of Animal Science; 2001. p. 223–36. Publ. No. 26.

61. Weber WJ, Wallace CR, Hansen LB, et al. Effects of genetic selection for milk yield on somatotropin, insulin-like growth factor-I, and placental lactogen in Holstein cows. J Dairy Sci 2007;90:3314–25.
62. Butler WR. Nutritional interactions with reproductive performance in dairy cattle. Anim Reprod Sci 2000;60-61:449–57.
63. Weber WJ, Kolath SJ, Lucy MC, et al. Effect of genetic potential for milk yield on the onset of reproductive activity and corpus luteum function in Holstein cows. J Dairy Sci 2003;86(Suppl 1) [abstract: 238].
64. Sangsritavong S, Combs DK, Sartori R, et al. High feed intake increases liver blood flow and metabolism of progesterone and estradiol-17beta in dairy cattle. J Dairy Sci 2002;85:2831–42.
65. Bello NM, Stevenson JS, Tempelman RJ. Invited review: milk production and reproductive performance: modern interdisciplinary insights into an enduring axiom. J Dairy Sci 2012;95:5461–75.
66. Berry DP, Wall E, Pryce JE. Genetics and genomics of reproductive performance in dairy and beef cattle. Animal 2014;8(Suppl 1):105–21.
67. Parker Gaddis KL, Cole JB, Clay JS. Genomic selection for producer-recorded health event data in US dairy cattle. J Dairy Sci 2014;97:3190–9.
68. Carthy TR, Ryan DP, Fitzgerald AM, et al. Genetic parameters of ovarian and uterine reproductive traits in dairy cows. J Dairy Sci 2014;98:4095–106.
69. Bamber RL, Shook GE, Wiltbank MC, et al. Genetic parameters for anovulation and pregnancy loss in dairy cattle. J Dairy Sci 2009;92:5739–53.
70. Darwash AO, Lamming GE, Woolliams JA. Estimation of genetic variation in the interval from calving to postpartum ovulation of dairy cows. J Dairy Sci 1997; 80:1227–34.
71. Schnabel RD, Sonstegard TS, Taylor JF. Whole genome scan to detect QTL for milk production, conformation and functional traits in two U.S. Holstein families. Anim Genet 2005;36:408–16.
72. Weigel KA, Van Tassell CP, O'Connell JR, et al. Prediction of unobserved single nucleotide polymorphism genotypes of Jersey cattle using reference panes and population-based imputation algorithms. J Dairy Sci 2010;93:2229–38.
73. Dassonneville R, Brondum RF, Druet T, et al. Effect of imputing markers from a low-density chip on the reliability of genomic breeding values in Holstein populations. J Dairy Sci 2011;94:3679–86.
74. Schaeffer LR. Strategy for applying genome-wide selection in dairy cattle. J Anim Breed Genet 2006;123:218–23.
75. Olson KM, VanRaden PM, Tooker ME. Multibreed genomic evaluations using purebred Holsteins, Jerseys, and Brown Swiss. J Dairy Sci 2012;95:5378–83.
76. Weigel KA, Hoffman PC, Herring W, et al. Potential gains in lifetime net merit from genomic testing of cows, heifers, and calves on commercial dairy farms. J Dairy Sci 2012;95:2215.
77. Claus MPL, Bijma P, Veerkamp RF. Evaluation of genomic selection for replacement strategies using selection index theory. J Dairy Sci 2015;98:6499–509.

Beef Heifer Development

Robert L. Larson, DVM, PhD, ACT, ACVPM-Epi[a],*, Brad J. White, DVM, MS[a],
Shelie Laflin, DVM[b]

KEYWORDS

- Beef heifer • Puberty • Reproductive soundness examination of heifers
- Estrous synchronization • Artificial insemination

KEY POINTS

- In order to become pregnant early in the breeding season as a heifer, deliver a live calf, and become pregnant early in the breeding season as a first-calf (primiparous) cow, management of heifer development must optimize nutrition, heifer maturity at the onset of breeding, bull fertility, and overall reproductive success.
- Examination of yearling heifers before breeding can provide information on the current pubertal status of the group and allow better predictions regarding success of the breeding season.
- Data used in the evaluation of breeding soundness of replacement heifers include body weight, days of age, reproductive tract maturity, and potentially pelvic area; the optimum timing of a reproductive soundness examination will depend on the nutrition, breeding, and marketing plans for specific herds.
- Using the Kansas State University 3-point system (R, I, and P), veterinarians classify prebreeding heifers as ready, intermediate, and problem.

INTRODUCTION

Replacement heifer management has a large influence on the reproductive success of beef herds. Overall herd productivity increases when a high percentage of heifers become pregnant early in the first breeding season and a high percentage of first-calf heifers (primiparous cows) conceive early in the breeding season for a second pregnancy.[1–4] In order to become pregnant early in the breeding season as a heifer (nulliparous), deliver a live calf, and become pregnant early in the breeding season as a first-calf (primiparous) cow, management of heifer development must optimize nutrition, heifer maturity (puberty) at the onset of breeding, bull fertility, and overall reproductive success.

The authors have received grants, or research contracts, from the National Cattlemen's Beef Association, the United States Department of Agriculture, Zoetis Animal Health, Merck & Company, CEVA Biomune, Boehringer Ingelheim Vetmedica, and Merial Animal Health.
[a] Department of Clinical Sciences, College of Veterinary Medicine, Kansas State University, 1800 Denison Avenue, Manhattan, KS 66506, USA; [b] 14075 Carnahan Road, Olsburg, KS 66520, USA
* Corresponding author.
E-mail address: RLarson@vet.ksu.edu

PUBERTY

- Puberty is reached when a beef heifer is able to express estrous behavior and ovulate a fertile oocyte.
- Maturing of the neuroendocrine system induces the maturation and ovulation of the first oocyte as well as the hormonal changes that induce the first expression of behavioral estrus.
  - A gradual increase in gonadotropic (luteinizing hormone and follicle-stimulating hormone) activity causes the neuroendocrine system to mature.[5,6]
- The first ovulation is usually not accompanied by external indications of estrus.[7] It is generally thought that a certain amount of progesterone is needed for a period of time preceding ovulation in order to induce estrus behavior and for the following cycle to be of normal length.
  - Fertility to a mating associated with the pubertal estrus is reduced compared with the fertility of subsequent estrous cycles[8]; therefore, heifers should reach puberty at least 21 days before the first day of the breeding season.
- Once the heifer has gone through a cycle with corpora luteal (CL) development or has been exposed to sufficient progesterone levels from other sources (eg, progesterone-impregnated intravaginal insert or feed-grade progestogen), the following cycles are normal.[9]

PUBERTY: INFLUENCE OF AGE

- The onset of puberty is primarily influenced by age and weight within the breed.[10–12]
- The average age at which cohorts of beef heifers reach puberty has been reported to range from 292 days to 678 days (9.6–22.0 months); with the average age at puberty for cohorts of the Bos taurus breed and Bos taurus–crossbred heifers commonly used in North America reported to be from 303 days to 429 days (10–14 months) (**Table 1**).
- Although reporting average age at puberty provides valuable information, this value represents a level at which approximately 50% of the heifers have reached puberty. Usually a percentage of the replacement heifer cohort reaching puberty much higher than 50% is desired by the time of the start of the breeding season.
- In order for primiparous cows (first-calf heifers) to give birth to their first calf at about 22 to 23 months of age so that they have 90 to 100 days between calving and the start of the breeding season, they must become pregnant by 388 to 418 days (12.7–13.7 months) of age and should reach puberty at least 21 days before the first day of the breeding season, that is, by 367 to 397 days (12.0–13.0 months) of age.
  - Crossbred heifers will reach puberty at a younger age than heifers that lack heterosis.[21]
  - Because of differences in nutritional management and genetic selection, replacement heifers from different herds are expected to vary around the age-at-puberty estimate reported by Freetly and Cundiff[19] (1997), so that in many herds, the expected date to reach puberty is close to or after the desired onset of breeding for herd replacements.
- Knowing information such as the age when you expect 90% (or an appropriate target percentage based on overall herd goals) of a herd's heifers to reach puberty and the length of time required for 90% of primiparous cows to resume fertile cycles after calving allows you to determine how much pressure to place on age when selecting replacement heifer candidates (**Table 2**).

Table 1
Mean age at which cohorts of beef heifers reach puberty

Heifer Description	Criterion for Puberty	Age at Puberty (Mean or Median)
Angus-Simmental (n = 33) Gunn et al,[13] 2015	Plasma P_4 concentration (q 7 d) Puberty = 7 d before P_4 >2 ng/mL	Mean Control: 303 ± 10 d (SEM) DDG Tx: 330 ± 10 d (SEM)
Bos indicus × *Bos taurus* (n = 120) Waters et al,[14] 2015	Plasma P_4 concentration (q 7 d) Puberty = d P_4 >0.5 ng/mL (followed by P_4 concentrations consistent with normal estrous cycle)	Mean Hay only Tx: 446 d CornSBM Tx: 423 d Perennial peanut Tx: 439 d
Hereford × Angus × Brahman (n = 40) Cardoso et al,[15] 2014	Serum P_4 concentration (q 3–4 d) Puberty = 3 consecutive samples ≥1 ng/mL P_4	Median (estimated from **Fig. 1**) Low control: not calculable High control: 305 d Tx 1: 315 d Tx 2: 349 d
Brahman × British (n = 78) Moriel et al,[16] 2014	Serum P_4 concentration (q 10 d) Puberty = first day of 2 consecutive samples ≥1.5 ng/mL P_4	Control: 397 d Tx 1: 292 d Tx 2: 347 d Tx 3: 379 d
Brahman (n = 6) and shorthorn (n = 6) Rodrigues et al,[17] 2002	CL detection by transrectal ultrasound examination and serum P_4 concentration (q 7 d) Puberty = first day CL detected and confirmed by ≥1 ng/mL P_4 and CL maintained for at least 2 successive examinations	Brahman: 678 d Shorthorn: 507 d
Various breeds Freetly et al,[18] 2011	Visual observation for estrous behavior twice daily Puberty = first detected behavioral estrus	Hereford (n = 28): 349 d Angus (n = 38): 347 d Belgian Blue (n = 25): 340 d Brahman (n = 34): 407 d Boran (n = 8): 384 d Tuli (n = 9): 365 d
Various breeds Freetly and Cundiff,[19] 1997	Visual observation for estrous behavior twice daily Puberty = first detected behavioral estrus	Hereford (n = 149): 355 d; 90% Puberal by 390–401 d Angus (n = 128): 351 d; 90% Puberal by 376–384 d Belgian Blue (n = 235): 347 d; 90% Puberal by 372–375 d Piedmontese (n = 72): 348 d; 90% Puberal by 386–394 d Brahman (n = 173): 426 d; 90% Puberal by 440–463 d Boran (n = 186): 396 d; 90% Puberal by 434–442 d Tuli (n = 234): 371 d; 90% Puberal by 412–432 d

(continued on next page)

Table 1
(continued)

Heifer Description	Criterion for Puberty	Age at Puberty (Mean or Median)
Various breeds Ferrell,[20] 1982	Visual observation for estrous behavior twice daily Puberty = first detected behavioral estrus	Angus (n = 76): 410 d Hereford (n = 84): 429 d Red poll (n = 61): 355 d Brown Swiss (n = 47): 317 d Charolais (n = 36): 388 d Simmental (n = 91): 348 d Low postweaning gain: 387 d Medium postweaning gain: 365 d High postweaning gain: 372 d

Abbreviations: CornSBM, corn-soybean meal; DDG, dried distillers grain; P_4, progesterone; SEM, standard error of the mean; Tx, treatment.

Age at Start of Breeding For Heifers Born in the First 21 Days of the Mature Cow Calving Season

First Day of Breeding Season for Mature (Multiparous) Cows (mm/dd/yyyyy)	6/22/2017
Desired Minimum Length of Postpartum Period to Ensure High % of First-Calf Heifers (Primiparous Cows) Resume Fertile Cycles (days)	100
Length of Breeding/Calving Season for Replacement (Nulliparous) Heifers (days)	30
First Day of Calving Season for First-Calf Heifers (Primiparous Cows)	2/12/2018
First Day of Calving Season for Mature (Multiparous) Cows	4/1/2018
First Day of Breeding Season for Replacement (Nulliparous) Heifers	**5/5/2017**
Last day of Breeding Season for Nulliparous (Replacement) Heifers (283 d gestation)	6/4/2017
Number of Days to Start Breeding Replacement Heifers Ahead of Cows	48 d
Age at the Start of the Breeding Season for Heifers Born During the First 21 Days of the Mature Cow Calving Season	**379–399 d**

Fig. 1. Calculator to determine date to start the breeding season for replacement (nulliparous) heifers and the expected age at the start of breeding for heifers born early in the preceding calving season.

Table 2
Maximum day of the calving season for birth of replacement heifer candidates based on herd-specific expectations for age at 21 days after puberty and length of postpartum anestrus following first calving

Age at Puberty (d)	Length of Postpartum Anestrus Following First Calving			
	90 d	100 d	110 d	120 d
350	67th	57th	47th	37th
370	47th	37th	27th	17th
390	27th	17th	7th	—
410	7th	—	—	—
430	—	—	—	—
450	—	—	—	—

- **Table 2**'s calculations should be interpreted as follows:
  - If you have data to support that 90% of the heifers from a ranch will reach puberty by 390 days of age and you expect that 90% of first-calf heifers (primiparous cows) will have resumed fertile cycles by 100 days' post partum, then you would only keep as replacement candidates heifers that were born by the 17th day of the mature cow calving season.
  - If you have data to support that 90% of the heifers from a ranch will reach puberty by 370 days of age and you expect that 90% of primiparous cows (first-calf heifers) will have resumed fertile cycles by 90 days' post partum, then you would only keep as replacement candidates heifers that were born by the 47th day of the mature cow calving season.
- In order to select for young age at puberty (or at least avoid selecting for older age at puberty), crossbred heifers should be selected when possible and selection of sires for herd replacements should be influenced by expected progeny differences (EPDs) for scrotal circumference and heifer pregnancy.[21,22]
  - Scrotal circumference is measured in centimeters and is used as an indication of the age of puberty onset. Larger scrotal circumference at yearling age is associated with a younger age at puberty for that bull as well as for his bull and heifer offspring. In theory, the larger a bull's scrotal circumference, the earlier his daughters will reach puberty and the higher probability that they will become pregnant early enough to calve at 2 years of age.
  - Heifer pregnancy is an economically relevant trait EPD that reports the probability that a bull's daughters will conceive to calve at 2 years of age. This EPD is reported as a percentage whereby a higher value indicates the progeny with a higher probability of calving at 2 years of age.
- If herd replacements are known or suspected to reach puberty at a relatively older age (due to breed, lack of heterosis, or management decisions to have a low rate of weight gain from weaning to breeding), then a greater number of heifers must be developed and exposed to breeding so that even if a relatively small percentage of heifers become pregnant in a short breeding season, the number of replacements is sufficient to meet herd goals.
- In order to meet the management goal to breed replacement heifers at about 388 to 418 days (12.7–13.7 months) of age while recognizing that the biological constraint of age at puberty in many cohorts approaches the target breeding

age, the heifer breeding season must be restricted to 30 to 45 days or less in many herds.

- o Depending on the length of the breeding season and whether or not estrous synchronization is used, heifers will have 1 to 3 mating opportunities and subsequently an expectation of approximately 60% to 95% of the cohort becoming pregnant.
- o An accurate estimation of pregnancy success for heifers is necessary in order to determine the appropriate number of heifers to enter the breeding season (and previously the number selected to enter the replacement heifer cohort at weaning).

CONSTRAINTS THAT DICTATE SELECTION CRITERIA FOR REPLACEMENT HEIFER CANDIDATES AT WEANING

- Primiparous cows (first-calf heifers) have a longer period of postpartum anestrus following the birth of their first calf compared with the length of anestrus following subsequent pregnancies; this period is expected to average about 80 to 100 days for primiparous cows in good body condition.[23,24]
- The nulliparous (replacement) heifer breeding season must end approximately 20 days before the start of the multiparous (mature) cow breeding season to ensure sufficient days post partum for most of the cohort to resume fertile estrous cycles by the start of the breeding season for their second pregnancy (**Fig. 1**).
  - o If the last day of the breeding season for replacement heifers is scheduled so that the last heifer is expected to calve 20 days before the start of the mature cow calving season, all primiparous cows (first-calf heifers) will have at least 100 days between calving and the start of breeding.
- Heifer calves born in the first 3 weeks of the mature cow calving season will be 379 to 399 days of age at the start of a 30-day heifer breeding season that is scheduled to allow 100 days between the end of calving and the start of the next breeding season or 364 to 384 days of age for a 45-day heifer breeding season (Document S1, **Table 3**).

Table 3
Replacement heifer age at the start of breeding depends on several management decisions

Length of Heifer Breeding Season (d)	Age of Heifers Born in First 3 wk of Mature Cow Calving Season at the Start of the Heifer Breeding Season (d)	Age of Heifers Born in Second 3 wk of Mature Cow Calving Season at the Start of the Heifer Breeding Season (d)
Breeding season management: The start of the heifer breeding season is scheduled so that there are 90 d between end of calving as heifers and start of breeding as mature cows		
30	389–409	368–388
45	374–394	353–373
60	359–379	338–358
Breeding season management: The start of the heifer breeding season is scheduled so that there are 100 d between end of calving as heifers and start of breeding as mature cows		
30	379–399	358–378
45	364–384	343–363
60	349–369	328–348

- Heifers that are born in the first 21 to 42 days of the calving season are more likely than later-born heifers to reach puberty before a controlled 30- to 45-day breeding season scheduled to allow 90 to 100 days between the last calf being born and the start of the breeding season for the cohort's second pregnancy (see **Table 3**).
- Heifers that reach puberty later than 399 days of age will not be cycling at the start of a 30-day breeding season scheduled to provide 100 days between calving and the start of the breeding season for a second pregnancy, even if born on the first day of the mature cow breeding season.

PUBERTY: INFLUENCE OF WEIGHT

- Weight is an important factor determining the onset of puberty.
- Ensuring that the nutritional program is meeting average daily gain requirements for the period from weaning to breeding is critical for a successful heifer development program.
  - Differences between actual weights and target weights at critical midpoints between weaning and breeding can be used to influence the recommendation to increase or decrease the energy content of the diet so that target weight will be met by the start of breeding.
  - The use of ionophores, anthelmintics, and progestogen-based synchronization protocols will help ensure that heifers reach target weights and puberty before the start of the breeding season.[25–31]
- The target weight to reach puberty is based on research that calculates the ratio between the average weight of heifers in a cohort divided by the average mature weight of the multiparous cows in the herd that produced the heifers.
  - Using this calculation, it has been reported that heifer cohorts fed diets to reach approximately 55% to 65% have better reproductive performance than heifer cohorts fed to reach lower weight ratios.[32–34]
- The question confronting managers developing replacement heifers and their veterinary advisors is as follows: What cohort-level average daily weight gain between weaning and breeding is needed (and consequently, what diet needs to be fed) in order to have a sufficient number of heifers able to become pregnant during a 30- to 45-day or less breeding season?
- Because the actual weight at puberty and average daily weight gain on a specific diet for individual heifers varies, the targeted weight gain for the cohort will be greatly influenced by the percentage of the group needed to reach puberty by the target date ahead of breeding.
  - A relatively low targeted weight gain is used by some producers to reduce feed costs for the replacement heifer cohort with the understanding that a percentage far less than 90% (eg, 50%) of the heifer will have fertile cycles at the start of the breeding season.
  - Other producers may desire that a high percentage (eg, 90%) of the heifers have fertile cycles at the start of breeding, and they will formulate diets to reach a higher targeted weight gain so that nearly all the heifers in the cohort will meet or exceed the weight necessary for each individual to attain puberty (and accept the higher feed costs).
  - Because the breeding season for replacement heifers needs to be relatively short (ie, 30–45 days or less), producers targeting lower weight gain from weaning to breeding will need to have a larger number of heifers in the replacement cohort in order to end up with adequate numbers of pregnant heifers compared with producers targeting higher weight gain.

- Research has indicated that heifer weight gain does not have to be consistent between weaning and breeding to achieve successful reproductive performance.[35–37]
  - Diets can be planned so that slower rates of weight gain can be targeted for an initial period after weaning followed by higher rates of gain in the weeks leading up to breeding, as long as a sufficient percentage of the replacement cohort reaches body weights consistent with puberty onset.
  - Although this management technique can produce reproductive success, more management acumen is required to ensure that targets are met during the higher gain period as this system creates a smaller margin for errors.
- The 1996 National Research Council's (NRC) estimations of energy (Mcal) and metabolizable protein requirements for *Bos taurus* beef heifers from weaning through early pregnancy should be used as a guideline in formulating rations for developing heifers, but adjustments may need to be made to achieve the desired gains.[38]
  - Factors such as amount of activity required for grazing, environmental temperature, breed, and compensatory gain may decrease or increase the actual nutritional requirements when compared with the NRC's estimates.[39]
  - Using the NRC's estimates for forage nutrient content reveals that replacement heifers consuming moderate- or poorer-quality forages cannot meet the NRC's requirements to meet targeted rates of weight gain. Therefore, except in situations whereby very high-quality forage is available, replacement heifers consuming moderate-quality forages must be supplemented with more energy-dense feeds.[38]

EVALUATION OF REPRODUCTIVE SOUNDNESS OF YEARLING HEIFERS

- Examination of yearling heifers before breeding can provide information on the current pubertal status of the group and allow better predictions regarding success of the breeding season. Data used in the evaluation of breeding soundness of replacement heifers include body weight, days of age, reproductive tract maturity, and, potentially, pelvic area.
- The optimum timing of a reproductive soundness examination will depend on the nutrition, breeding, and marketing plans for specific herds.
  - Evaluating heifers 6 weeks before the breeding season offers the most time to correct low body weight and corresponds to optimal timing of prebreeding vaccination but will provide less certainty about the percentage of heifers that will be cycling when the breeding season starts.
  - Evaluating heifers immediately before synchronization or just before bull turnout provides very accurate information about the percentage of cycling heifers but affords no opportunity to make adjustments that may increase that number.
  - Confirming that a high percentage of replacement heifers are cycling before the start of the breeding season as well as identifying and removing freemartins, very immature heifers, and pregnant heifers will increase the success of an estrous synchronization and artificial insemination (AI) program.
- Potential replacement heifers should undergo a thorough physical examination, including determination of body weight and palpation of the reproductive tract.
  - Palpation of the reproductive tract to determine the presence of a CL or large follicles on the ovaries and to estimate the size of the uterus is done in order to determine if a heifer is cycling.

- The use of pelvic area measurement at 1 year of age has been described extensively since the late 1970s,[40,41] but its value to decrease the risk of calving difficulty should not be overestimated.
  - Veterinarians have used pelvic area measurements of yearlings because the major cause of dystocia is a disproportionately large calf compared with the heifer's pelvic area.
  - The correlation between the yearling and 2-year-old pelvic area is 0.70; therefore, measuring pelvic area as a yearling is beneficial for predicting pelvic size at the time of parturition.[40]
  - Critics of using pelvic area measurements to decrease calving difficulty point out that pelvic area is also positively correlated to mature cow size and calf birth weight and that selection based on pelvic area alone did not significantly reduce the risk of dystocia in groups of heifers.[42–46]
  - Rather than using pelvic area measurement to select for maximum pelvic size, this tool should be used to set a minimum pelvic size as a culling criterion (such as 130–150 cm^2 at 1 year of age) without assigning preference for heifers that exceed the minimum.
  - Pelvic area tends to increase more rapidly near the time of puberty than during the prepubertal period. This knowledge is used when concluding that a heifer that is cycling and is of adequate yearling weight but who has a small pelvis (<130 cm^2) has a high probability of dystocia due to having a small pelvis at the time of calving as a 2 year old. However, a heifer with the same pelvic area that has not reached puberty and has not reached her target weight may very well have an adequate pelvis at calving if management changes are made so that she reaches puberty and becomes pregnant.
- The Kansas State University replacement heifer evaluation system combines several of these assessments into a single 3-point classification system (ready, intermediate, and problem) to facilitate communication between the veterinarian and producer concerning heifer breeding management (**Table 4**).
  - *Ready*: adequate weight and body condition, no structural flaws that impede fertility or longevity, palpable CL or large follicle with good uterine tone consistent with normal estrous cycles, and a normally shaped pelvis with a minimum pelvic area of 130 cm^2. (This cutoff is considered to be a minimum for cycling moderate-framed heifers. Producers and their veterinarians may choose a higher [eg, 150 cm^2] cutoff for cycling heifers in herds with larger-framed heifers.)
  - *Intermediate*: adequate weight and body condition, no structural flaws that impede fertility or longevity, some uterine tone and small palpable follicles but may not be cycling at the start of the breeding season
  - *Problem*: heifers that are not adequately heavy or with frame size that does not meet herd goals, structural flaws that impede fertility or longevity, very immature reproductive tracts, ovarian abnormalities, eye lesions that impede vision, heifers with an abnormally shaped pelvis, freemartins, and, in most situations, pregnant heifers
- These classifications are interpreted as follows:
  - *Ready*: These heifers are ready to breed by AI or bull exposure.
    - If heifers are evaluated immediately before the initiation of an estrous synchronization protocol for AI breeding, the producer and veterinarian may elect to only include ready heifers to ensure the greatest response to synchronization and the highest percent of heifers bred with AI that conceive with the AI mating.

Table 4
The Kansas State University replacement heifer evaluation scoring system used at a time approaching the breeding season to classify potential replacement heifers as ready, intermediate, or problem

Score	BCS		Weight		Reproductive Tract		Pelvic Area		Pelvic Shape
R	≥5	&	55%–65% of mature wt	&	Cycling: CL present and/or >10 mm follicles with good uterine tone	&	>130 cm² or herd-specific cutoff	&	Normal
I	≥5	&	50%–60% of mature wt	&	Not cycling but palpable ovarian structures and slight to good uterine tone	&	>130 cm²	&	Normal
P	<5	or	<50% of mature wt	or	Immature uterus with no palpable follicles or follicles <8 mm, freemartin, or pregnant	or	<130 cm² or herd-specific cutoff	or	Abnormal

Abbreviations: BCS, body condition score; I, intermediate; P, problem; R, ready; wt, weight.

- o *Intermediate*: These heifers are expected to have good reproductive success with a 30- to 60-day exposure to bulls but may have only moderate success with an AI mating at the start of the breeding season. Whether or not to expose intermediate heifers to AI breeding, bull-exposure only, or to manage them as stocker heifers will be based on the length of time between prebreeding evaluation and the start of the breeding season and other herd-specific management and marketing goals and options.
  - ■ If the heifers are evaluated 4 to 6 weeks ahead of AI breeding, the veterinarian and producer may elect to include some or all of the intermediate heifers in the group to be synchronized based on criterion, such as age or weight.
  - ■ If natural service is to be used, the length of time between evaluation and the start of breeding will influence the pregnancy success of intermediate heifers.
- o *Problem*: These heifers are not ideal candidates for replacement heifers.
  - ■ In order for a high percentage of heifers to become pregnant with an AI mating or to become pregnant in the first 21 days of the breeding season if using natural service, at least 80% of the heifers must be cycling by the start of breeding, with many herds setting a goal of at least 90% cycling.
  - ■ Approximately 70% to 90% of cycling heifers are expected to express estrus and/or ovulate a viable oocyte at the time predicted by a properly administered synchronization protocol.[47–50]
  - ■ Beef heifers that are bred with AI at an appropriate time relative to ovulation of a fertile oocyte have a 60% to 80% probability of establishing a pregnancy that can be detected at 50 days of gestation or later.[47,49,51]
  - ■ **Table 5** illustrates that the maximum percentage of pregnancies with an AI mating following estrous synchronization is 48% to 72% if all heifers have fertile estrous cycles and 38% to 58% if 80% of heifers have fertile estrous cycles.

Table 5
Maximum percentage of synchronized heifers that maintain an AI pregnancy based on the initial percent cycling, the efficacy of the synchronization protocol, and the pregnancy success per mating

Percentage of Cycling (Capable of Ovulating) (%)	Percentage of Cycling Heifers (Heifers Capable of Ovulating) that Actually Ovulate at a Time Predicted by a Properly Administered Ovulation Synchronization Protocol (%)	Pregnancy Success per Mating of Ovulating Heifer with Fertile Semen (%)	Expected Percentage of Heifers Exposed to a Synchronization Protocol that Maintain an AI Pregnancy (%)
100	80	60	48
		70	56
		80	64
	90	60	54
		70	63
		80	72
90	80	60	43
		70	50
		80	58
	90	60	49
		70	57
		80	65
80	80	60	38
		70	45
		80	51
	90	60	43
		70	50
		80	58
70	80	60	34
		70	39
		80	45
	90	60	38
		70	44
		80	50
60	80	60	29
		70	34
		80	38
	90	60	32
		70	38
		80	43

- ■ **Table 5** illustrates that if the percentage of heifers that could respond to a synchronization protocol decreases to less than 80%, the percentage of synchronized heifers that could possibly conceive and maintain and AI pregnancy becomes quite low and the synchronization and breeding cost per AI pregnancy becomes high.
- A review of estrous and ovulation synchronization protocols reported that the percentage of synchronized beef heifers that become pregnant with AI averaged 50% to 60%, which is aligned with the estimates from **Table 5** for situations when 90% to 100% of heifers have the ability to respond to a synchronization protocol and are bred with fertile semen by a competent technician.[48]
  - ○ If the percent of heifers exposed to synchronization and AI that become pregnant decreases to less than expectations, then a lower-than-expected percentage of cycling heifers should be an important rule-out to consider.

DETERMINATION OF MINIMUM NUMBER OF HEIFERS TO SAVE AT WEANING

- The minimum number of heifers that should be retained at weaning as potential replacements depends on the following (**Table 6**):
  - ○ The number of pregnant replacements desired to meet herd size goals
  - ○ The expected percentage of the starting cohort that will meet herd-specific goals for prebreeding heifer evaluation classification (eg, 100% ready or 70% ready, and 30% intermediate, and so forth)
  - ○ The expected response to synchronization protocol (if used) of heifers retained for breeding
  - ○ The expected pregnancy success per mating
- The percentage values from **Table 5** (or herd-specific values based on previous herd performance) can be used to calculate the minimum number of heifers to save at weaning using the following equation:

Number desired as replacements ÷ % pregnant in first 2 mating opportunities (or % pregnant with AI) = minimum number of heifers to save at weaning

Examples

50 replacements needed (pregnant with AI) *high input strategy* ÷ 51% expected to be pregnant to AI mating = ≥98 heifers retained at weaning

50 replacements needed (pregnant in first 2 opportunities) *moderate input strategy* ÷ 50% expected to be pregnant from first 2 mating opportunities = ≥100 heifers retained at weaning

BULL FERTILITY

- All bulls used to breed heifers should be evaluated to be certain that their EPDs for birthweight or direct calving ease are consistent with the ranch's goals.
- To ensure that bulls can deliver fertile semen to the reproductive tract of heifers, a thorough breeding soundness examination to evaluate semen quality, structural soundness, and health of all breeding bulls should be done before the start of the breeding season.
- Once the breeding season begins, producers should spend time observing activity in the breeding pasture to make sure that bulls are searching out

Table 6
The percentage of heifers retained at weaning as potential replacements that obtain desired pregnancy classification based on most likely estimate (and estimated range) for meeting prebreeding cutoff, synchronization success, and mating success

	Expected Percentage of Heifers that Meet Herd-Specific Evaluation Cutoff (R and/or I) (%)	Expected Response to Synch Protocol (%)	Expected Pregnancy Success per Mating (%)	Percentage of Heifers Pregnant with AI (%)	Percentage of Heifers Pregnant in First 2 Mating Opportunities (%)
High-input development strategy	85 (80–90)	85 (80–90)	70 (60–80)	51 (38–65)	77 (70–84)
Moderate- to low-input development strategy	55 (50–60)	85 (80–90)	70 (60–80)	33 (24–43)	50 (44–56)

Abbreviations: I, intermediate; R, ready; Synch, synchronization.

heifers that are in heat and they are able to mount and complete the act of breeding.

- o It is particularly important the first 30 days of the breeding season to visually evaluate bull performance and estimate the percentage of heifers being bred each day.
- o Chin ball markers on bulls, tail head paint on cows, and other mounting detection aids can be valuable tools to evaluate the number of mating acts per day or per week in a breeding pasture (depending on frequency of observation).[52]
- o If 80% to 100% of the heifers are cycling at the start of the breeding season, on average 4% to 5% should be bred each day.

DETERMINING SUCCESS OF ESTROUS SYNCHRONIZATION AND ARTIFICIAL INSEMINATION PROGRAM

- Heifers are ideal candidates for utilization of estrous synchronization and AI. Because they are not nursing calves and are often housed by themselves away from the mature cows, application of synchronization protocols and handling for insemination are much more convenient than with mature cows.
  - o If heifers have reached puberty and the synchronization system was applied appropriately, 70% to 90% or more of heifers should display estrus within the time window predicted by the synchronization system. If results do not meet this goal, the percentage of heifers that are pubertal, the accuracy of estrous detection, and the success of administering the synchronization system should all be investigated.
  - o If estrous response to synchronization is poor, alternate or additional synchronization systems can be implemented, the period of estrous detection and AI can be extended, or the date for the start of the natural breeding season can be altered.
  - o If heifers are synchronized and bred with AI, bulls should be held out of the breeding pasture for an appropriate length of time (eg, 2 weeks) following the last day of AI breeding so that AI pregnancy rate can be accurately determined early in gestation via fetal aging by palpation or ultrasound examination.
  - o Sixty percent to 70% or more of the heifers identified in estrus and bred artificially should become pregnant with AI. Failure to meet this goal could indicate inaccurate determination of estrus, poor semen delivery by the AI technician, poor semen quality, or poor condition of the heifers (stress, high environmental temperature, losing weight).

DETERMINING SUCCESS OF BREEDING SEASON

- The final culling of prospective replacement heifers is done once pregnancy status is determined soon after the end of the breeding season.
- By selecting only those heifers that maintain a pregnancy from an AI mating or with natural service during a short breeding season, producers can be assured of selecting heifers that reach puberty at a young age and conceive early in the breeding season.
- By determining pregnancy status shortly after the breeding season so that fetal age can be estimated accurately (eg, between 40 and 100 days' gestation), the veterinarian can determine the pregnancy percentage for the first 30 days of breeding (AI and first return to estrus).
- Identification of heifers that are not pregnant allows the producer to determine the best marketing plan for those animals. In addition, if more pregnant heifers

are available than are needed as replacements, the excess can be marketed to other ranches needing pregnant animals.

MONITORING BODY CONDITION SCORE IN MIDGESTATION TO LATE GESTATION

- Because body condition at the start of the second breeding season is a good predictor of breeding season success, it is important that the ranch's goal be met for the body condition score (BCS) (5–6 on a 9-point scale) and body weight (85% of mature weight).
- Adding body condition to a growing heifer that is lactating is very difficult; therefore, adequate BCS at calving is necessary to have adequate BCS at breeding.
- Growing, pregnant heifers require either high-quality forage sufficient to meet all nutritional demands or a supplementation strategy that adds adequate calories to the available forage base to meet their nutrient needs.

EVALUATING CALVING INFORMATION

- Data collected at calving are very valuable for evaluating overall heifer development management.
- The prediction of AI pregnancy percentage should be compared with the percentage of calves born in the first 2 weeks of the calving season. (Note: If the calving season start is based on 283 days after the date of AI, it is not uncommon that calves will be born before the start of the calving season.)
  - Failure to have a high percentage of calves born when predicted by palpation will allow the palpator to recalibrate his or her criteria for fetal aging and to determine the stage of pregnancy where he or she is most accurate to improve future predictions of calving date.
- The percentage of heifers confirmed to be pregnant but that fail to calve should not exceed herd-specific goals (eg, 2%), and an investigation should be initiated if the goal is not met.
  - High gestational loss should initiate a focus on biosecurity and vaccination protocols for diseases that cause pregnancy wastage.
- Calving ease scores should reflect herd-specific goals for the percentage of heifers experiencing dystocia (eg, <15%); levels exceeding that goal indicate a need to examine both growth of the heifers and birth weight EPDs of the bulls used as sires.
  - Excessive occurrence and severity of dystocia indicate that either heifers were underdeveloped or, more likely, the calf birth weight was excessive because of genetic predisposition by either the dam or sire.
  - Because each sire will affect many calves, accurate predictions of the sires' influence on birth weight by using EPDs is critical to avoiding excessive dystocia.

SUMMARY

Proper selection and development of replacement heifers that results in a high percentage of heifers becoming pregnant early in the first breeding season, having a calf with little or no assistance, and then rebreeding early in the second breeding season are essential for efficient and profitable beef cattle production. Veterinary involvement in the selection process and continued evaluation of heifer replacements throughout the first 2 years of life can greatly assist beef producers in meeting their production goals.

SUPPLEMENTARY DATA

Supplementary data related to this article can be found at http://dx.doi.org/10.1016/j.cvfa.2016.01.003.

REFERENCES

1. Lesmeister JL, Burfening PJ, Blackwell RL. Date of first calving in beef cows and subsequent calf production. J Anim Sci 1973;36:1–6.
2. Patterson HH, Adams DC, Klopfenstein TJ, et al. Supplementation to meet metabolizable protein requirements of primiparous beef heifers: II. Pregnancy and economics. J Anim Sci 2003;81:563.
3. Funston RN, Musgrave JA, Meyer TL, et al. Effect of calving distribution on beef cattle progeny performance. J Anim Sci 2012;90:5118–21.
4. Cushman RA, Kill LK, Funston RN, et al. Heifer calving date positively influences calf weaning weights through six parturitions. J Anim Sci 2013;91:4486–91.
5. Niswender GD, Farin CE, Braden TD. Reproductive physiology of domestic ruminants. In: Proceedings, Society for Theriogenology. 1984. p. 116–36.
6. Foster DL, Yellon SM, Olster DH. Internal and external determinants of the timing of puberty in the female. J Reprod Fertil 1985;75:327–44.
7. Dodson SE, McLeod BJ, Haresign W, et al. Endocrine changes from birth to puberty in the heifer. J Reprod Fertil 1988;82:527–38.
8. Byerley DJ, Staigmiller RB, Berardinelli JG, et al. Pregnancy rates of beef heifers bred either on puberal or third estrus. J Anim Sci 1987;65:646–50.
9. Gonzalez-Padilla E, Wiltbank JN, Niswender GD. Puberty in beef heifers. I. The interrelationship between pituitary, hypothalamic and ovarian hormones. J Anim Sci 1975;40:1091–104.
10. Wiltbank JN, Kasson CW, Ingalls JE. Puberty in crossbred and straightbred beef heifers on two levels of feed. J Anim Sci 1969;29:602–5.
11. Oeydipe EO, Osori DIK, Aderejola O, et al. Effect of level of nutrition on onset of puberty and conception rates of Zebu heifers. Theriogenology 1982;18:525–39.
12. Nelsen TC, Short RE, Phelps DA, et al. Nonpuberal estrus and mature cow influences on growth and puberty in heifers. J Anim Sci 1985;61:470–3.
13. Gunn PJ, Schoonmaker JP, Lemenager RP, et al. Feeding distiller's grains as an energy source to gestating and lactating beef heifers: impact on female progeny growth, puberty attainment, and reproductive processes. J Anim Sci 2015;93:746–57.
14. Waters KM, Black TE, Mercadante VRG, et al. Effects of feeding perennial peanut hay on growth, development, attainment of puberty, and fertility in beef replacement heifers. Prof Anim Sci 2015;31:40–9.
15. Cardoso RC, Alves BRC, Prezotto LD, et al. Use of a stair-step compensatory gain nutritional regimen to program the onset of puberty in beef heifers. J Anim Sci 2014;92:2942–9.
16. Moriel P, Johnson SE, Vendramini JMB, et al. Effects of calf weaning age and subsequent management system on growth and reproductive performance of beef heifers. J Anim Sci 2014;92:3096–107.
17. Rodrigues HD, Kinder JE, Fitzpatrick LA. Estradiol regulation of luteinizing hormone secretion in heifers of two breed types that reach puberty at different ages. Biosci Rep 2002;66:603–9.
18. Freetly HC, Kuehn LA, Cundiff LV. Growth curves of crossbred cows sired by Hereford, Angus, Belgian Blue, Brahman, Boran, and Tuli bulls, and the fraction of mature body weight and height at puberty. J Anim Sci 2011;89:2373–9.

19. Freetly HC, Cundiff LV. Postweaning growth and reproduction characteristics of heifers sired by bulls of seven breeds and raised on different levels of nutrition. J Anim Sci 1997;75:2841–51.

20. Ferrell CL. Effects of postweaning rate of gain on onset of puberty and productive performance of heifers of different breeds. J Anim Sci 1982;55:1272–83.

21. Martin LC, Brinks JS, Bourdon RM, et al. Genetic effects on beef heifer puberty and subsequent reproduction. J Anim Sci 1992;70:4008–17.

22. Moser DW, Bertrand JK, Benyshek LL, et al. Effects of selection for scrotal circumference in Limousin bulls on reproductive and growth traits of progeny. J Anim Sci 1996;74:2052–7.

23. Ciccioli NH, Wettemann RP, Spicer LJ, et al. Influence of body condition at calving and postpartum nutrition on endocrine function and reproductive performance of primiparous beef cows. J Anim Sci 2003;81:3107–20.

24. Berardinelli JG, Joshi PS. Introduction of bulls at different days postpartum on resumption of ovarian cycling activity in primiparous beef cows. J Anim Sci 2006;83:2106–10.

25. Short RE, Billows RA, Carr JB, et al. Induced or synchronized puberty in beef heifers. J Anim Sci 1976;43:1254–8.

26. Bushmich SL, Randel RD, McCartor MM, et al. Effect of dietary monensin on ovarian response following gonadotropin treatment in prepuberal heifers. J Anim Sci 1980;51:692–7.

27. Moseley WM, Dunn TG, Kaltenbach CC, et al. Relationship of growth and puberty in beef heifers fed monensin. J Anim Sci 1982;55:357–62.

28. Sprott LR, Goehring TB, Beverly JR, et al. Effects of ionophores on cow herd production: a review. J Anim Sci 1988;66:1340–6.

29. Larson RL, Corah LR, Spire MF, et al. Effect of treatment with ivermectin on reproductive performance of yearling beef heifers. Theriogenology 1995;44:189–97.

30. Purvis HT, Whittier JC. Effects of ionophore feeding and anthelmintic administration on age and weight at puberty in spring-born beef heifers. J Anim Sci 1996; 74:736–44.

31. Lucy MC, Billings HJ, Butler WR, et al. Efficacy of an intravaginal progesterone insert and an injection of PGF2a for synchronization of estrus and shortening the interval to pregnancy in postpartum beef cows, peripubertal beef heifers, and diary heifers. J Anim Sci 2001;79:982–95.

32. Patterson DJ, Corah LR, Kiracofe GH, et al. Conception rate in Bos taurus and Bos indicus crossbred heifers after postweaning energy manipulation and synchronization of estrus with melengestrol acetate and fenprostalene. J Anim Sci 1989;67:1138–47.

33. Patterson DJ, Perry RC, Kiracofe GH, et al. Management considerations in heifer development and puberty. J Anim Sci 1992;70:4018–35.

34. Funston RN, Martin JL, Larson DM, et al. Physiology and endocrinology symposium: nutritional aspects of developing replacement heifers. J Anim Sci 2012;90: 1166–71.

35. Clanton DC, Jones LE, England ME. Effect of rate and time of gain after weaning on the development of replacement beef heifers. J Anim Sci 1983;56:280–5.

36. Lynch JM, Lamb GC, Miller BL, et al. Influence of timing of gain on growth and reproductive performance of beef replacement heifers. J Anim Sci 1997;75: 1715–22.

37. Freetly HC, Ferrell CL, Jenkins TG. Production performance of beef cows raised on three different nutritionally controlled heifer development programs. J Anim Sci 2001;79:819–26.

38. National Research Council. Nutrient requirements of beef cattle. 7th edition. Washington, DC: National Academy Press; 1996.
39. Larson RL. Heifer development – reproduction and nutrition. In: Olson KC, editor. Veterinary clinics of North America: food animal practice bovine nutrition, vol. 23(1). , Philadelphia: W.B. Saunders Company; 2007. p. 53–68.
40. Neville WE, Mullinix BG, Smith JB, et al. Growth patterns for pelvic dimensions and other body measurements of beef females. J Anim Sci 1978;47:1080–8.
41. Deutscher GH. Using pelvic measurements to reduce dystocia in heifers. Mod Vet Pract 1985;66:751–5.
42. Laster DB. Factors affecting pelvic size and dystocia in beef cattle. J Anim Sci 1974;38:496–503.
43. Price TD, Wiltbank JN. Predicting dystocia in heifers. Theriogenology 1978;9: 221–49.
44. Basarab JA, Rutter LM, Day PA. The efficacy of predicting dystocia in yearling beef heifers: I. Using ratios of pelvic area to birth weight or pelvic area to heifer weight. J Anim Sci 1993;71:1359–71.
45. Naazie A, Makarechian MM, Berg RT. Factors influencing calving difficulty in beef heifers. J Anim Sci 1989;67:3243–9.
46. Van Donkersgoed J, Ribble CS, Townsend HGG, et al. The usefulness of pelvic measurements as an on-farm test for predicting calving difficulty in beef heifers. Can Vet J 1990;31:190–3.
47. Wood-Follis SL, Kojima FN, Lucy MC, et al. Estrus synchronization in beef heifers with progestin-based protocols I. Differences in response based on pubertal status at the initiation of treatment. Theriogenology 2004;62:1518–28.
48. Day ML, Grum DE. Breeding strategies to optimize reproductive efficiency in beef herds. Vet Clin North Am Food Anim Pract 2005;21:367–81.
49. Tauck SA, Wilkinson JRC, Olsen JR, et al. Comparison of controlled internal drug release device and melengesterol acetate as progestin sources in an estrous synchronization protocol for beef heifers. Theriogenology 2007;68:162–7.
50. Leitman NR, Busch DC, Mallory DA, et al. Comparison of long-term CIDR-based protocols to synchronize estrus in beef heifers. Anim Reprod Sci 2009;114: 345–55.
51. BonDurant RH. Selected diseases and conditions associated with bovine conceptus loss in the first trimester. Theriogenology 2007;68:461–73.
52. Davis AJ, Lester TD, Backes EA, et al. Sequential use of estrous-detection patches as a reproductive-management tool. Prof Anim Sci 2015;31:50–6.

Dairy Heifer Development and Nutrition Management

Matthew S. Akins, PhD Dairy Science*

KEYWORDS

- Dairy heifer • Development • Growth • Nutrition

KEY POINTS

- High rates of milk feeding decrease age at breeding, first calving, and increase first-lactation milk yield.
- Adequate prepubertal growth rate is needed to attain a breeding age for a 22-month to 24-month first calving age.
- Proper nutritional management postbreeding is needed to control growth rate and minimize cost and nutrient inputs.

INTRODUCTION

Raising dairy heifers requires significant resources (feed, time, facilities) that make up about 25% of a dairy farm's production costs. Of these costs, feed typically comprises about 50% of the total cost of raising dairy heifers.[1] The goal of raising dairy heifers is to have optimal growth to calve between 22 and 24 months of age while minimizing inputs (feed, time, labor) and nutrient output in manure. Understanding impacts of nutritional management on heifer development is essential to raising heifers that are efficient and profitable. This article focuses on current feeding strategies and impacts on calf and heifer growth, feed efficiency, nutrient use/output, and future lactation performance.

HEIFER GROWTH

Calving first-lactation cows at 22 to 24 months of age with an optimal body weight is most favorable for decreasing feed costs for heifer rearing and increasing productive life.[2] Calving at this age requires adequate growth rates to attain target weights at breeding and calving. The desired weights at breeding, precalving, and postcalving are 55%, 94%, and 85% of mature body weight (MBW), respectively, to maximize future milk yield.[3] Desired growth rate thus depends on the desired age at calving and estimated body weight at calving (94% of MBW) to calculate the number of

Disclosure: The author has nothing to disclose.
Department of Dairy Science, University of Wisconsin-Madison, 1675 Observatory Dr, Madison, WI 53706, USA
* 2615 Yellowstone Drive, Marshfield, WI 54449.
E-mail address: msakins@wisc.edu

days for growth and the total weight gain before calving. Typical recommended body weight gain from birth to calving (included conceptus gain) is 0.8 kg per day for Holstein heifers with a breed average MBW of 682 kg and a calving age of 24 months.

- The calculation to derive the gain needed from birth to precalving is:

((682 kg MBW $\times$ 0.94) – 42 kg birth weight)/730 days = 0.82 kg gain per day

However, MBW is variable depending on breed and genetic variance of mature weight, which can be as large as differences between breeds.[4] To determine MBW of heifers can be difficult and simply using an average body weight of mature cows (in third or greater lactation) as a starting point may not reflect the mature body size of the heifers. Hoffman[4] suggested to use a surrogate MBW (MBWs) to more accurately estimate MBW of the heifer. The MBWs is the 0 to 2- day postcalving dam body weight multiplied by an adjustment factor to adjust to a fourth-lactation MBW if the cow is in lactation 1 to 3. This value should better reflect genetic inheritance of body size from the dam.

Factors to adjust in 0 to 21-day postcalving cows:

First lactation	1.176
Second lactation	1.087
Third lactation	1.042

An example calculation for a 13-month-old heifer (breeding age):

Heifer weight = 400 kg; dam weight beginning of second lactation = 670 kg

400-kg heifer/(670-kg dam $\times$ 1.087) = 400-kg heifer/728-kg dam MBWs = 54.9% of MBW

Overall, heifer growers should focus on growing heifers with an adequate rate of gain without excessive body condition.

Maintaining optimal gains ensures favorable heifer development. Inadequate gains extend the breeding and calving ages, causing additional feed costs of rearing. Higher rates of growth may allow breeding and calving at target age but excess gain (especially adipose tissue) may cause dystocia or calving difficulties and other transition cow metabolic diseases. Also, excess gain as a prepubertal heifer between 3 and 10 months of age has been thought to cause accumulation of adipose deposits in the mammary gland, reducing mammary excretory tissue and subsequent milk production.[5] However, recent research shows that feeding for higher prepubertal weight gain does not negatively affect mammary development or lactation performance.[6,7]

Breed and genetic variance on each farm leads to heifers having different weights at different ages. Regular measuring of weight (ideally using an electronic scale) and height at approximately 12 months of age and before calving provides important information for managing and evaluating heifer growth and breeding and calving size/age. Weighing at 12 months of age also allows herd managers to evaluate whether the heifer is large enough for subsequent breeding starting at approximately 13 months of age. **Fig. 1** shows growth curves for heifers with 3 different MBW causing different growth rates needed to reach their MBW. A Universal Growth Chart estimation tool has been developed by Pat Hoffman, Emeritus Professor at the University of Wisconsin-Madison (http://fyi.uwex.edu/heifermgmt/growth-charts) to assess body weight based on percentage of estimated MBW, which is more useful than simply using a growth

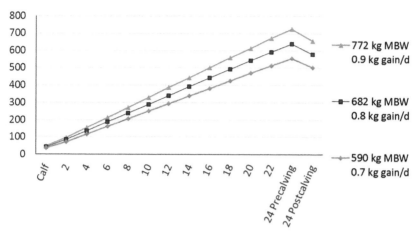

Fig. 1. Growth curves for heifers with estimated MBW of 590, 682, and 772 kg. Legend includes average daily gain needed to attain precalving weight. (*Courtesy of* P.C. Hoffman, MS Dairy Science, Marshfield, WI: Universal Heifer Growth Chart; http://fyi.uwex.edu/heifermgmt/growth-charts.)

chart with breed average data. The spreadsheet tool can be used to estimate the body weight that heifers should reach each month of growth depending on the estimated MBW.

HEIFER DEVELOPMENT: NEWBORN CALF TO WEANING

Before discussing development of calves, a short review of the importance of colostrum is needed. As most producers, nutritionists, and veterinarians know, proper colostrum management is necessary to provide passive immunity to newborn calves. Three main factors are important to managing colostrum: timing, quantity, and quality. Colostrum should be given as soon as possible after calving (preferably within 3 hours). Intestinal absorption ability of colostrum immunoglobulins decreases rapidly, with only 50% absorption by 9 hours after birth. Calves should be fed colostrum at 12% to 15% of body weight (for a 40-kg [90 lb] calf this would equal 3.8 L [4 quarts]). A second feeding of 2.0 L (2 quarts) of colostrum at 12 hours after birth is generally recommended. Colostrum quality refers to both cleanliness and immunoglobulin content. Colostrum should be free from blood, dirt, and manure, and be from cows not testing positive with *Mycoplasma paratuberculosis*. Good-quality colostrum should contain at least 50 g of immunoglobulins per liter measured using a colostrum meter or a refractometer. Samples measured using a Colostrometer must be at room temperature for accuracy. If colostrum is found to be of poor quality and no frozen source of quality colostrum is available, a colostrum supplement (to supplement colostrum with low immunoglobulin content) or colostrum replacer (as the only feed if usable colostrum is not available) can be used.

Calves, defined as animals individually fed liquid feed diets, are able to have the highest lean muscle growth compared with all other stages of heifer development. The goal for calf growth is to double the weight of the calf by weaning, so, for a calf weighing 42 kg at birth, the calf should weigh 84 kg by weaning. To reach this goal at a 6-week weaning age the calf must gain 1 kg per day and, if the weaning age is 8 weeks, the calf must gain 0.75 kg per day. The ability to attain this goal depends on the liquid feeding nutrition program (covered later in the article). For calves, muscle and skeletal growth should be the primary sources of weight gain, with minimal fat deposition. The amount of fat and muscle growth are highly dependent on the feeding rates of liquid feed and metabolizable energy and protein content of the milk replacer. If the diet is a conventional milk replacer with 20% protein and the calf is fed at a higher intake level with hopes to increase growth, the protein content will be inadequate to meet protein gain needs and the additional energy will cause excess fat gain. In another circumstance, if calves are fed an intensive program of milk replacer (ie, 28% protein) at lower levels of intake, the calves will have insufficient energy intake to use the protein for muscle growth.

Although body weight gain is often of primary consideration when discussing heifer development, digestive system (mainly the reticulorumen) development is essential for transition of calves from liquid to solid feed diets. Calves are born with a small, nonfunctional rumen that has minimal epithelial papillae and muscle development. Liquid feed does not initiate rumen development of either epithelial papillae or muscle growth. Solid feed fed to calves (mainly calf starter) containing high levels of highly fermentable carbohydrates (starch and sugars) is necessary for growth of the rumen papillae. This requirement is caused by the rumen microbial population fermenting starch and sugars to volatile fatty acids. One of the volatile fatty acids, butyric acid, is used preferentially by the rumen epithelial tissue for growth of papillae.[8] Growth of rumen papillae is important for calf digestive system development because rumen papillae are essential for absorption of volatile fatty acids. Feeding of forages to heifers increases rumen muscular development because of increased stimulation of the rumen contractions needed to move the rumen digesta. However, forages are not thought to be needed until after weaning because they may restrict starter intake and do not enhance the rumen papillae development needed for volatile fatty acid absorption.

NUTRITIONAL STRATEGIES FOR CALVES

During this phase of development, calves are functionally considered to be nonruminant animals with minimal to no dry feed intake the first 2 weeks of life. As nonruminants, calves receive their nutrients through liquid feed, which can have various forms and nutrient contents. Much recent research has shown that increasing growth rate of young calves leads to earlier breeding and calving, greater productive life, and greater first-lactation milk production.[2,9] An excellent review of calf nutrition from birth to weaning by Drackley[10] explains in detail the calf's nutrient requirements, liquid feeding options, milk replacer ingredients, and practical feeding regimes.

Producers have the option to feed a conventional limit fed, accelerated growth, or a moderate (between conventional and intensive) liquid feeding program to attain desired rates of growth before weaning. The conventional program is a strategy to feed liquid feed at approximately 8% to 10% of body weight, whereas the intensive program offers liquid feed at 16% to 20% of body weight. Typical formulation of conventional milk replacer is 20% protein and between 15% and 20% fat on an as-fed basis and is reconstituted to 12.5% solids. Intensive milk replacers are usually 26% to 28% protein on an as-fed basis with fat content similar to conventional milk replacer and are reconstituted between 12.5% and 17.5% solids. Pasteurized whole or waste milk is also an option and is often economical for large dairies that have enough waste milk to feed their calves. The greater liquid feed intake of intensive feeding programs is thought to be closer to what calves would eat if suckling from their mothers. The conventional program typically results in calves that have increased calf starter intake at an earlier age than calves on the intensive feeding program, but calves fed a conventional feeding program have lower energy and protein intakes from liquid feed compared with calves on an intensive program, resulting in lower growth rates, especially in the first 2 weeks of life[2,9] (**Table 1**). Calves fed an intensive feeding program have significantly greater daily gains from birth to weaning. Costs of feeding an intensive program are higher compared with conventional programs; however, heifers are bred and calve about 15 to 30 days earlier, which increases productive time. In addition, heifers fed an intensive feeding program have been shown to have increased first-lactation milk yield. The increase in first-lactation milk production may be further improved when the intensive program feeds whole milk compared with milk replacer. Calves fed ad-libitum whole milk and fed a higher protein diet from 150 to 320 days of age had increased first-lactation milk production compared with calves fed ad-libitum milk replacer. This finding was attributed to increased mammary fat pad mass, which had a paracrine and endocrine effect on mammary gland development[11] (**Table 2**). Feeding additional protein during the prepubertal period had a larger impact on milk yield than feeding whole milk[11] (**Table 3**). Expected growth rates of calves on conventional or intensive programs are 0.5 to 0.6 kg/d and 0.6 to 0.8 kg/d, respectively.[10] Postweaning nutrition to maintain higher gains of 0.9 kg/d are recommended until breeding age to attain an earlier breeding age.

An alternative to hand-feeding liquid diets that has gained much interest is the use of automatic milk feeding stations. Automatic feeders allow calves to consume liquid feed (ie, milk replacer, saleable milk, or waste milk) in more frequent meals than individual manual feeding systems. Calves are able to access the feeder a set number of times per day and eat a set meal size per visit. Managers can set the total feeding amount allowed, number of visits, and meal size per visit. The feed allowance per visit and total feed allowed per day affect the feeding behavior of calves. When the total feed allowance was 4 L per day compared with 8 L per day with 4 feeding visits allowed per day, the calves fed the lower amount had more unrewarded visits (no feed offered when visiting feeder) and more nonnutritive suckling after a feeding,[12] caused by the calves' hunger not being satisfied by the low feeding amount allowed and low amount allowed per visit. A manager can set a larger meal size and a low minimum number of visits to allow the calves greater feeding pattern flexibility.[13] To help diagnose health issues, the feeding system is able to alert managers to assess

Table 1
Effect of intensive milk replacer feeding on heifer development and lactation performance

	Treatment		
	Conventional	Intensive	P Value[a]
Milk Replacer Intake (kg DM)[a]	0.60	1.03	<.01
Starter Intake (kg DM)[a]	0.39	0.20	<.01
Starter Intake 6–8 weeks (kg DM)	2.33	2.29	.58
Average Daily Gain 2–42 d (kg)	0.44	0.64	<.01
Hip height at 42 d (cm)	83.6	86.3	<.01
Age at Puberty (d)	301	270	<.01
Body Weight at Puberty (kg)	307	287	<.01
First-lactation Average Milk Yield Through 150 DIM (kg/d)	33.1	33.3	.86
First Lactation PA Corrected Projected 305-d Milk Yield (kg)	9712	10,128	.08

Abbreviations: DIM, days in milk; DM, dry matter; PA, parent averages used as covariate.
[a] Milk replacer and starter intake were from preweaning period (birth to 6 weeks of age).
Data from Davis Rincker LE, VandeHaar MJ, Wolf CA, et al. Effect of intensified feeding of heifer calves on growth, pubertal age, calving age, milk yield, and economics. J Dairy Sci 2011;94:3554–67.

Table 2
Effect of feeding ad-libitum milk replacer or whole milk on heifer development and milk production

	Treatment		P Value
	Milk Replacer	Whole Milk	
Milk Intake (kg DM)	1.19	1.09	<.01
Starter Intake (kg DM)	0.17	0.18	.62
Body Weight at Weaning (kg)	82.7	85.8	.03
Average Daily Gain to Weaning (kg/d)	0.733	0.807	.01

Data from Moallem U, Werner D, Lehrer H, et al. Long-term effects of ad libitum whole milk prior to weaning and prepubertal protein supplementation on skeletal growth rate and first-lactation milk production. J Dairy Sci 2010;93:2639–50.

calves for disease when individuals have fewer than the expected number of visits to the feeders; however, regular observation for calf health is still needed with these systems. Group feeding reduces socialization problems associated with housing changes at weaning; however, these systems can also increase disease incidence if proper facility ventilation and cleanliness are not maintained.

Transition of calves from a diet that combines both liquid and solid feed to a diet that consists of only solid feed requires adequate dry feed intake (typical recommendations are at least 1.2 kg starter intake per day for 3 consecutive days before weaning) to maintain growth rates after weaning. It is recommended to allow a 1-week time frame to reduce liquid feedings to once per day, during which time starter intake is stimulated and rumen development is increased so that the calves are prepared for weaning. Intensive feeding programs may require 2 weeks to reduce liquid feedings to allow increased starter intake to transition calves before weaning. The same calf starter should be used before and after weaning to reduce feed changes and encourage feed intake.

A controversial topic in calf feeding is the optimum time to start feeding forages, with the common recommendation to wait until after weaning to offer high-quality

Table 3
Effect of feeding ad-libitum milk replacer or whole milk and increased dietary protein during prepubertal period (150–320 days of age) on heifer development and milk production

	Treatment				P Value		
	MRC	MRP	WMC	WMP	Milk	Protein	M × P
Age at First AI (d)	452	456	426	434	.05	.61	.87
Age at First Calving (d)	750	740	705	745	.24	.39	.15
Body Weight at Calving (kg)	532[ab]	521[b]	535[ab]	559[a]	.10	.57	.14
4% Fat-corrected Milk Yield (kg)	28.5[bc]	27.6[c]	29.1[b]	31.0[a]	.001	.27	.03

Means within rows with different superscript letters (a–c) differ ($P<.05$).

Abbreviations: AI, artificial insemination; MRC, ad-libitum milk replacer with no added protein during prepubertal period; MRP, ad-libitum milk replacer with 2% added protein during prepubertal period; WMC, ad-libitum whole milk with no added protein during prepubertal period; WMP, ad-libitum whole milk with 2% added protein during prepubertal period.

Data from Moallem U, Werner D, Lehrer H, et al. Long-term effects of ad libitum whole milk prior to weaning and prepubertal protein supplementation on skeletal growth rate and first-lactation milk production. J Dairy Sci 2010;93:2639–50.

hay. Forages are less digestible than concentrates such as calf starter mixes and can reduce intake of starter and thus energy intake if fed before weaning. Cellulose digestion is limited in calves because of their limited capacity for rumen digesta, limited microbial fermentation, and rumen pH less than 6, which reduces cellulolytic bacteria fermentation.[14] However, recent research with calves fed an intensive liquid feeding program showed improved dry feed intake when offered both calf starter and chopped orchard grass hay compared with being offered only calf starter.[15] Rumen weight, size, and pH were also increased when feeding hay, but no differences in rumen thickness, papillae length, body weight, or size were found. Additional research is needed to evaluate feeding forages (including silages such as corn silage that contain high levels of fermentable starch) before weaning.

HEIFER DEVELOPMENT: WEANING TO BREEDING

After weaning, heifer development continues with high rates of protein/muscle weight gain and low rates of adipose gain desired. During this period, heifers can be fed to gain 0.9 kg/d to reduce days until breeding, and thus calving, compared with lower rates of daily weight gain. The farm's goal for age at first calving dictates when the heifers need to be bred in order to meet that goal. For instance, if the farm wants heifers to calve at 22 months of age, then the heifers must be bred by 13 months of age. Heifer body weight at breeding should be 55% of MBW. Thus, if the weaning weight, breeding weight, and goal for age at breeding are known, the growth rate from weaning to breeding can be calculated. If a heifer has an estimated MBW of 682 kg, a weaning weight of 82 kg at 2 months of age, and a weight at breeding (13 months of age) of 375 kg, then the heifer must gain 0.9 kg per day.

From about 3 to 9 months of age, mammary development occurs at a faster rate than in other organs (allometric growth) and can be affected by nutrition during this period. When fed excess energy, epithelial tissue cell proliferation was decreased and additional adipose tissue was deposited in the mammary gland, which was associated with reduced later milk production.[5] More recent work has shown that additional energy during the postweaning time frame increased mammary parenchymal DNA but no improvement in milk production was observed.[7] Prebreeding heifer diets should be formulated with adequate metabolizable protein to meet the demand for lean growth. Excess energy intake should be avoided prebreeding to reduce adipose tissue deposition. Heifer body condition should be observed for excess adipose deposition, especially when feeding for faster weight gains to allow for earlier breeding and calving. Nutrient recommendations for an 0.8-kg gain per day for various weight class heifers are provided in **Table 4**. Additional details on nutrient requirements for metabolizable protein, minerals, and vitamins can be found in the 2001 *Nutrient Requirements of Dairy Cattle*.[16] Producers should consult with a nutritionist to balance diets that meet specific animal groups' needs because the National Research Council recommendations do not consider MBW or environmental effects (temperature, wind, mud) that affect nutrient needs.

Research into controlled or restricted growth rates during the prepubertal rearing period has shown improvements in lactation performance compared with ad-libitum prepubertal feeding. Lammers and colleagues[17] fed prepubertal heifers differing amounts of the same diet (16% crude protein; 2.7 Mcal/kg of metabolizable energy) resulting in gains of 0.7 kg and 1 kg per day. The heifers with 0.7-kg daily gain had 7% greater milk production than those with 1-kg daily gain, which was attributed to different mammary development (**Table 5**). No differences in age or weight at first calving were found because the heifers fed to gain 0.7 kg/d had significant

Table 4
Diet energy and protein requirements for large-breed dairy heifers gaining 0.8 kg/d in a thermoneutral environment

	Heifer Body Weight (kg)			
	150	300	450	600 (240 d Pregnant)
DM Intake (kg/d)	4.2	7.1	11.3	13.0
Crude protein (% of DM)[a]	15.9	12.3	11.0	12.9
Rumen-undegradable Protein (% of CP)	4.5	2.6	1.4	3.1
Rumen-degradable Protein (% of CP)	10.4	9.7	9.6	9.8
Total Digestible Nutrients (% of DM)	67.7	63.4	57.7	64.0
Metabolizable Energy (Mcal/kg)	2.45	2.28	2.08	2.31
Calcium (% of DM)	0.74	0.50	0.37	0.46
Phosphorus (% of DM)	0.36	0.24	0.18	0.23

Abbreviations: CP, crude protein; DM, dry matter.
[a] Crude protein required only if rumen-degradable and undegradable protein balanced.
Data from NRC. Nutrient requirements of dairy cattle: seventh revised edition. Washington, DC: National Academy Press; 2001. p. 276–9.

compensatory growth posttreatment. Ford and Park[18] assessed a stair-step feeding system with periods of restricted feeding followed by feeding a high-energy diet to enhance compensatory growth. The investigators fed heifers at 70% of ad-libitum intake of a high-protein diet (17% crude protein and 2.35 Mcal/kg metabolizable energy) to allow similar protein, mineral, and vitamin intakes as the controls but lower energy intakes during 3 specific time periods of isometric growth in which the mammary gland develops at similar rates to other tissues. They then followed the growth restriction by feeding a high-energy diet (12% crude protein and 3.05 Mcal/kg metabolizable energy) during periods of allometric mammary development. This stair-step feeding pattern led to improved milk production in first (21% greater) and second (15% greater) lactations. The increase was attributed to altered growth hormone levels and increased mammary development, especially during periods of compensatory growth during gestation. The 3-step method described would be difficult for producers to implement so the investigators are now investigating a simpler 1-step system during the last trimester of gestation because the most critical stage for mammary development occurs at that time.

Table 5
Effect of accelerated prepubertal gain (19–39 weeks of age) on weight and age at first calving, and first-lactation performance

	Treatment		
	0.7 kg/d	1 kg/d	P Value
Puberty Age (mo)	334	311	.01
Body Weight at Puberty (kg)	294	306	NS
Body Weight at Calving (kg)	632	620	NS
Age at Calving (mo)	22.9	22.9	NS
4% Fat-corrected milk yield (kg)	8040	7750	.01

Abbreviation: NS, no significant treatment effect.
Data from Lammers BP, Heinrichs AJ, Kensinjer RS. The effects of accelerated growth rates and estrogen implants in prepubertal Holstein heifers on estimates of mammary development and subsequent reproduction and milk production. J Dairy Sci 1999;82:1753–64.

Determining the proper timing of heifer breeding ensures that heifers are of adequate size for carrying a calf to term and to minimize later negative effects (dystocia and low milk production) when heifers calve earlier than 22 months of age. However, overly cautious age at first breeding can delay conception and the start of lactation. Consideration of both age and body size is useful to ensure that heifers are bred in a timely manner and are of proper size. Prescreening heifers at 12 months of age for body weight provides valuable information to indicate whether individuals are ready for breeding (at or greater than a certain goal weight at breeding)[19]; for example, having a goal of heifers weighing at or greater than 390 kg at 12 months of age to be eligible for breeding. This specific weight goal depends on the MBW and the percentage of MBW at breeding (55%–60% of MBW).

In addition to muscle, skeletal, and mammary growth during this time, the rumen is still developing by increasing in size and microbial populations. As the rumen size increases, heifers are able to consume high-forage, lower cost diets because of increased volume and retention time of slowly fermented fiber. At weaning, heifers are usually eating only a starter concentrate mix with minimal fiber content. After weaning, forages should be slowly increased in the heifers' diet to avoid decreasing concentrate intake and weight gain. High-quality, fine-stemmed hay is preferred to encourage forage intake. Silages are generally not recommended until 3 months of age because of lower dry matter intakes, possible mold contamination, and poor ruminal use of highly degradable protein and nonprotein nitrogen by young heifers. Research by Dennis and colleagues[20] showed that heifers (approximately 4 months of age) fed grass hay had increased growth compared with those fed grass baleage because of increased dry matter intake of the grass hay diet. Additional research is needed to evaluate the possibilities of feeding silages to preweaned and postweaned calves and associated impacts on growth and future production. Total mixed rations containing forage and concentrates are useful to reduce sorting of forages to ensure that heifers eat the desired diets. A useful method to transition heifers to a total mixed ration is to slowly replace part of the concentrate/hay diet with the total mixed ration each day over 2 to 4 weeks.

HEIFER DEVELOPMENT: BREEDING TO CALVING

Heifer development after breeding should focus on maintaining adequate growth rates while minimizing excess body condition gains. As heifers mature, the rate of lean tissue deposition decreases while adipose deposition rate increases. Heifers can quickly become overconditioned even on moderate-quality forages fed ad libitum or if diets with higher energy contents are not limited appropriately. Excess adipose tissue deposition during this period results in negative effects on heifers as they transition to lactation. These negative effects include increased metabolic problems,[21] dystocia,[22] and lower milk production.[23] Body condition scoring is a simple method for managers to monitor the condition of the cow and heifer herd, with a body condition score of 3.5 desired at calving.

NUTRITIONAL STRATEGIES FOR OPTIMUM HEIFER DEVELOPMENT

After weaning, most nutritional strategies focus on growing heifers at an adequate rate to breed and calve at the desired age with the least amount of feed and cost inputs. Ensuring heifers are bred at the correct weight and age range for calving between 22 and 24 months of age also ensures that producers are not feeding heifers for an extended period of time. An excellent reproductive program that results in heifers being bred at the correct age and weight with a high service and conception rate ensures that heifers calve within a producer's first calving age goal. A poor reproductive program that has a low service rate and conception rate causes a wide range in calving ages and additional days on feed, which significantly increases costs. A useful tool to evaluate a heifer reproductive program was developed by Pat Hoffman and Victor Cabrera from the University of Wisconsin-Madison Department of Dairy Science (http://dairymgt.uwex.edu/tools/heifer_pregnancy_rate/index.php). Producers enter each heifer's first calving age and the tool calculates average age at first calving, graphs the distribution of calving ages, and calculates the number of excess days on feed and the costs associated with these additional growing days.

Improving heifer feed efficiency has received much interest from producers and researchers in an attempt to reduce feed inputs and manure output. In addition to targeting high feed efficiency, heifer nutritional programs must minimize risk of overconditioning. Limit-feeding heifers to only the energy amount needed and not allowing ad-libitum intake greatly improves feed efficiency and helps control body condition. Another option for bred heifers is to feed forages with lower nutritive values with higher neutral detergent fiber (NDF) content because these heifers have lower requirements for energy and protein compared with lactating cows. Feeding higher fiber diets has the potential to reduce ad-libitum feed intake because heifers have an intake limit of approximately 1% of body weight as NDF.[24] Several alternative forages and low-nutritive-value roughages can be used, which control energy intake and fat gain but can result in reduced feed efficiency. The use of these strategies should be based on the producer's management potential, facility stocking rate/bunk space, and feed costs.

Limit-feeding is a strategy to feed heifers to meet nutrient requirements (amounts of energy, protein, minerals) but at lower feed intake by feeding a diet with a greater nutrient density. Reasons for using limit-feeding include control of heifer overconditioning, improved feed efficiency by reducing feed usage with similar weight gains, and reduced fecal output. A limit-fed diet has a higher nutrient density that is offered in a daily amount to meet the nutrient amount required by the heifer for maintenance and growth. For example, if a heifer requires 5 kg of total digestible nutrients (TDN) and the diet contains 70% TDN on a dry matter basis, then the heifer only needs to be fed 7.1 kg of dry matter in the diet. This system is different from an ad-libitum feeding system, in which a less nutrient-dense diet is fed and the animals are allowed to eat as much as they are able to eat to satisfy their gut fill. Feeding an ad-libitum diet leads to lower feed efficiency and possibly excess body weight and condition gain if the diet is not balanced correctly for lower energy content. Hoffman and colleagues[25] fed bred heifers diets with either 67.5%, 70%, or 73.9% TDN, dry matter basis. The different energy contents were formulated by increasing dry corn and soybean meal and decreasing corn silage and oatlage. The 67.5% TDN diet was fed ad libitum and the 70% and 73.9% TDN diets limit-fed at 90% or 80% of their ad-libitum intake. The limit-fed heifers had similar weight gains with 10% to 20% less dry matter intake, 10% to 25% less manure excretion, and 30% higher feed efficiency (**Table 6**). Nitrogen and phosphorus excretion were similar between the ad-libitum and limit-fed heifers because the diets were fed so heifers had similar intakes of both nutrients. Zanton and Heinrichs[26] compared feeding an ad-libitum high-forage (75% forage) diet and a limit-fed high-concentrate (75% concentrate) diet to prepubertal heifers for 35 weeks. The limit-fed high-concentrate diet was fed so the heifers received nutrient amounts that were similar to the ad-libitum diet. Results were similar to those of Hoffman and colleagues,[25] with similar weight gains, skeletal growth, and improved feed efficiency for the limit-fed diet (**Table 7**). However, feeding the higher concentrate limit-fed diet caused increased paunch girth, which was thought to be caused by greater fat deposition. Also, the limit-fed heifers had increased milk fat yield and

Table 6
Effect of limit-feeding on bred heifer growth and first-lactation milk yield

	Treatment			
	C100	L90	L80	Contrast C vs L (*P* Value)[a]
Intake (kg DM)	10.0	9.1	7.8	.002
DM Excretion (kg)	3.5	3.1	2.6	.10
Average Daily Gain (kg/d)	0.754	0.872	0.835	NS
Feed Efficiency (kg DM/kg Gain)	12.8	10.4	9.9	.09
3.5% Fat-corrected Milk (kg/d)	32.3	31.6	32.9	NS

Treatments: C100, ad-libitum feed allowance; L80, fed 80% of C100 diet; L90, fed 90% of C100.
Abbreviation: DM, dry matter.
[a] Contrast comparing the ad-libitum fed diet (C100) versus the mean of the limit-fed diets (L90 and L80).
Data from Hoffman PC, Simson CR, Wattiaux M. Limit feeding of gravid Holstein heifers: effect on growth, manure nutrient excretion, and subsequent early lactation performance. J Dairy Sci 2007;90:946–54.

fat-corrected milk yield, which was thought to be caused by increased body fat available for mobilizing into milk. There is some concern that limit-feeding has some negative carryover effects on rumen volume and milk yield. However, Kruse and colleagues[27] found no differences in rumen volume, digesta weight, postcalving body weight, or milk production of heifers fed ad-libitum or limit-fed diets at either 85% or 80% of ad-libitum intakes.

The cost of using a limit-feeding strategy needs to be considered because the diet possibly contains additional purchased ingredients (energy and protein sources) leading to increased feed costs. Bach and Ahedo[28] in 2008 calculated the feed costs for the limit-fed rations used by Hoffman and colleagues[25] and found that the ad-libitum ration was $1.70 per day, whereas the 90% and 80% limit-fed diets were $2.10 and 2.70 per day respectively. Use of linear programming to reformulate the limit-fed diets with lower cost byproduct feeds to decrease feed cost may result in limit-fed diets with more similar costs to a high-forage diet. However, the feed costs do not consider the important aspect of reducing manure excretion and possibly lower nutrient excretion compared with a high-forage ad-libitum diet.

Table 7
Effect of controlled feeding of a high-forage diet or high-concentrate diet on prepubertal heifer growth and first-lactation milk yield

	Treatment		
	HF	HC	*P* Value
Intake (kg DM)	5.96	5.32	<.001
Prepubertal Daily Gain (kg/d)	0.828	0.827	.94
Feed Efficiency (kg Gain/kg DM)	0.142	0.156	<.002
Body Weight at Calving (kg)	536	560	.17
Body Weight Loss to Nadir (kg)	43	76	.01
305-d 4% Fat-corrected Milk (kg)	8343	9681	.02

Both diets fed to attain 0.8 kg daily prepubertal gain.
Abbreviations: DM, dry matter; HC, diet with 75% concentrate; HF, diet with 75% forage.
Data from Zanton GI, Heinrichs AJ. The effects of controlled feeding of a high-forage or high-concentrate ration on heifer growth and first-lactation milk production. J Dairy Sci 2007;90:3388–96.

Implementation of limit-feeding programs requires precise feeding management to ensure that animals are fed correct feed amounts and to void overfeeding or underfeeding heifers. Use of a mixer wagon with weigh scales is necessary and regular analysis of dry matter content of wet feeds (at least weekly and whenever feeds change) is needed to adjust ratios of as-fed ingredients in the diet because small changes in dry matter content change the amounts of nutrients fed. Working with a nutritionist is needed to balance limit-fed diets according to heifer requirements and adjust intake amounts as heifers increase intake as they increase in size. After feeding a limit-fed diet, animals have aggressive feeding behavior, with most of the feed being consumed within 1 to 2 hours. A feed push-up should be done within 1 hour so that heifers are not reaching for feed, which could cause increased shoulder abrasions and inner hoof wear on the front hoofs caused by pushing forward to reach feed. Having adequate bunk space is important when feeding limit-fed diets to ensure that all heifers can eat at the same time. If inadequate space is available, submissive heifers may have lower intakes and insufficient weight gain.

Feeding a high-forage diet with higher NDF and lower energy density is also an option for producers to control weight gain and prevent overconditioning of heifers. However, corn silage–based diets can have excess energy for bred heifers, causing overconditioning and subsequent negative lactation effects. Heifers are only able to consume approximately 1% of body weight at NDF[24] and this can be used to formulate diets to control intakes and weight gain, especially for bred heifers. Use of high-fiber forages such as straw or mature forages with high-energy feedstuffs has the potential to reduce diet dry matter and energy intake. Coblentz and colleagues[29] evaluated eastern gamagrass, straw, and corn stover as options to increase diet NDF content and dilute energy content. The control diet contained corn silage and alfalfa silage and was 44% NDF, 66.8% TDN, and 13.9% crude protein, dry matter basis. Treatment diets contained the diluting forages to increase NDF to about 50%, decrease TDN to approximately 60%, and maintain protein between 13.6% and 13.8%. Heifers fed diets with the diluting forages had lower feed and energy intake leading to a more desirable average daily gain of between 0.8 and 1.0 kg/d, compared with 1.16 kg/d for those fed a corn silage/alfalfa silage diet (**Table 8**).

Table 8
Effect of feeding a corn silage/alfalfa silage diet with or without forage dilution on bred heifer growth

	Treatment			Contrast *P* Value (Control vs Mean of EGH, WS, CF)
	Control	EGH	WS	CF	
Intake (kg DM)	11.06	10.55	9.48	10.09	<.001
Digestible NDF (kg)[3]	2.92	3.04	2.82	2.91	.98
TDN Intake (kg)[4]	7.39	6.22	5.66	5.97	<.001
Fecal DM Output (kg/d)	3.76	4.12	3.48	3.58	.62
Average Daily Gain (kg/d)	1.16	0.98	0.79	0.97	<.001
Final Body Condition Score	3.7	3.6	3.3	3.5	.001
Feed Efficiency (kg DM/kg Gain)	9.6	10.8	12.1	10.5	.002

Control was a corn silage-alfalfa silage diet.
Abbreviations: CF, control diet diluted with chopped corn fodder; DM, dry matter; EGH, control diet diluted with eastern gamagrass haylage; NDF, neutral detergent fiber; TDN, total digestible nutrients; WS, control diet diluted with chopped wheat straw.
Data from Coblentz WK, Esser NM, Hoffman PC, et al. Growth performance and sorting characteristics of corn silage-alfalfa haylage diets with or without forage dilution offered to replacement Holstein dairy heifers. J Dairy Sci 2015;98:8018–34.

Use of the diluting forages reduced body condition score, which may help reduce metabolic and dystocia issues at calving. In addition, use of eastern gamagrass haylage resulted in minimal sorting, which is often a problem with using straw or corn fodder and can lead to variable intake and weight gains between animals within a pen. Further research is needed to identify forages that can dilute diet energy, lead to minimal sorting, and are economical to produce.

SUMMARY

Heifer development and production are vital parts of a dairy farm and deserve close attention to ensure proper growth and subsequent lactation performance. The main goal of heifer production is to raise heifers to calve between 22 and 24 months of age while minimizing costs and nutrient excretion and potentially improving subsequent milk production. The optimal first calving age is 22 to 24 months of age, with early calving (especially before 22 months of age) leading to lower first-lactation milk yield, whereas calving after 24 months of age results in excess days on feed and cost of heifer rearing. Feeding higher milk or milk replacer amounts preweaning improves subsequent milk production compared with conventional feeding programs. Prepubertal rates of gain should be based on desired first calving age and estimated MBW and the proper nutrition program balanced for that gain. Excessive energy intake leading to overconditioning should be avoided, especially postbreeding because of potential dystocia and metabolic disease. Understanding of heifer development principles is useful to improve heifer rearing practices and management.

REFERENCES

1. Zwald A, Kohlman TL, Gunderson SL, et al. Economic costs and labor Efficiencies associated with raising dairy replacements on Wisconsin dairy farms and custom heifer raising operations. Madison, WI: University of Wisconsin-Extension; 2007.
2. Raeth-Knight M, Chester-Jones H, Hayes S, et al. Impact of conventional or intensive milk replacer programs on Holstein heifer performance through six months of age and during first lactation. J Dairy Sci 2009;92(2):799–809.
3. Van Amburgh M, Meyer M. Target growth and nutrient requirements of post-weaned dairy heifers. In: Dairy calves and heifers: integrating biology and management. Syracuse (NY): Natural Resource, Agriculture, and Engineering Services; 2005. p. 128–38.
4. Hoffman PC. Innovations in dairy replacement heifer management. Reno, NV: Western Dairy Management Conference; 2007. p. 237–48.
5. Sejrsen K, Huber JT, Tucker HA, et al. Influence of nutrition on mammary development in pre- and postpubertal heifers. J Dairy Sci 1982;65(5):793–800.
6. Radcliff RP, Vandehaar MJ, Skidmore AL, et al. Effects of diet and bovine somatotropin on heifer growth and mammary development. J Dairy Sci 1997;80(9):1996–2003.
7. Radcliff RP, Vandehaar MJ, Chapin LT, et al. Effects of diet and injection of bovine somatotropin on prepubertal growth and first-lactation milk yields of Holstein cows. J Dairy Sci 2000;83(1):23–9.
8. Heinrichs AJ, Lesmeister KE. Rumen development in the dairy calf. In: Garnsworthy PC, editor. Calf and heifer rearing. Nottingham (United Kingdom): Nottingham University Press; 2005. p. 53–65.

9. Davis Rincker LE, VandeHaar MJ, Wolf CA, et al. Effect of intensified feeding of heifer calves on growth, pubertal age, calving age, milk yield, and economics. J Dairy Sci 2011;94(7):3554–67.

10. Drackley JK. Calf nutrition from birth to breeding. Vet Clin North Am Food Anim Pract 2008;24:55–86.

11. Moallem U, Werner D, Lehrer H, et al. Long-term effects of ad libitum whole milk prior to weaning and prepubertal protein supplementation on skeletal growth rate and first-lactation milk production. J Dairy Sci 2010;93(6):2639–50.

12. Jensen MB. Computer-controlled milk feeding of group-housed calves: the effect of milk allowance and weaning type. J Dairy Sci 2006;89(1):201–6.

13. Jensen MB. Short communication: milk meal pattern of dairy calves is affected by computer-controlled milk feeder set-up. J Dairy Sci 2009;92(6):2906–10.

14. Anderson KL, Nagaraja TG, Morrill JL. Ruminal metabolic development in calves weaned conventionally or early. J Dairy Sci 1987;70(5):1000–5.

15. Khan MA, Weary DM, von Keyserlingk MA. Hay intake improves performance and rumen development of calves fed higher quantities of milk. J Dairy Sci 2011; 94(7):3547–53.

16. National Research Council. Nutrient requirements of dairy cattle: seventh revised edition. Washington, DC: National Academy Press; 2001.

17. Lammers BP, Heinrichs AJ, Kensinger RS. The effects of accelerated growth rates and estrogen implants in prepubertal Holstein heifers on estimates of mammary development and subsequent reproduction and milk production. J Dairy Sci 1999;82(8):1753–64.

18. Ford JA, Park CS. Nutritionally directed compensatory growth enhances heifer development and lactation potential. J Dairy Sci 2001;84(7):1669–78.

19. Vanderwerff L, Hoffman PC. Building a better breeding criteria for dairy heifers. Madison, WI: University of Wisconsin-Madison; 2013. Available at: http://fyi. uwex.edu/heifermgmt/heifer-management/. Accessed October 25, 2015.

20. Dennis TS, Tower JE, Nennich TD. Effects of feeding hay and baleage to prepubertal dairy heifers during the grower period. Prof Anim Sci 2012;28(6):648–56.

21. Grummer RR, Hoffman PC, Luck ML, et al. Effect of prepartum and postpartum dietary energy on growth and lactation of primiparous cows. J Dairy Sci 1995; 78(1):172–80.

22. Hoffman PC, Brehm NM, Price SG, et al. Effect of accelerated postpubertal growth and early calving on lactation performance of primiparous Holstein heifers. J Dairy Sci 1996;79(11):2024–31.

23. Waltner SS, McNamara JP, Hillers JK. Relationships of body condition score to production variables in high producing Holstein dairy cattle. J Dairy Sci 1993; 76(11):3410–9.

24. Hoffman PC, Kester KL. Estimating dry matter intake of dairy heifers. Madison, WI: University of Wisconsin-Madison; 2012. Available at: http://fyi.uwex.edu/ heifermgmt/heifer-management/. Accessed October 23, 2015.

25. Hoffman PC, Simson CR, Wattiaux M. Limit feeding of gravid Holstein heifers: effect on growth, manure nutrient excretion, and subsequent early lactation performance. J Dairy Sci 2007;90(2):946–54.

26. Zanton GI, Heinrichs AJ. The effects of controlled feeding of a high-forage or high-concentrate ration on heifer growth and first-lactation milk production. J Dairy Sci 2007;90(7):3388–96.

27. Kruse KA, Combs DK, Esser NM, et al. Evaluation of potential carryover effects associated with limit feeding of gravid Holstein heifers. J Dairy Sci 2010;93(11): 5374–84.

28. Bach A, Ahedo J. Record keeping and economics of dairy heifers. Vet Clin North Am Food Anim Pract 2008;24(1):117–38.
29. Coblentz WK, Esser NM, Hoffman PC, et al. Growth performance and sorting characteristics of corn silage-alfalfa haylage diets with or without forage dilution offered to replacement Holstein dairy heifers. J Dairy Sci 2015;98(11):8018–34.

Evaluating Information Obtained from Diagnosis of Pregnancy Status of Beef Herds

 CrossMark

Robert L. Larson, DVM, PhD, ACT, ACVPM-Epi*, Brad J. White, DVM, MS

KEYWORDS

- Reproductive profile • Fetal aging • Breeding soundness examination
- Pregnancy loss

KEY POINTS

- Diagnosis of pregnancy status for beef herds is commonly done at a time point in midgestation that is early enough to allow accurate estimation of fetal age but late enough to facilitate evaluation of the first 3 21-day periods of the breeding season.
- Breaking the fetal age estimation data collected at the time of pregnancy diagnosis into separate reproductive profiles based on categories of cow age, breed, breeding pasture, or other management groups is often necessary to accurately identify deficiencies in herd reproductive efficiency and to direct the investigation to the correct subset of the cow herd.
- By starting with the flow of beef cows through the reproductive system and gathering fetal age estimation at the time of pregnancy diagnosis, veterinarians can use reproductive profiles and other readily available information to systematically go through a decision tree to diagnose reproductive inefficiency and to advise producers which areas of improved reproductive efficiency are available for their herds.

INTRODUCTION

Good reproductive efficiency and low pregnancy wastage are critical for economic sustainability of beef cow-calf herds. Two standard measurements of reproductive success for beef cowherds are the percentage of cows exposed to bulls at the start of the breeding season that are identified as pregnant at a midgestation evaluation and the percentage of pregnant cows that give birth to a live calf. In addition to these standard performance assessments, converting fetal age data to a reproductive

The authors have received grants, or research contracts, from the National Cattlemen's Beef Association, the United States Department of Agriculture, Zoetis Animal Health, Merck & Company, CEVA Biomune, Boehringer Ingelheim Vetmedica, and Merial Animal Health.
Department of Clinical Sciences, College of Veterinary Medicine, Kansas State University, 1800 Denison Avenue, Manhattan, KS 66506, USA
* Corresponding author.
E-mail address: RLarson@vet.ksu.edu

profile (or pregnancy distribution) that displays pregnancy percentages by 21-day periods can provide enhanced information to assist in the diagnostic work-up for suboptimal reproductive efficiency and to guide the design of intervention strategies. The value of fetal age data can be amplified by further segregating reproductive profiles by animal age and/or other management groups when evaluating a herd with reproductive or production shortfalls.[1–4]

FLOW OF COWS THROUGH POTENTIAL REPRODUCTIVE STATES DURING A PRODUCTION CYCLE

From a reproductive standpoint, mature female cattle should pass through a series of states each year (**Fig. 1**):

- Starting in late pregnancy, a cow moves from the state of pregnancy before calving to the state of being nonpregnant but not having fertile ovulations once parturition has completed (see **Fig. 1**).
- Beef cows have a period of time after calving, called postpartum anestrus, when they do not display the behavioral aspects of estrus necessary to initiate mating and they do not ovulate fertile eggs. Postpartum anestrus in multiparous (mature) cows averages about 50 to 80 days if the cows are in good body condition[5,6] and requires an estimate of 70 to 100 days to reach a herd goal of 90% of cows that resume fertile cycles.
  - This period is longer if cows are thin and following the first (primiparous) pregnancy (average of 80–100 days)[7,8] compared with later (multiparous) pregnancies (50–80 days).

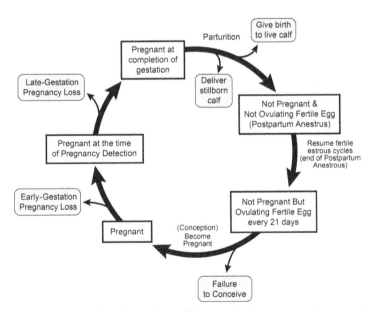

Fig. 1. Female beef cattle flow through specific reproductive states: not pregnant and not ovulating fertile oocytes, not pregnant and ovulating fertile oocytes every 21 days, pregnant, pregnant at the time of pregnancy detection, and pregnant at the completion of gestation. There are several alternative pathways in this system, including failure to conceive, early-gestation pregnancy loss, late-gestation pregnancy loss, and delivery of a stillborn calf.

- ○ A cow will resume ovulating fertile eggs every 21 days once the postpartum anestrus period is passed and she enters the state of being nonpregnant and having fertile 21-day estrous cycles (see **Fig. 1**).
- If a fertile, cycling cow is in the presence of a fertile bull, the subsequent mating has about a 60% to 70% probability of a pregnancy that can be detected 50 days later and consequently a calf being born at the end of gestation.[9]
  - ○ Following approximately 30% of mating between a fertile cow and a fertile bull, either fertilization fails to take place or fertilization occurs but the early embryo is not maintained. When fertilization fails or an embryo is lost before day 14 of gestation, the cow will express estrus and ovulate a fertile oocyte about 21 days after her last estrus and have another 60% to 70% probability of conceiving and maintaining a pregnancy.
- On mating with a fertile bull, and subsequent conception and maintenance of a pregnancy, cows move to the state of being pregnant until parturition (see **Fig. 1**).
  - ○ There are several alternative pathways in this system, including failure to conceive, early-gestation pregnancy loss, late-gestation pregnancy loss, and delivery of a stillborn calf.

CREATING HERD REPRODUCTIVE PROFILES FROM INFORMATION OBTAINED FROM DIAGNOSIS OF PREGNANCY STATUS OF BEEF HERDS

Diagnosis of pregnancy status for beef herds is commonly done at a time in midgestation that is early enough to allow accurate estimation of fetal age but late enough to facilitate evaluation of the first 3 21-day periods of the breeding season.[10] The stage of gestation in which estimation of fetal age begins to become less accurate varies between veterinarians; however, accuracy of gestational staging to 21-day cycles tends to decline at gestational lengths more than 100 days.

A pregnancy evaluation done 105 days after the start of the breeding season allows veterinarians comfortable with determining pregnancy status starting at 40 days of gestation to describe cows with estimated gestational lengths of 85 to 105 days, 64 to 84 days, and 43 to 63 days as conceiving in the first, second, and third 21-day periods, respectively (**Fig. 2**).

The ability to estimate fetal age accurately enough to place cows within fairly tight stages or 21-day periods of the breeding season is a great advantage for veterinarians providing advice to cow-calf clients when evaluating the nutritional and reproductive status of the herd's recent past and in planning to optimize the upcoming nutritional and marketing options for the herd.

If fetal age estimates are not available, recording the date of calving for each individual (or, at least, the number of calves born each 21-day period) also allows producers to generate calving distribution profiles; however, by analyzing pregnancy distribution soon after the end of the breeding season, information is generated 6 to 7 months earlier.

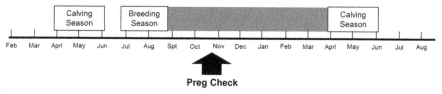

Fig. 2. Approximate timing of diagnosis of pregnancy (Preg) status in beef herds in relationship to the beginning of the breeding season.

The most common method of analyzing pregnancy data is to break the breeding season into 21-day periods. Then, for further diagnostic power, the breeding season can be broken down another level, into 2 or more categories by 21-day periods.

Categories analyzed can include age, breed, pasture, or other management groups. Gestational age data can be collected and displayed while on-farm by using hand-written grids (**Fig. 3**) or with computer-generated spreadsheets (**Fig. 4**, Document S1).

For a 60 to 65 day breeding season, the ideal profile should resemble **Fig. 5**. Producers should strive for nutritional and management systems that allow 60% to 65% of the exposed cows to become pregnant in the first 21 days of the breeding season.[11] Most of the remaining cows should become pregnant in the second 21-day period. Also, 5% or less of the herd should be nonpregnant at the end of the 60 to 65 day breeding period.

Beef Cattle Veterinary Services
Anywhere, USA

Pregnancy Distribution Evaluation

Farm DIAMOND BAR J   Dr. H.O. JOHNSON   Date 10/3/16

Breeding Season Starts 6/5/16   Ends 8/20/16 # Head 89

Categories	1st 21 Days	2nd 21 Days	3rd 21 Days	4th 21 Days	Open	
	110-90	69-89	48-68	27-47	<40	
MATURE COWS	THL THL THL THL THL THL THL THL II 42	THL THL III 13	THL 5	II 2	THL 5	= 67
1st CALF	III 3	III 3	I 1		III 3	= 10
HEIFERS	THL III 8	III 3			I 1	= 12
	53	19	6	2	9	

Report

Categories	1st 21 Days		1st 63 Days		Total	
	#	%	#	%	#	%
Overall	53/89	59.6	78/89	87.6	80/89	89.9
1) MATURE COWS	42/67	62.7	60/67	89.5	62/67	92.5
2) 1st CALF	3/10	30	7/10	70	7/10	70
3) HEIFERS	8/12	66.7	11/12	91.7	11/12	91.7
4)						

Comments:
　　3 BULLS AT TURN-OUT, 1 REMOVED 7/8/16 (INJURY)

Fig. 3. Example of form for hand-written data collection and display.

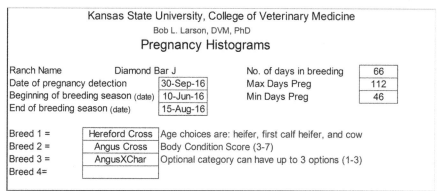

Kansas State University, College of Veterinary Medicine
Bob L. Larson, DVM, PhD

Pregnancy Histograms

Ranch Name	Diamond Bar J		No. of days in breeding	66
Date of pregnancy detection	30-Sep-16		Max Days Preg	112
Beginning of breeding season (date)	10-Jun-16		Min Days Preg	46
End of breeding season (date)	15-Aug-16			

Breed 1 =	Hereford Cross	Age choices are: heifer, first calf heifer, and cow
Breed 2 =	Angus Cross	Body Condition Score (3-7)
Breed 3 =	AngusXChar	Optional category can have up to 3 options (1-3)
Breed 4=		

Total pregnancy %

% preg	% open
82.09	17.91

Number preg	Number open
55	12

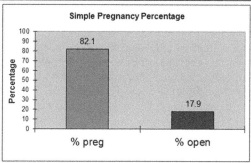

Percentage by age in each 21-d interval

	Heifer	1st Calf Heifer	Cow
First	62.50	50.00	45.16
Second	18.75	20.00	29.03
Third	6.25	5.00	12.90
Fourth	0.00	0.00	0.00
Fifth	0.00	0.00	0.00
Open	12.50	25.00	12.90
Preg	87.50	75.00	87.10
Total #	16	20	31

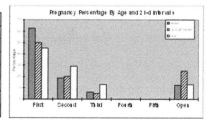

Fig. 4. Example of spread-sheet generated data display.

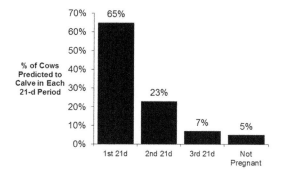

Fig. 5. Pregnancy distribution goal for a 63-day breeding season.

Once fetal age data is collected and organized for analysis, conclusions or further questions may present themselves. If the data meet the criteria in **Fig. 5**, the breeding season can be considered a success and further diagnostics are probably not warranted. If, however, the profile is less than ideal, further evaluation should be done to determine the cause.

INVESTIGATION OF LESS-THAN-IDEAL HERD REPRODUCTIVE PROFILES

If a client is concerned that too few calves are born live from the cows that entered the breeding season, a veterinarian looking at the flow of cows through the reproductive cycle (see **Fig. 1**) will recognize that the potential pathways that result in calves not being born alive include failure to conceive, early-gestation pregnancy loss, late-gestation pregnancy loss, and birth of stillborn calves.

Fortunately, the most likely rule-outs for the various alternate pathways that result in cows that enter the breeding season failing to give birth to live calves are mostly mutually exclusive.

In contrast to only evaluating low overall pregnancy success, the reproductive profile can provide information to narrow the list of potential causative factors for the reproductive loss. For example, when low pregnancy success is identified, there are many potential causes but they fall into several broader categories (**Fig. 6**). The reproductive profile can help identify which broad category is most likely.

FAILURE TO CONCEIVE
Failure to Conceive: Cow Problems

Failure to conceive due to cow or heifer problems related to displaying the behavioral characteristics of estrus necessary to induce mating, ovulating a fertile oocyte, or

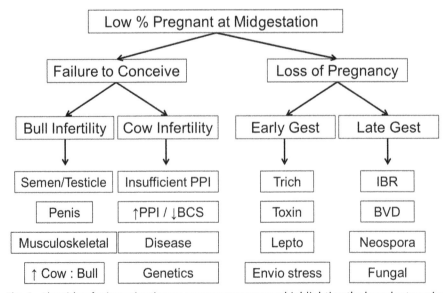

Fig. 6. Algorithm for investigating poor pregnancy success highlighting the broad categories of largely mutually exclusive rule-out lists. BCS, body condition score; BVD, bovine viral diarrhea; Enviro, environment; Gest, gestation; IBR, infectious bovine rhinotracheitis; Lepto, *Leptospira* sp; PPI, postpartum interval; Trich, *Trichomonas fetus*.

maintaining an early embryo is due to factors that occur before or during the breeding season (**Fig. 7**).

Because gestation lasts about 283 days, cows must become pregnant again within 82 days after calving to maintain a 365-day calving interval. Because of the biologic constraints listed previously (70–100 day or more period until 90% of cows have retained postpartum fertility and 60%–70% expected successful pregnancies from mating of fertile bulls and cows), the number of cows cycling at the start of the breeding season is greatly influenced by the immediately preceding calving distribution (and calving distributions of previous years).

Cow problem factors include:

- The term momentum is used to describe the reality of beef herd reproduction that last year's breeding and calving season pattern is an important predictor of this year's breeding season pattern.
- Although calving distributions can become much less than ideal in a single year, it is very difficult to improve calving distributions in a single year (or even over several years).
- Herds that have 50% of cows cycling by the end of the first 21 days of the breeding season are expected to have 30% to 35% of the herd become pregnant in the first 21 days (60%–70% pregnancy success from the mating of fertile cows to fertile bulls).
  - Herds may only have 50% cycling at the start of the breeding season because only one-half of the herd calved early enough to complete the period of post-partum anestrus by the end of the first 21 days of breeding.
  - The 30% to 40% of cycling, fertile cows that failed to maintain a pregnancy from the first mating will have a second 60% to 70% probability of establishing a successful pregnancy 21 days later. The previously cycling cows will be joined by the portion of the herd that resumes cycling during the second 21 days. This results in approximately another 30% of the herd establishing a pregnancy during the second 21 days of breeding.
  - Herds that have approximately 50% of cows cycling by the end of the first 21 days of the breeding season will have a flat pregnancy distribution that will require 4 or more 21-day periods to reach 95% of the herd establishing a successful pregnancy (**Fig. 8**).
  - A herd with a previously front-end loaded distribution similar to **Fig. 5** that calves in thin body condition and/or that loses body condition after calving will have prolonged periods of postpartum anestrous and can have a pregnancy distribution similar to **Fig. 8** within a year or 2 once the percentage

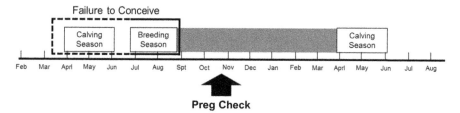

Fig. 7. In situations when failure to conceive leads to a poor reproductive profile, the problem occurred before the time of pregnancy diagnosis and the causes must have occurred during the breeding season (bull problems) or during the breeding season because of factors starting at or before calving (cow problems). In addition, few, if any, cows have palpable evidence of an involuting uterus or a retained placenta indicating pregnancy loss.

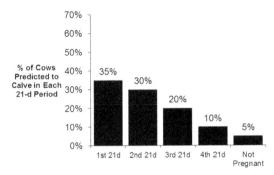

Fig. 8. Typical reproductive profile for herd with 50% of cows cycling by the end of the first 21 days of the breeding season.

of cows that have resumed fertile cycles by the end of the first 21 days of breeding drops to 50% or fewer.

o If the breeding season is confined to 60 to 65 days, approximately 15% of the herd is expected to be nonpregnant, even though the cows are fertile and mated to fertile bulls (see **Fig. 8**).

o This profile is expected to be repeated the following breeding season because nearly all the cows that calve in the first 21-day period and about one-half the cows that calve in the second 21-day period are expected to resume fertile cycles by the end of the first 21 days of the next breeding season (35% + 15% = 50%), the same percentage of cycling cows that created the current distribution.

o If a reproductive profile similar to **Fig. 8** is due to a high percentage of the herd not resuming fertile cycles until the second or later 21-day period of breeding, palpation of the reproductive tracts of the nonpregnant cows should not reveal evidence of pregnancy loss (ie, involuting uterus).

o The magnitude of nonpregnant cows at the end of the breeding season will depend on the length of the breeding season and the percentage of the herd that are cycling by the end of the first 21 days of breeding.

  ▪ Even if the breeding season is limited to 63 days and postpartum anestrus is prolonged, at least 80% of the cows are expected to be pregnant if the problem is confined to issues of cows resuming fertile estrous cycling during the breeding season.

  ▪ A magnitude of nonpregnant cows that exceeds 20% of the herd is not likely due to cow problems alone, and either bull problems or a combination of cow problems and bull problems should be investigated.

Failure to Conceive: Bull Problems

Because bulls are responsible for establishing viable pregnancies in multiple cows, bull failure can result in a high percentage of the herd being nonpregnant, particularly if the breeding season is limited to 60 to 65 days.

Bull problem considerations include:

- Any time that reproductive efficiency during a breeding season suddenly decreases, bull problems should be considered likely.
- Single-bull breeding pastures are particularly prone to a high percentage of nonpregnant cows if bulls do not successfully breed cycling, fertile cows.

- ○ The magnitude of pregnancy loss due to an infertile bull in a single sire pasture can be extremely high and combined with sudden onset may be pathognomonic for a bull problem.
- Bull problems at a point after the start of the breeding season
  Decrease in percent of open cows becoming pregnant from one 21-day period to the next does not have to be as obvious or drastic as that depicted in **Fig. 9** for bull problems to be the most likely cause of reproductive inefficiency.
  - ○ Populations of fertile, cycling cows are not likely to have a sudden decrease in the percentage having fertile cycles because reduction in cow fertility due to body condition change usually requires several weeks and severe disruptions in nutrient intake.
  - ○ Because the breeding season depicted in **Fig. 9** starts with good reproductive success, the bulls associated with this problem would have passed a breeding soundness examination of bulls (BSEB) before the start of breeding. In addition, a BSEB done after the breeding season may or may not provide indications of subfertility, depending on the type of insult and the length of time between the insult and the BSEB.
- Bull problems at the start of the breeding season
  A herd with too few bulls for the number of cycling cows, a herd with a single bull recovering from an injury or disease, or a herd with a group of bulls that are subfertile at the start of breeding (eg, peripubertal bulls) but that regain or obtain normal fertility as the breeding season progresses may or may not include a history of passing a BSEB before the start of the breeding season. However, if a BSEB is used after the breeding season as part of the reproductive inefficiency investigation, the bulls are likely to pass (**Fig. 10**).
  - ○ A BSEB should be performed before the start of the breeding season on all bulls in the breeding program. Although a satisfactory BSEB does not eliminate bull subfertility as a rule-out for poor breeding performance, a questionable breeder as determined by BSEB may affect the cow-to-fertile bull ratio if not replaced. Failure to obtain a BSEB on all bulls leaves bull fertility at the start of the breeding season as an unknown variable among possible rule-outs when investigating poor herd-level reproductive performance.

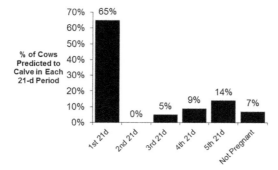

Fig. 9. Pregnancy distribution in a single-bull herd in which cows are cycling at the start of the breeding season. The bull is successfully mating cows but an acute onset of bull infertility occurs at the end of the first 21 days of the breeding season (eg, injury, disease) followed by a period of partial recovery.

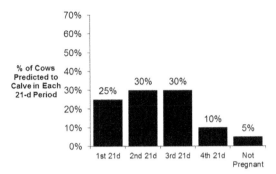

Fig. 10. Pregnancy distribution of a herd with fertile, cycling cows, but subfertile bulls at the start of the breeding season; however, bulls obtain or recover normal fertility, or the ratio between fertile bulls and cycling cows improves as cows become pregnant as the breeding season progresses. The percent of nonpregnant cows becoming pregnant each 21-day period (1st through 4th) is 25%, 40%, 67%, and 67%, respectively.

- A BSEB (including a through physical examination) at the time the breeding season problem is discovered may supply information about penile, testicular, foot and leg, or other musculoskeletal health problems during the breeding season. However, lack of identifiable disease pathologic condition during an examination following the breeding season does not rule out a physical (locomotion, mounting, intromission) or semen quality problem and an associated cow-to-bull ratio inadequacy that impaired successful mating earlier in the breeding season.
- Multiple-bull breeding pastures are resilient to breeding failure due to the inability of a single bull to successfully mate cows. However, because of potential problems arising from injuries due to bull-on-bull fighting, social dominance by subfertile bulls, and isolation of groups of cows without 1 or more bulls present in an extensive breeding pasture, multiple-bull pastures can also have poor reproductive efficiency due to bull problems and have reproductive profiles similar to **Fig. 9** or **10**.
- The reproductive profile depicted in **Fig. 8** can be due to cows not cycling at the start of the breeding season or due to bull problems that result in suboptimum breeding success such that only 40% to 50% of mating with fertile, cycling cows result in a viable pregnancy.
- If a reproductive profile similar to **Figs. 8** and **9**, or **10** is due to bull subfertility or inability to successfully mate, palpation of the reproductive tracts of the nonpregnant cows should not reveal evidence of pregnancy loss (ie, involuting uterus).
- The magnitude of nonpregnant cows at the end of the breeding season will depend on the number of cycling cows per fertile bull and the length of the breeding season. However, any reproductive profile that indicates that 15% or more of cows are not pregnant after the first 63 days of the breeding season is sufficiently suggestive of bull problems to justify further investigation of bull fertility.

EARLY-GESTATION PREGNANCY LOSS

Infection with the protozoa *Trichomonas fetus* (Trich) is an important cause of early-gestation pregnancy loss in North America because it is present in many cattle-dense areas of the continent and because it can cause a high percentage of exposed

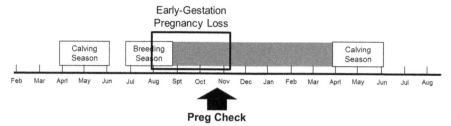

Fig. 11. In situations when early-gestation pregnancy loss leads to negative effects on the reproductive profile, the problem occurs after the breeding season started and probably before the time of pregnancy diagnosis. The overall pregnancy percentage and the distribution of pregnancies are expected to be affected by early-pregnancy loss. In addition, some of the nonpregnant cows are likely to exhibit palpable evidence of an involuting uterus as evidence for recent pregnancy loss.

cows to lose their pregnancies (**Fig. 11**). The pregnancy profile of a herd infected with Trich will vary depending on what the profile would have been without infection and the timing of Trich introduction into the herd.

If Trich entered the herd before the start of the breeding season, so that a high percentage bulls are already infected, the cows will become pregnant at a time similar to last year's breeding season. However, infected cows are likely to lose their pregnancies approximately 15 to 80 days into gestation, at which time the embryo or fetus dies and is resorbed or aborted. A period of cow infertility is expected to last for another 2 to 6 months as a result of infection. The magnitude of loss is expected to approach 30% to 50% of exposed cows (**Fig. 12**).

If Trich entered the herd during the breeding season, or only a few bulls were infected at the start of the breeding season but the number of infected bulls increased as the breeding season progressed, then the reproductive profile is greatly influenced by what the profile would have been without Trich exposure and the speed at which additional bulls become infected (**Fig. 13**).

If few bulls are Trich-infected at the start of breeding, only a few cows that become pregnant during the first 21 days are mated by Trich-infected bulls so few pregnancies

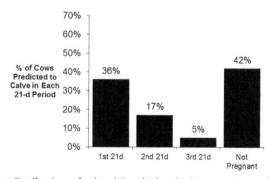

Fig. 12. Pregnancy distribution of a herd in which a high percentage of bulls are infected with Trich at the start of the breeding season. About 40% (30% to 50%) of the cows that become pregnant during each 21-day cycle will lose their pregnancy. Most cows that become pregnant in the first 2 21-day cycles will be nonpregnant by the time of pregnancy diagnosis; however, some later-conceiving cows may resorb or abort the fetus due to Trich after the time of pregnancy diagnosis.

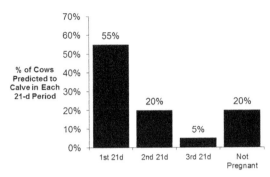

Fig. 13. Pregnancy distribution of a herd in which few bulls are infected with Trich at the start of the breeding season but during the breeding season, many become infected.

are lost from this portion of the breeding season. By the second 21 days of breeding, more bulls have become infected with Trich and cows mated by positive bulls may lose their pregnancies. And, by the third 21 days, many cows are mated by Trich-infected bulls and about 40% (30% to 50%) of these cows will lose their pregnancy.

Most cows that become pregnant from mating by Trich-infected bulls in the first 2 21-day cycles will be nonpregnant by the time of pregnancy diagnosis, but some later-conceiving cows may not abort due to Trich until after the time of pregnancy diagnosis.

If any disease-causing organism or toxin causes early-gestation loss, palpation of the reproductive tracts of the nonpregnant cows relatively soon after pregnancy loss should reveal evidence of that loss in some of the affected cows (ie, involuting uterus).

The magnitude of nonpregnant cows at the end of the breeding season will depend on when in the breeding season the herd becomes infected with Trich and the percentage of the bulls in the breeding pasture that become infected. If a high percentage of bulls are infected for most of the breeding season, the magnitude of pregnancy loss is expected to be very high (eg, 20%–50% fewer pregnancies than expected) and evidence of pregnancy loss is likely to be found on palpation of the nonpregnant cows' uteri.

Other causes of early-gestation pregnancy loss (eg, *Campylobacter fetus* subspecies *venerialis*, bluetongue virus, *Leptospira borgpetersenii* serovar *hardjo* type *hardjo-bovis*, bovine viral diarrhea virus [BVDv]) will have a similar effect on the reproductive profile but the magnitude of pregnancy loss is not expected to be as high as with Trich.[9,12]

LATE-GESTATION PREGNANCY LOSS

Infectious, toxic, and nutritional causes of pregnancy loss that are expected to be most commonly expressed in midgestation to late gestation include bovine herpes virus 1 (infectious bovine rhinotracheitis [IBR]), BVDv, *Neospora caninum*, *Leptospira* sp, epizootic bovine abortion, pine-needle toxicosis, and others (**Fig. 14**).[12,13]

Pregnancy losses in midgestation to late gestation are likely to occur after the time of pregnancy diagnosis; therefore, the profile as determined at the time of pregnancy diagnosis will look similar to the proceeding calving pattern. If some losses occurred before the time that pregnancy status is determined, evidence of that loss is likely to be found on palpation of the nonpregnant cows' uteri.

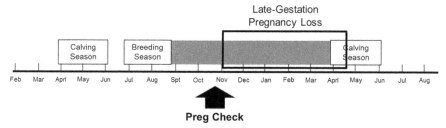

Fig. 14. In situations when late-gestation pregnancy loss leads to pregnancy wastage, the problem likely reveals itself after pregnancy diagnosis; therefore, the reproductive profile based on data collected at pregnancy diagnosis may not be affected. Evidence of abortion or failure to calve in cows that were diagnosed as pregnant in midgestation indicates a late-gestation pregnancy loss problem. Comparison of calving profiles to pregnancy profiles can be very helpful in the investigation.

The magnitude of pregnancy loss due to midgestation to late-gestation infection, toxins, or nutrition will depend on the agent, toxin, or nutrient involved, the percentage of the herd that is most susceptible at the time of the insult, and the immune status of the herd. Except in unusual situations of concurrent high susceptibility and exposure, the percent of cows that lose their pregnancy is expected to be relatively low and much lower than losses associated with bull failure or Trich exposure.

STILLBIRTH LOSS

Pregnancy losses in at the end of gestation will, by definition, occur after the time of pregnancy diagnosis and, therefore, the reproductive profile is not affected (**Fig. 15**). Available records gathered at the time of calving, as well as questions directed to the cow-calf producer that specifically define the number of stillborn calves or calves that die shortly after birth, will determine whether excessive calf losses should be investigated.

SECOND-LEVEL ANALYSIS OF GESTATION-AGE DATA

To capture more information from reproductive profiles, the distribution of breeding dates can be analyzed not only by 21-day intervals but also by category within those intervals. The herd depicted by **Fig. 16** has an overall pregnancy proportion of 91%, which is less than the goal of 95% following a 63-day breeding season but is not alarming. In addition, the percentage of the herd that became pregnant during the first

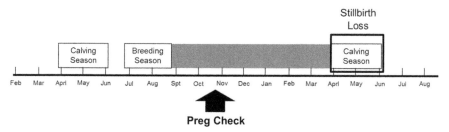

Fig. 15. In situations when stillbirth loss leads to pregnancy wastage, the reproductive profile based on data collected at pregnancy diagnosis would not be affected.

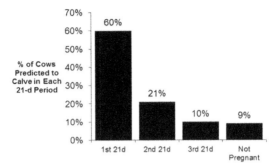

Fig. 16. A nearly ideal pregnancy distribution in a herd with a hidden breeding season problem.

21 days of the breeding season is near the goal of 65%. From these observations, one could conclude that the herd has normal fertility and that there are no reproductive management problems.

A closer examination of the information gathered while determining pregnancy status of the herd reveals a much different conclusion. The herd depicted in **Fig. 16** consists of heifers (nulliparous heifers), first-calf heifers (primiparous cows), and mature (multiparous) cows. Estrous synchronization and artificial insemination was used in the heifers. The rest of the cowherd was exposed to 5 bulls that had each passed a BSEB before the start of the breeding season. The data in are further analyzed by breaking it into 4 separate evaluations for each 21-day period: the overall proportion of pregnancy, the proportion of pregnancy for the heifers, the proportion of pregnancy for first-calf heifers (primiparous cows), and the proportion of pregnancy for the mature (multiparous) cows (**Fig. 17**). Although the overall pregnancy distribution for this herd is not alarming, a very poor reproductive profile for the first-calf heifers (primiparous cows) indicates that management for this herd is not satisfactory. Not only are more than one-half of the open animals from the first-calf heifer group, the percentage pregnant during the first 21 days of the breeding season for this group is also unacceptable. Breaking the fetal age estimation data collected at the time of pregnancy diagnosis (or calving date data collected at calving) into separate reproductive profiles based on cow age category, breed, breeding pasture, or other management group is often necessary to accurately identify deficiencies in herd reproductive efficiency and to direct the investigation to the correct subset of the cow herd.

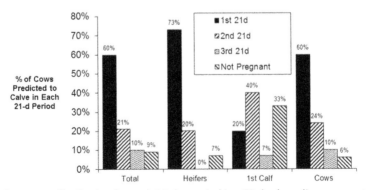

Fig. 17. Pregnancy distribution for each 21-day period in a 63-day breeding season, analyzed by age group.

SUMMARY

Pregnancy distributions are 1 of several important pieces of diagnostic data used by veterinarians evaluating beef herd reproduction.

- Information obtained at the time of diagnosis of pregnancy status to evaluate beef herd reproduction
  - Reproductive profile (pregnancy distribution)
    Pregnancy distributions created from data collected at the time of pregnancy diagnosis often do not provide definitive answers in herd fertility investigations because 1 or more factors may cause or may combine to cause a specific distribution and a single cause may manifest itself as more than 1 reproductive profile. However, pregnancy distributions are a powerful diagnostic tool in the investigation of beef cow herd reproductive performance.
  - Characteristics of nonpregnant uteri per palpation
    Palpable evidence of cows with an involuting uterus or a retained placenta provide proof of recent pregnancy loss that could be the remnants of a herd problem of early-gestation loss or the beginnings of late-gestation pregnancy loss.
- Additional information to evaluate beef herd reproduction
  - Comprehensive BSEB before the start of the breeding season, including determination of bull-to-cow ratio in breeding pastures (or confirmation of absence of BSEB)
  - Calving distribution of the just-completed calving season
  - Pregnancy distribution (or calving distribution) from previous year (1 or more) reproductive performance
  - Breeding soundness examination (BSE) of replacement (nulliparous) heifers before breeding season (eg, percent cycling, reproductive tract score, body weight, pelvic area)
  - Estimation of the percentage of first-calf heifers (primiparous cows) that have resumed fertile cycles by the start of the breeding season for their second pregnancy by palpation or ultrasound examination for presence of corpus luteum, observation for expression of estrus (with or without heat detection aids), or measurement of progesterone levels in blood
  - Estimation of the risk of herd exposure to Trich, BVDv, IBR, pine-needle toxicosis, or other abortion-causing agents and biosecurity and management factors that contribute to increased or decreased risk
  - If midgestation to late-gestation pregnancy loss is identified as the problem, a rule-out list of infectious agents or toxins that cause late-gestation losses can be investigated with specific diagnostic tests for the most likely rule-outs.
  - If early-gestation pregnancy loss is identified as the problem, then physical examination findings and diagnostic tests specific for infectious, toxic, and physiologic insults that are associated with early-gestation loss can be initiated.
  - If failure-to-conceive is identified as the problem, BSEB, BSE findings of replacement heifers, and herd records can be used to indicate whether a bull-infertility or cow-infertility problem is the most likely cause.
    - Once the distinction of which sex is mostly likely associated with the conception failure, specific diagnostic tests or examination of records can be used to investigate the principal bull or cow problem.

By starting with the flow of beef cows through the reproductive system and gathering fetal age estimation at the time of pregnancy diagnosis, veterinarians can use reproductive profiles and other readily available information to systematically go through a decision tree to diagnose reproductive inefficiency and to advise producers which areas of improved reproductive efficiency are available for their herds.

SUPPLEMENTARY DATA

Supplementary data related to this article can be found at http://dx.doi.org/10.1016/j.cvfa.2016.01.005.

REFERENCES

1. Spire MF. Breeding season evaluation of beef herds. In: Howard JF, editor. Current veterinary therapy. 2nd edition. Philadelphia: WB Saunders; 1986. p. 808–11.
2. Randle RF. Production medicine considerations for enhanced reproductive performance in beef herds. Vet Clin North Am 1993;9:404–15.
3. Larson RL. Evaluating information obtained from pregnancy examination in beef herds. Vet Med 1999;94:566–76.
4. White BJ. Beef herd record analysis. In: Hopper R, editor. Bovine reproduction. Oxford (United Kingdom): Wiley-Blackwell; 2015. p. 364–9.
5. Cushman RA, Allan MF, Thallman RM, et al. Characterization of biological types of cattle (Cycle VII): influence of postpartum interval and estrous cycle length on fertility. J Anim Sci 2007;85:2156–62.
6. Lents CA, White FJ, Ciccioli NH, et al. Effects of body condition score at parturition and postpartum protein on estrous behavior and size of the dominant follicle in beef cows. J Anim Sci 2008;86:2549–56.
7. Ciccioli NH, Wettemann RP, Spicer LJ, et al. Influence of body condition at calving and postpartum nutrition on endocrine function and reproductive performance of primiparous beef cows. J Anim Sci 2003;81:3107–20.
8. Berardinelli JG, Joshi PS. Introduction of bulls at different days postpartum on resumption of ovarian cycling activity in primiparous beef cows. J Anim Sci 2006;83:2106–10.
9. BonDurant RH. Selected diseases and conditions associated with bovine conceptus loss in the first trimester. Theriogenology 2007;68:461–73.
10. Bretzlaff K. A pictorial guide to bovine pregnancy diagnosis. Vet Med 1987;82: 295–304.
11. Kasari T, Gleason D. Herd management practices that influence total beef calf production – part I. Comp Cont Ed Pract Vet 1996;18(7):823–32.
12. Larson RL. Diagnosing the cause of bovine abortion and other perinatal deaths. Vet Med 1996;91:478–86.
13. Anderson ML. Infectious causes of bovine abortion during mid- to late-gestation. Theriogenology 2007;68:474–86.

Synchronization and Artificial Insemination Strategies in Beef Cattle

Graham Clifford Lamb, PhD[a],*, Vitor R.G. Mercadante, PhD[b]

KEYWORDS

- Estrus synchronization • Artificial insemination • Beef cattle • Economics

KEY POINTS

- Development of fixed-time artificial insemination (TAI) estrus-synchronization protocols limit animal handling and eliminate detection of estrus to provide users an opportunity to more readily incorporate artificial insemination (AI) into their herds.
- Annually, the Beef Reproduction Task Force (http://beefrepro.unl.edu) updates recommended estrus-synchronization protocols for beef cows and heifers.
- The development of the AI Cowculator economic decision-aid tool allows producers an opportunity to determine whether they should consider AI rather than purchasing herd sires.
- As a result of continued use of intensive reproductive management tools, such as estrus synchronization and AI, producers will note a benefit in calving distribution, enhanced pregnancy rates, and increased subsequent calf value.

INTRODUCTION

Advances in reproductive biotechnologies and enhanced understanding of the dynamics of the bovine estrous cycle have made possible the development of protocols to manipulate the estrous cycle and control ovulation using natural and/or artificially synthesized hormones. Utilization of estrus or ovulation synchronization and fixed-timed artificial insemination (TAI) has facilitated the widespread utilization of artificial insemination (AI) and can greatly impact the economic viability of cow-calf systems by enhancing weaning weights.[1] Implementation of TAI programs by beef producers, however, depends largely on 2 key factors:

1. Limited frequency of handling cattle; and
2. Elimination of detection of estrus by using TAI.

The authors have nothing to disclose.
[a] North Florida Research and Education Center, University of Florida, 3925 Highway 71, Marianna, FL 32446, USA; [b] Department of Animal and Poultry Sciences, Virginia Tech, 3470 Litton Reaves Hall, Blacksburg, VA 24061, USA
* Corresponding author.
E-mail address: gclamb@ufl.edu

Vet Clin Food Anim 32 (2016) 335–347
http://dx.doi.org/10.1016/j.cvfa.2016.01.006
vetfood.theclinics.com

Currently only 7.6% of beef operations in the United Sates use AI as a reproductive management tool,[2] whereas 72.5% of all pregnancies in dairy females are the result of AI.[3] When queried as to their reluctance to use AI, more than 53% of operations cited labor concerns or complicated estrous synchronization protocols as primary reasons for not implementing this reproductive technology.[2] During the past decade, TAI protocols have been developed that eliminate detecting estrus and yield satisfactory pregnancy rates. Most of these TAI protocols depend largely on the use of exogenous progesterone (P4), gonadotropin-release hormone (GnRH) to induce ovulation, and luteolysis via administration of prostaglandin $F_{2\alpha}$ (PGF).[4,5]

EARLY ESTROUS SYNCHRONIZATION PROTOCOLS

A single injection of PGF to induce luteolysis followed by detection of estrus and AI in heifers was one of the first attempts to synchronize estrus.[6] Conception rates did not differ between control (21 days of detection of estrus) and treated heifers. However, induction of luteolysis via injection of PGF can be achieved only during diestrus, when a corpus luteum (CL) is present[7] and injection of PGF in females during metestrus failed to induce luteolysis due to the refractoriness of the young CL during this phase of the estrous cycle.[6] In addition, no estrus response would be observed in anestrus or prepubertal females, because of the absence of a CL.[8]

Administration of GnRH to cows successfully increased concentrations of luteinizing hormone (LH) and ovulation of the dominant follicle was achieved within 24 to 32 hours after GnRH injection.[9,10] A combination of a GnRH injection followed by PGF injection 7 days later was used to synchronize the follicular wave and induce luteolysis, respectively, allowing a concentration of estrus activity and increased number of females exposed to AI.[9] A second injection of GnRH 48 hours after PGF injection was introduced to induce ovulation of the dominant follicle, allowing TAI to be performed, excluding the necessity of detection of estrus. This TAI protocol was termed "Ovsynch."[9] In the Ovsynch protocol, the first GnRH injection is administered to induce ovulation of the dominant follicle, resetting the follicular wave. However, the ovulation response to the first injection of GnRH was 31% in anestrous beef cows[11] and varies according to the day of the estrous cycle,[12,13] diameter of the dominant follicle,[14] and stage of follicular development.[9] When ovulation from the first GnRH fails, the second GnRH injection may cause the dominant follicle to ovulate at unexpected intervals before AI impairing fertilization and pregnancy success.[15]

CURRENT ESTROUS SYNCHRONIZATION PROTOCOLS

Later, the inclusion of P4, supplemented by a controlled internal drug release (CIDR) device, to prevent ovulation before PGF injection was extensively investigated.[4,15–17] Comparing conception rates between protocols with or without exogenous sources of P4 indicated that fertility was improved when the device was applied (7-day CO-Synch + CIDR protocol).[4,15,18] In addition, pregnancy rates of anestrus cows synchronized with the CIDR were similar to cyclic cows.[15,16,19] However, follicles that fail to ovulate to the first GnRH in the 7-day CO-Synch + CIDR protocol[4,18] may become persistent during the 7-day period in which the CIDR is present, thereby reducing fertility to TAI. The proestrus phase in the 7-day CO-Synch + CIDR protocol may be defined as the interval from the administration of PGF to the second injection of GnRH, which may have a duration of 60 to 72 hours.[4,15,17] Recently, in an attempt to improve fertility, research focused on increasing the length of the proestrus in estrous synchronization protocols from 66 hours (7-day CO-Synch + CIDR) to 72 hours (5-day CO-Synch + CIDR).[17,20,21]

Extensive research has been done and is still being conducted by several research groups to enhance the understanding of physiologic processes involved in the estrous cycle and to enhance fertility and pregnancy success of TAI protocols. In an effort to combine expertise in reproductive physiology and estrous synchronization and encourage research cooperation across the United States, the Beef Reproduction Task Force (BRTF) was formed in 2002. The BRTF is a multistate team of reproductive physiology experts from 7 to 9 universities across the United States (http://beefrepro. unl.edu/). The objectives of the BRTF are as follows:

- Improve the understanding of the physiologic processes of the estrous cycle, the procedures available to synchronize estrus and ovulation, and the proper application of these systems.
- Improve the understanding of methods to assess male fertility and how it affects the success of AI programs.

Every year the BRTF releases an updated chart of recommended estrous synchronization and TAI protocols that have been tested and are proven to be effective for beef cows and heifers, including different protocols for *Bos taurus* and *Bos indicus* cattle (**Figs. 1** and **2**). These charts are an excellent source of information and serve as a guideline for beef producers and industry leaders in the United States.

FACTORS AFFECTING PREGNANCY SUCCESS OF ESTROUS SYNCHRONIZATION PROTOCOLS
Anestrous and Concentration of Progesterone

Postpartum anestrous is the major contributor to infertility in cattle.[22] The resumption of cyclicity, with the development of a functional CL that is capable of producing P4, earlier in the postpartum period increases the number of estrous cycles and the chances of a cow becoming pregnant during the breeding season. Reducing the postpartum interval may be accomplished by managing nutrition, body condition score (BCS), disease, and the suckling interaction between cow and calf.[23] Resumption of postpartum estrous cycles relies on increasing LH pulse frequency and overall concentration of LH in blood and the increasing LH secretion stimulates follicle growth and ovulation.[24]

It has been suggested that a decrease in concentrations of P4 and an increase in E_2 at the initiation of synchronization protocol may be important in initiating an increase in LH release and consequently ovulation in cattle.[25] In beef cows, presynchronization (PGF administered 3 days before initiating a 6-day CO-Synch + CIDR TAI protocol) improved follicle turnover in response to the first GnRH and subsequent pregnancy success compared with a 5-day CO-Synch + CIDR treatment.[26] In addition, heifers were more likely to display estrus and had better follicle turnover after the first GnRH when presynchronized with PGF.[26] Recently, it has been reported that suckled beef cows with concentrations of P4 of 4 ng/mL or more at the initiation of a synchronization protocol had a 7.6% increase in pregnancy to TAI than cows with concentrations of P4 of 0.5 ng/mL or less.[27] In that same study, pregnancy to TAI for cows with concentration of P4 at CIDR insertion of 0.50 to 3.99 ng/mL did not differ from cows with concentration of P4 of 0.5 ng/mL or less. In contrast, beef cows with reduced concentrations of P4 at the onset of TAI protocols have been shown to enhance pregnancy to TAI success.[26]

Follicle Development

Several ovulation-synchronization protocols use GnRH at the time of CIDR insertion to induce ovulation and reset follicular waves to improve pregnancy outcomes.[5]

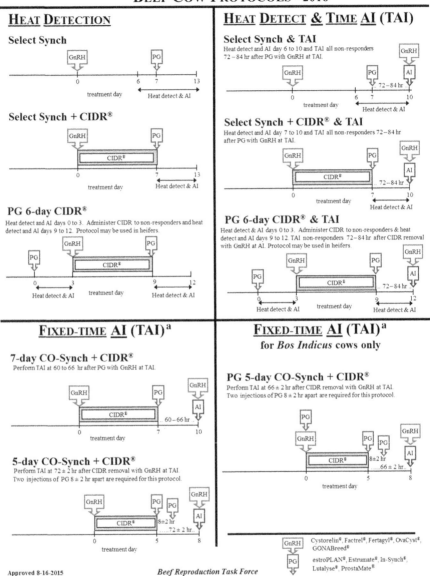

Fig. 1. BRTF chart of recommended estrous synchronization and TAI protocols for beef cows. [a] The time listed for *"Fixed-time AI"* should be considered as the approximate average time of insemination. This should be based on the number of cows to inseminate, labor, and facilities. (*Courtesy of* Beef Reproduction Task Force, University of Nebraska-Lincoln, Lincoln, NB; with permission.)

Ovulation induced by GnRH is dependent on the stage of follicular maturity when GnRH injection occurs[28] and ovulation of follicles smaller than 11 mm in diameter resulted in compromised pregnancy rates to TAI.[29] In addition, replacement beef heifers were more likely to become pregnant when follicles induced to ovulate with

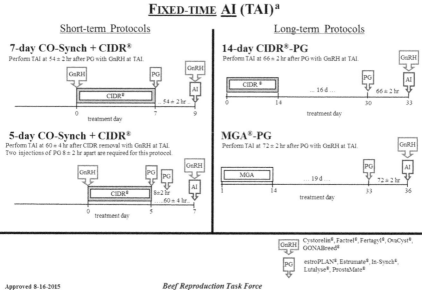

BEEF HEIFER PROTOCOLS - 2016

Fig. 2. BRTF chart of recommended estrous synchronization and TAI protocols for beef heifers. [a] The times listed for "*Fixed-time AI*" should be considered as the approximate average time of insemination. This should be based on the number of heifers to inseminate, labor, and facilities. (*Courtesy of* the Beef Reproduction Task Force, University of Nebraska-Lincoln, Lincoln, NB; with permission.)

GnRH ranged from 10.7 to 15.7 mm in diameter.[30] Nonetheless, recent studies investigating the effects of different follicle ages by manipulating the duration of proestrus and comparing mature larger follicles with young smaller follicles in beef cows and heifers determined that the age and maturity of the ovulatory follicle did not influence pregnancy to TAI outcome.[31,32]

Body Condition Score

Body condition score during the peripartum period also affects fertility. Previously, we[15] demonstrated that a single unit increase in BCS, especially from poor BCS to adequate BCS, resulted in a 23% point increase in the proportion of cows pregnant to TAI. Cows calving in poor BCS experience longer postpartum intervals to first estrus than those cows calving in moderate to good BCS.[33] The quantity of fat tissue is an indicator of BCS and energy reserves, but is not only an energy source tissue but also an important endocrine organ that synthesizes several hormones.[34] Leptin is synthesized mainly by white adipose tissue, commonly referred to as fat tissue[35] and it regulates body energy metabolism and food intake.[36] Concentrations of leptin are positively correlated with amplitude and frequency of LH pulses.[37] In addition, the interval from parturition to first ovulation was positively correlated with the leptin nadir, indicating that a delay in the rise of leptin in blood is associated with an increase in the interval to first ovulation.[38] Furthermore, in a review combining data from 3269 suckled cows exposed to estrous synchronization protocols, as BCS increased from 3.5 or less to 6.0 or more, the percentage of cows cycling increased linearly by 18% $\pm$ 2% for each unit increase in BCS, and pregnancy rates were greater in cows that calved during the first 7 weeks of the calving season, even though they had a lower overall BCS than later-calving cows.[39]

Days Postpartum and Parity

The effects of days postpartum (DPP) on pregnancy rate to TAI in suckled beef cows have also been previously shown, with improved fertility in multiparous cows and when DPP was greater than 50 days.[4,15,27] Differences in pregnancy responses of primiparous versus multiparous cows can be attributed to more than the continual presence of a suckling calf that prolongs anestrus and delays the reinitiation of estrous cycles.[40] In a review of several studies including 3269 suckled cows, regardless of parity, cyclic activity increased curvilinearly from 9% at 30 days or less to a peak of 70% at 81 to 90 days postpartum.[39]

Recent Findings on Factors Affecting Pregnancy Success of CO-Synch Programs

In a retrospective study[41] to determine the effect of the P4 environment preceding the onset of the estrus-synchronization or ovulation-synchronization program in addition to the well-documented influence of parity, BCS, and DPP on resulting pregnancy rates per AI, experimental data were combined from 73 herd-year studies consisting of more than 8500 suckled beef cows exposed to 5-day or 7-day CO-Synch–like programs. The P4 environment preceding synchronization was assessed using 3 different methods based on P4 concentrations measured in blood samples collected at 10 and 0 days before initiating the CO-Synch program and its tested variants.

Few head-to-head multiple-location or single-herd comparisons of the 5-day versus 7-day CO-Synch + CIDR programs are available. Overall, results have favored the 5-day CO-Synch + CIDR program over the 7-day program; with either increased pregnancy outcome in the 5-day program,[17,42] or similar pregnancy rates between both programs.[21] Nonetheless, results substantiated by data analyzed by Stevenson and colleagues (2015)[41] detected no advantage for the 5-day duration CO-Synch + CIDR program compared with the 7-day program. In addition, pregnancy rates after timed AI were superior for treatments that included a progestin source (ie, melengestrol acetate, norgestomet, or P4) compared with programs that included GnRH + PGF or PGF alone.

The most desirable pregnancy outcomes indicated in the review[41] were noted in older, early calving cows in better body condition, and the poorest outcomes were in primiparous, late-calving cows in the poorest body condition (**Table 1**). Progesterone status at the onset of synchronization was not critical to pregnancy outcome in multiparous cows, whereas pregnancy rate per AI was suppressed in primiparous cows starting in a low-P4 environment (proestrus, metestrus, estrus, or anestrus), reinforcing the necessity of developing heifers adequately for early puberty to increase the proportion that calve early in the calving season,[43] which is related to their postpartum reproductive performance.

Economic Implications of Combining Artificial Insemination with Estrus Synchronization

Possible outcomes from the combined use of estrous synchronization and TAI include shortened calving season, increased calf uniformity, and earlier births during the calving season. Previous models have evaluated the economic benefits derived from estrous synchronization and TAI based on heavier weaned calves with a potential increased return of $25 to $40 per calf born from AI breeding for producers who decide to dedicate the time and effort required to successfully implement an AI protocol.[44] In an analysis that investigated the incorporation of TAI compared with natural mating in a cow/calf production setting, 84% of cows exposed to TAI subsequently weaned a calf compared with 78% of cows in the natural mating group.[1] Calving distribution also differed, resulting in the mean calving day from initiation of the calving season to be 26.8 days for cows exposed to TAI and 31.3 days for cows exposed to natural mating.[1] According to these data, not only are more calves weaned per cow exposed to estrous synchronization and TAI, but calves may be older at weaning and have had the opportunity to gain more weight.

This increase in weaning weight may have the greatest potential to offset the cost of estrous synchronization and TAI systems. Although the improvement in genetics is a significant and long-term improvement, many producers have a desire for an immediate recovery of costs. Such costs can be recovered with the increase in total pounds of calf produced. The increase in total pounds produced was due to cows producing more weaned calves, which tend to be older and heavier. It is clear that the benefits of

Table 1
Influence of parity, days postpartum, and body condition score on resulting pregnancy rate per artificial insemination in 8500 suckled beef cows exposed to variation of the CO-Synch program

Parity	Days Postpartum	Body Condition Score	n	Pregnancy Rate
Multiparous	>72	>5	2154	51.7[a]
	>72	≤5	2054	43.8[b]
	≤72	>5	1056	44.2[b]
	≤72	≤5	1676	41.8[b]
Primiparous	>72	>5	496	43.8[a]
	>72	≤5	623	43.5[a]
	≤72	>5	166	40.7[a,b]
	≤72	≤5	284	33.3[b]

[a,b] Within parity, means without a common superscript differ ($P<.05$).
Adapted from Stevenson JS, Hill SL, Bridges GA, et al. Progesterone status, parity, body condition, and days postpartum before estrus or ovulation synchronization in suckled beef cattle influence artificial insemination pregnancy outcomes. J Anim Sci 2015;93:2119; with permission.

estrous synchronization in combination with AI will continue to be realized and incorporated into beef production systems, with a subsequent improvement in efficiency of beef cattle operations.

Artificial Insemination Cowculator

Using this economic model of estrous synchronization and AI, we developed the AI Cowculator Smartphone Application. The AI Cowculator may be downloaded free of charge and is a decision-aid tool to assist producers to determine whether they should consider TAI rather than purchasing herd sires for their cow herds. Producers and members of the allied industry are encouraged to download the AI Cowculator and use this tool to assist in making bull buying and breeding season decisions. Since inception, the AI Cowculator has been downloaded 3429 times in 42 states and 4 countries. Features of the application include the following:

1. Simple calculator including 18 entries divided into 3 categories (natural service sires costs, herd-related costs, and AI-related costs) to assist producers decide whether to use AI or purchase a herd sire.
2. Push-pin locator that allows users to locate representatives who perform AI services or suppliers of semen and AI supplies.
3. Resources icon that allows users to access helpful resources for reproduction planning including future cattle prices.
4. Gallery of pictures and estrus-synchronization protocols recommended by experts in the field.
5. Social media icon that directs to Facebook and Twitter pages with relevant reproductive management information and technical assistance, and allows users to share their results.

Utilization of Fixed-Timed Artificial Insemination to Reduce Breeding Season Length and Its Effects on Subsequent Calf Value: A Case Study

An example of the influence of using reproductive technologies, such as estrous synchronization and TAI on the subsequent value of the calf crop is reflected in a case study conducted at the University of Florida–North Florida Research and Education Center (NFREC) located in Marianna, FL. The development of TAI protocols has resulted in the opportunity for increased application of AI in commercial cattle operations; however, the long-term production and economic impact of implementing a TAI protocol in beef cattle operations has not been evaluated. This case study was conducted during an 8-year period in which we evaluated the impacts of TAI to reduce the length of the breeding season and its effects on subsequent calving distribution, calf value, and breeding season pregnancy rates.

The NFREC consists of a beef herd containing 300 cows of Angus, Brangus, and Braford breed origin. During the 2006 and 2007 breeding seasons, the cows were exposed to a 120-day breeding season by natural service. In 2008, and every subsequent breeding season to 2013, all females were exposed to TAI using either the 5-day or 7-day CO-Synch + CIDR protocols with the goal of reducing the breeding season to 70 days, to expose every female in the herd to TAI, improve fertility, and calf crop uniformity and weaning weights. To achieve this, it was decided that all females in the operation would be exposed to the following criteria:

1. Replacement heifers must become pregnant during the first 25 days of the breeding season
2. Every cow will be exposed to estrous synchronization and TAI

3. Each cow must produce a live calf every year and calve without assistance or they will be culled
4. Every cow must provide the resources for the genetic potential of the calves and each calf she produces must be genetically capable of performing
5. No supplemental feeding was offered to cows that failed to maintain body condition
6. Any cow with an undesirable temperament or disposition was culled.

Initially, calving season length resulted in cows being inseminated in 3 TAI groups (in the 2008 and 2009 breeding seasons), subsequently reduced to 2 TAI groups (in the 2010 and 2011 breeding seasons), and eventually to a single TAI group (in the 2012 and 2013 breeding seasons; **Fig. 3**). Following the initial TAI for each group, females

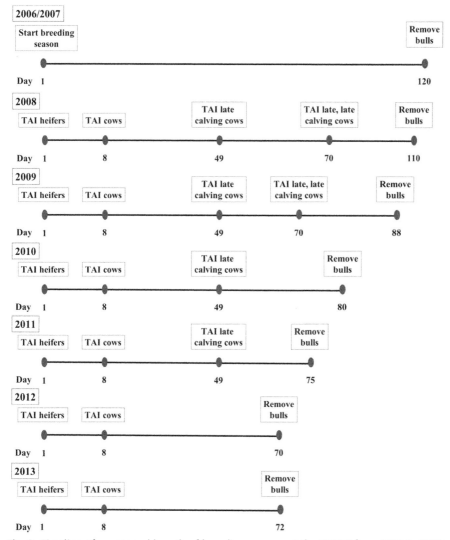

Fig. 3. Timeline of events and length of breeding seasons at the NFREC from 2006 to 2013.

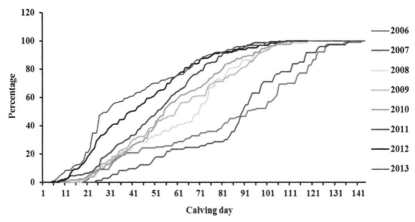

Fig. 4. Cumulative calving percentage during each calving season at the NFREC from 2006 to 2013.

were detected for estrus and inseminated artificially after an observed estrus until day 23 after TAI. On day 23 after TAI, bulls were introduced and cows were naturally mated for the remainder of the breeding season. All bulls passed a breeding soundness examination before being introduced to females.

As a result of incorporating estrous synchronization and TAI, in addition to other reproductive management practices, the breeding season was reduced from 120 to 70 days in the course of 5 years. Furthermore, currently almost all cows calve before initiation of the subsequent breeding season and are exposed to a single TAI on the first day of the breeding season. The effect of using estrous synchronization and TAI on calving distribution can be observed in **Fig. 4**. In 2006 and 2007, before initiation of the TAI program, it took 90 days for 50% of the calves to be born. In 2013, however, it took less than 30 days for 50% of the calves to be born. Mean calving date from the first calf born during each calving season was reduced from 80.9 days from the 2007 breeding season to 38.7 days from the 2013 breeding season. In addition, overall pregnancy rates, including AI and natural service, increased from 81% and 86% in the 2006 and 2007 breeding seasons, respectively, to 92% and 93% in 2012 and 2013, respectively (**Table 2**).

Table 2
Breeding season length, final pregnancy rate, mean calving day, and change in calf value at weaning, after initiation of an estrous synchronization and fixed-timed artificial insemination program at the North Florida Research and Education Center

Year	2006	2007	2008	2009	2010	2011	2012	2013
Breeding season length, d	120	120	110	88	80	75	70	72
Pregnancy rate, %	81	86	84	86	82	94	92	93
Mean calving day	79.2	80.9	59.2	56.2	53.7	47.2	39.5	38.7
Difference from 2006/2007, d	0	0	21.7	24.7	27.2	33.7	41.4	42.2
Per calf increase in value, $[a]	0	0	87	99	109	135	166	169
Herd increase in value, $1000[b]	0	0	21.9	25.5	26.8	38.1	45.8	47.1

[a] Assuming an average daily gain of 0.91 kg/d, a fixed calf value of $4.41/kg.
[b] Values are based on a 300-head cow operation and adjusted for the overall breeding season pregnancy rates for each year.

Assuming an average daily gain of 0.91 kg per day, a fixed calf value of $4.41/kg across years, the mean value per calf increased by $87 per calf resulting from the 2008 breeding season to $169 per calf resulting from the 2013 season. Overall, the net result of a more compact calving season with increased value of calves (in current dollars) by $169 per calf resulted in an increased net result of $47,151.00 per year for the 300-head herd and 94% pregnancy rate at the NFREC (see **Table 2**).

REFERENCES

1. Rodgers JC, Bird SL, Larson JE, et al. An economic evaluation of estrous synchronization and timed artificial insemination in suckled beef cows. J Anim Sci 2012;10:1297–308.

2. National Animal Health Monitoring System NAHMS. Part II. Reference of beef cow-calf management practices in the United States. Fort Collins (CO): USDA-APHIS; 2009.

3. National Animal Health Monitoring System NAHMS. Part IV. Reference of dairy cattle health and management practices in the United States. Fort Collins (CO): USDA-APHIS; 2009.

4. Larson JE, Lamb GC, Stevenson JS, et al. Synchronization of estrus in suckled beef cows for detected estrus and artificial insemination and timed artificial insemination using gonadotropin-releasing hormone, prostaglandin F2α, and progesterone. J Anim Sci 2006;84:332–42.

5. Lamb GC, Dahlen CR, Larson JE, et al. Control of the estrous cycle to improve fertility for fixed-time artificial insemination in beef cattle: a review. J Anim Sci 2010;88:E181–92.

6. Lauderdale JW, Seguin BE, Stellflug JN, et al. Fertility of cattle following PGF2α injection. J Anim Sci 1974;38:964–7.

7. Wiltbank MC, Shiao TF, Bergfelt DR, et al. Prostaglandin F2α receptors in the early bovine corpus luteum. J Anim Sci 1995;52:74–8.

8. Macmillan KL, Henderson NV. Analysis of the variation in the interval from an injection of prostaglandin F2α to oestrous as a method of studying patterns of follicle development during diestrus in dairy cows. Anim Reprod Sci 1983;6:245–54.

9. Pursley JR, Mee MO, Wiltbank MC. Synchronization of ovulation in dairy cows using PG and GnRH. Theriogenology 1995;44:915–23.

10. Carter ML, Dierschke DJ, Rutledge JJ, et al. Effect of gonadotropin-releasing hormone and calf removal on pituitary-ovarian function and reproductive performance in postpartum beef cows. J Anim Sci 1980;51:903–10.

11. Geary TW, Whittier JC, Hallford DM, et al. Calf removal improves conception rates to the ovsynch and CO-Synch protocols. J Anim Sci 2001;79:1–4.

12. Atkins JA, Busch DC, Bader JF, et al. Gonadotropin-releasing hormone-induced ovulation and luteinizing hormone release in beef heifers: effect of day of the cycle. J Anim Sci 2008;86:83–93.

13. Vasconcelos JLM, Silcox RW, Rosa GJM, et al. Synchronization rate, size of the ovulatory follicle, and pregnancy rate after synchronization of ovulation beginning on different days of the estrous cycle in lactating dairy cows. Theriogenology 1999;52:1067–78.

14. Mihm M, Baguisi A, Boland MP, et al. Association between the duration of dominance of the ovulatory follicle and pregnancy rate in beef heifers. Biol Reprod 1994;102:123–30.

15. Lamb GC, Stevenson JS, Kesler DJ, et al. Inclusion of an intravaginal progesterone insert plus GnRH and prostaglandin F2α for ovulation control in postpartum suckled beef cows. J Anim Sci 2001;79:2253–9.

16. Busch DC, Wilson DJ, Schafer DJ, et al. Comparison of progestin-based estrus synchronization protocols before fixed-time artificial insemination on pregnancy rate in beef heifers. J Anim Sci 2007;85:1933–9.

17. Bridges GA, Helser LA, Grum DE, et al. Decreasing the interval between GnRH and PG from 7 to 5 days and lengthening proestrus increases timed-AI pregnancy rates in beef cows. Theriogenology 2008;69:843–51.

18. Lamb GC, Larson JE, Geary TW, et al. Synchronization of estrus and artificial insemination in replacement beef heifers using gonadotropin-releasing hormone, prostaglandin F2α, and progesterone. J Anim Sci 2006;84:3000–9.

19. Stevenson JS, Thompson KE, Forbes WL, et al. Synchronizing estrus and (or) ovulation in beef cows after combinations of GnRH, norgestomet, and prostaglandin F2α with or without timed insemination. J Anim Sci 2000;78:1747–58.

20. Busch DC, Schafer DJ, Wilson DJ, et al. Timing of artificial insemination in postpartum beef cows following administration of the CO-Synch + controlled internal drug-release protocol. J Anim Sci 2008;86:1519–25.

21. Wilson DJ, Mallory DA, Busch DC, et al. Comparison of short-term progestin-based protocols to synchronize estrus and ovulation in postpartum beef cows. J Anim Sci 2010;88:2045–54.

22. Short RE, Bellows RA, Staigmiller RB, et al. Physiological mechanisms controlling anestrus and infertility in postpartum beef cattle. J Anim Sci 1990;68:799–816.

23. Crowe M. Resumption of ovarian cyclicity in post-partum beef and dairy cows. Reprod Domest Anim 2008;43:20–8.

24. Yavas Y, Walton JS. Induction of ovulation in postpartum suckled beef cows: a review. Theriogenology 2000;54:1–23.

25. Grant JK, Abreu FM, Hojer NL, et al. Influence of inducing luteal regression before a modified controlled internal drug-releasing device treatment on control of follicular development. J Anim Sci 2011;89:3531–41.

26. Perry GA, Perry BL, Krantz JH, et al. Influence of inducing luteal regression before a modified fixed-time artificial insemination protocol in postpartum beef cows on pregnancy success. J Anim Sci 2012;90:489–94.

27. Hill SL, Perry GA, Mercadante VRG, et al. Altered progesterone concentrations by hormonal manipulations before a fixed-time artificial insemination CO-Synch + CIDR program in suckled beef cows. Theriogenology 2014;82:104–13.

28. Bridges GA, Mussard ML, Burke CR, et al. Influence of the length of proestrus on fertility and endocrine function in female cattle. J Anim Sci 2010;117:208–15.

29. Perry GA, Smith MF, Lucy MC, et al. Relationship between follicle size at insemination and pregnancy success. Proc Natl Acad Sci U S A 2005;102:5268–73.

30. Perry G, Smith M, Roberts A, et al. Relationship between size of ovulatory follicle and pregnancy success in beef heifers. J Anim Sci 2007;85:684–9.

31. Abreu FM, Cruppe LH, Maquivar M, et al. Effect of follicle age on conception rate in beef heifers. J Anim Sci 2014;92:1022–8.

32. Abreu FM, Geary TW, Cruppe LH, et al. The effect of follicle age on pregnancy rate in beef cows. J Anim Sci 2014;92:1015–21.

33. Rutter LM, Randel RD. Postpartum nutrient intake and body condition: effect on pituitary function and onset of estrus in beef cattle. J Anim Sci 1984;58:265–74.

34. Kershaw EE, Flier JS. Adipose tissue as an endocrine organ. J Clin Endocrinol Metab 2004;89:2548–56.

35. Friedman JM, Halaas JL. Leptin and the regulation of body weight in mammals. Nature 1998;395:763–70.
36. Coleman DL. Obese and diabetes: two mutant genes causing diabetes-obesity syndromes in mice. Diabetologia 1978;14:141–8.
37. Kadokawa H, Blache D, Martin GB. Plasma leptin concentrations correlate with luteinizing hormone secretion in early postpartum holstein cows. J Dairy Sci 2006;89:3020–7.
38. Kadokawa H, Blache D, Martin GB. Relationships between changes in plasma concentrations of leptin before and after parturition and the timing of first post-partum ovulation in high-producing Holstein dairy cows. Reprod Fertil Dev 2000;12:405–11.
39. Stevenson JS, Lamb GC, Johnson SK, et al. Supplemental norgestomet, proges-terone, or melengestrol acetate increases pregnancy rates in suckled beef cows after timed inseminations. J Anim Sci 2003;81:571–86.
40. Williams GL. Suckling as a regulator of postpartum rebreeding in cattle: a review. J Anim Sci 1990;68:831–52.
41. Stevenson JS, Hill SL, Bridges GA, et al. Progesterone status, parity, body condition, and days postpartum before estrus or ovulation synchronization in suckled beef cattle influence artificial insemination pregnancy outcomes. J Anim Sci 2015;93:2111–23.
42. Whittier WD, Currin JF, Schramm H, et al. Fertility in Angus cross beef cows following 5-day CO-Synch + CIDR or 7-day CO-Synch + CIDR estrus synchroni-zation and timed artificial insemination. Theriogenology 2013;80:963–9.
43. Patterson DJ, Corah LR, Brethour JR, et al. Evaluation of reproductive traits in *Bos taurus* and *Bos indicus* crossbred heifers: relationship of age at puberty to length of the postpartum interval to estrus. J Anim Sci 1992;70:1994–9.
44. Johnson SK, Jones RD. A stochastic model to compare breeding system costs for synchronization of estrus and artificial insemination to natural service. Prof Anim Sci 2008;24:588–95.

Synchronization and Artificial Insemination Strategies in Dairy Herds

 CrossMark

Jeffrey S. Stevenson, MS, PhD

KEYWORDS

- Estrus • Ovulation • Gonadotropin-releasing hormone • $PGF_{2\alpha}$ • Timed AI

KEY POINTS

- Presynchronization of estrous cycles using prostaglandin $F_{2\alpha}$ ($PGF_{2\alpha}$) injections before the standard Ovsynch timed AI program produces a greater percentage of inseminations resulting in pregnancy.
- Presynchronization programs incorporating gonadotropin-releasing hormone (GnRH) and $PGF_{2\alpha}$ improve pregnancy outcomes at first service compared with standard Presynch $PGF_{2\alpha}$ programs.
- Resynchronization programs that include administering GnRH 7 days before starting a Resynch-Ovsynch program improve pregnancy outcomes compared with a standard Resynch-Ovsynch programs alone.
- In resynchronization programs, $PGF_{2\alpha}$ facilitates estrus expression and reduces the proportion of cows requiring timed AI; GnRH administration inhibits estrus expression and increases the proportion of cows requiring timed AI.
- Five-day timed AI programs can produce acceptable pregnancy outcomes in replacement dairy heifers.

INTRODUCTION

Overall pregnancy risk of lactating dairy cows in North America has decreased since the 1950s,[1] whereas annual milk yield per cow has increased nearly 4-fold from 5313 to 20,576 lb. Based on a sample of less-productive dairy cows in the United Kingdom, fertility also decreased from 1975 to 1982 and from 1995 to 1998.[2] During that period, conception risk after first services decreased from 56% to 40% despite similar intervals to first service, whereas calving intervals increased from 370 to 390 days. Given this potential inverse relationship between milk yield and fertility, it is no wonder that a genetic antagonism may exist between some reproductive traits and milk yield, which is manifested particularly in first lactation cows.

The author has nothing to disclose.
Department of Animal Sciences and Industry, Kansas State University, 1424 Claflin Road, Manhattan, KS 66506-0201, USA
E-mail address: jss@ksu.edu

Since 2000, an apparent change in the genetic estimate of daughter pregnancy rate has occurred.[3] For every unit increase or decrease in daughter pregnancy rate (a value derived from days open), the 21-day pregnancy rate (proportion of breeding eligible cows that become pregnant every 21 days) of a sire's daughters increase or decrease by 1%. During the past decade, while milk yield continues to increase, a dramatic increase of approximately 5% in daughter pregnancy rate has occurred, which should translate into a reduction of 20 days open for their daughters when they become cows.

Although benefits of improving reproduction are apparent, specific causes of poor reproductive performance are difficult to identify and not easily resolved. To improve reproductive efficiency, the limiting factors must be identified. In earlier days, detecting estrus was the major limitation to achieving a pregnancy. Today, to maximize the chances of a renewed pregnancy for every heifer and cow that calves requires attention to a number of important time-dependent components of the estrous cycle of cows during the voluntary waiting period and in the active AI breeding period. Some of these solutions are found in improved rates of detected estrus and strategic application of hormones to manipulate ovarian follicular growth, corpus luteum (CL) life span, ovulation, and time of semen placement in various fixed timed AI programs.

VOLUNTARY WAITING PERIOD

A number of physiologic changes, including uterine involution and recrudescence of ovarian follicular waves and normal estrous cycles, must occur early postpartum to facilitate good fertility at first AI breeding. Many factors affect these outcomes, including but not limited to body condition, energy balance (milk yield and dry matter intake), parity, season, and disease.[3]

A recent review[3] reported that most dairy cows have emergence of their first postpartum ovarian follicular wave between 5 and 10 days postpartum, with 50% to 80% of cows ovulating the first dominant follicle.

- First ovulation occurs between 15 and 25 days postpartum and is uncommonly preceded by estrus.
- More than 70% of cycles are short after first ovulation.
- First estrus occurs between 25 and 45 days postpartum. Most dairy cows have 2 follicular waves per cycle.
- Regulators of luteinizing hormone pulse frequency necessary to induce first postpartum ovulation include increasing energy balance, body condition and weight at calving, increasing dry matter intake, and absence of disease.

TIMED ARTIFICIAL INSEMINATION PROGRAMS BEFORE FIRST SERVICES FOR LACTATING DAIRY COWS
Ovsynch

The most common timed AI system is a 7-day Ovsynch (**Fig. 1**). Some variations have included a 5-day program with doses of prostaglandin $F_{2\alpha}$ ($PGF_{2\alpha}$) given on days 5 and 6 and timed AI on day 8 (0–16 hours after the second gonadotropin-releasing hormone [GnRH] injection; see **Fig. 1**). In the peer-reviewed literature,[4] hundreds of articles have cited the original Ovsynch article (Google Scholar = 860; Web of Science = 557), and numerous articles use the term Ovsynch in the title (n = 76) or in the abstract (n = 256). Obviously, the "Ovsynch" term and technology have become an integral part of bovine research and of the dairy cattle industry during the 20 years since the original

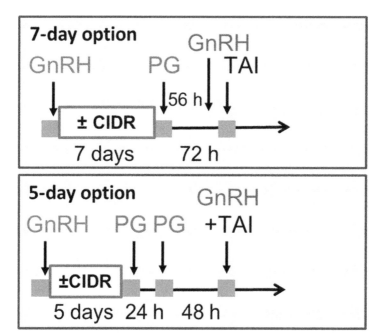

Fig. 1. The basic ovulation synchronization timed artificial insemination (AI) program is known as Ovsynch. It consists of a gonadotropin-releasing hormone injection (GnRH; 100 µg) to induce an luteinizing hormone surge to cause ovulation followed in 5 or 7 days with prostaglandin $F_{2\alpha}$ ($PGF_{2\alpha}$ [PG]; 1 injection for the 7-day program or 2 injections for the 5-day program; 24 hours apart) to lyse the corpus luteum or corpora lutea before a second dose of gonadotropin-releasing hormone (GnRH) is administered (56 hours after $PGF_{2\alpha}$ for the 7-day [Ovsynch-56] or 48 hours after the second $PGF_{2\alpha}$ for the 5-day program [Cosynch-72]) and timed AI (TAI) occurs at 72 hours after the first (5-day) or only (7-day) $PGF_{2\alpha}$ injection. Progesterone supplementation can be applied via an intravaginal progesterone-releasing controlled internal drug release (CIDR) insert.

publication. A recent review of ovulation synchronization for management of reproduction in dairy cows provides insights into current methods and limitations.[5]

Presynchronization Prostaglandin $F_{2\alpha}$ Programs

Early studies indicated that pregnancy outcomes at first AI service after calving might be improved when cows were at specific stages of the estrous cycle before initiating a timed AI program. Cows beginning the timed AI program on days 5 through 12 of the estrous cycle had greater ovulatory responses to GnRH administration and greater fertility than cows at other stages of the estrous cycle.[6] Early studies[7,8] tested whether estrous cycles could be staged in cows to meet this ideal by applying 2 injections of $PGF_{2\alpha}$ administered 14 days apart and then initiating the timed AI program 12 days after the second $PGF_{2\alpha}$ injection (named Presynch-12; **Fig. 2**). The Presynch-14 program also was superior to Ovsynch alone for timed AI pregnancy outcome.[9]

Various permutations of the standard Presynch have been applied (eg, Presynch-14, Presynch-11, and Presynch-10) where the 2 injections of $PGF_{2\alpha}$ were consistently administered 14 days apart, but the interval from the last injection to the onset of the timed AI program was either 14, 11, or 10 days, respectively (see **Fig. 2**). The interval

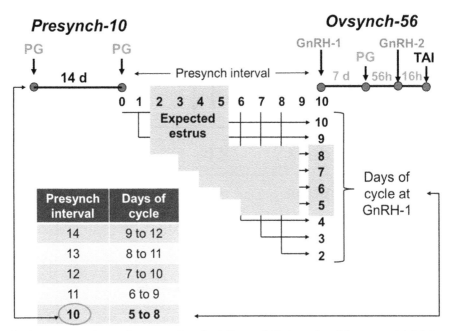

Fig. 2. Estrous cycles can be presynchronized (Presynch) in lactating dairy cows with 2 injections of prostaglandin $F_{2\alpha}$ (PG) administered 14 days apart to ensure that a large proportion of cows are between days 5 through 12 of the estrous cycle at the initiation of the timed artificial insemination (AI; Ovsynch) program for first postpartum AI. Various intervals between the second PG injection and the onset of Ovsynch have been attempted (10–14 days). Studies verify that 10 or 11 days are more ideal relative to pregnancy outcomes as shown by the stage of the estrous cycle at which a large proportion of cows are in at the onset of Ovsynch. Pregnancy risk is increased when presynchronization is applied compared with cows starting the Ovsynch program at random stages of the estrous cycle. Anovulatory cows (those that have not initiated estrous cycles before the presynchronization) can still become pregnant if they ovulate in response to gonadotropin-releasing hormone (GnRH-1 or GnRH-2).

between the second Presynch $PGF_{2\alpha}$ injection and the onset of Ovsynch determines the stage of the cycle at the onset of Ovsynch (see **Fig. 2**).

In nearly all published studies, these Presynch $PGF_{2\alpha}$ systems have produced improved pregnancy outcomes in cows than in those submitted to the timed AI program at random stages of the estrous cycle without Presynch (**Table 1**). Overall, lactating dairy cows exposed to Presynch $PGF_{2\alpha}$ programs for presynchronization have 42% greater odds of pregnancy compared with cows receiving only the timed

Table 1
Pregnancy risk in dairy cows exposed to a 7-day timed AI program (Ovsynch) at first postpartum AI with or without estrous cycles presynchronized (Presynch) before timed AI program

Program	Pregnancy Risk 32–45 d After AI		No. of Studies
	Study Average, %	Study Weighted Average, %	
Ovsynch alone	35.4	35.7 (828)[a]	4
Presynch + Ovsynch	46.5	46.5 (843)	4

[a] No. of cows.

AI program.[5] Furthermore, improved pregnancy outcomes were reported in cows treated with Presynch-11 than Presynch-14 before a timed AI program,[10] probably because more cows were at the ideal stage of the cycle after Presynch-11 treatment (see **Fig. 2**). Further shortening the interval between Presynch and Ovsynch, however, may reduce pregnancy outcomes.[11] An additional benefit of Presynch $PGF_{2\alpha}$ programs is the flexibility of choosing to inseminate cows detected in estrus after $PGF_{2\alpha}$ rather than waiting to inseminate after the Ovsynch protocol.[12–14]

Presynchronization Gonadotropin-releasing Hormone Programs

The major limitation to Presynch $PGF_{2\alpha}$ programs is their inability to improve fertility in anovular cows—those that have not initiated estrous cycles since calving, which may represent up to 41% of dairy cows at the end of the voluntary waiting period.[5] Including GnRH administration in addition to injections of $PGF_{2\alpha}$ increases the odds for pregnancy by 1.65 times[5] and has resulted in new presynchronization systems (eg, Double Ovsynch, PG-3-G, and G-6-G; **Fig. 3**). In some cases, Double Ovsynch[15,16] and PG-3-G[17] may produce greater pregnancy outcomes than the 2 standard Presynch $PGF_{2\alpha}$ variants (Presynch-12 or Presynch-10). The PG-3-G program produced improved timed AI pregnancy outcomes during summer than Presynch-10.[17] These Presynch GnRH programs cause a large proportion of cows to be at the most ideal stage of the cycle to initiate Ovsynch (days 6–8; **Fig. 4**).

Improved pregnancy outcomes of Presynch GnRH programs may be realized in herds where more cows are anovulatory when submitted to the timed AI programs before

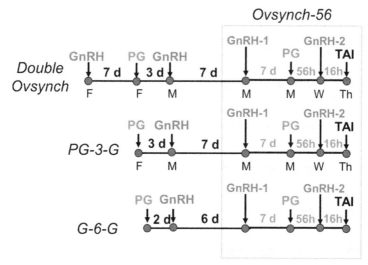

Fig. 3. Estrous cycles can be presynchronized in lactating dairy cows by 3 different presynchronization programs consisting of a combination of prostaglandin $F_{2\alpha}$ (PG) and gonadotropin-releasing hormone (GnRH) to ensure that a large proportion of cows are on days 5 through 8 of the estrous cycle at the initiation of the timed artificial insemination (AI; Ovsynch) program for first postpartum AI. The benefits of the preGnRH include initiating ovulation in anovulatory cows, improving follicular synchrony, and increasing progesterone concentrations in cows at the initiation of Ovsynch. Pregnancy risk is increased when presynchronization is applied compared with cows starting the Ovsynch program at random stages of the estrous cycle. Anovulatory cows (those that have not initiated estrous cycles before the presynchronization) can still become pregnant if they ovulate for the first time since calving in response to the pre-GnRH, GnRH-1, or GnRH-2. TAI, timed artificial insemination.

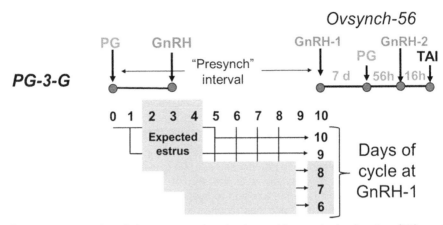

Fig. 4. An example of how presynchronization with prostaglandin $F_{2\alpha}$ (PG) and gonadotropin-releasing hormone (GnRH) can cause a large proportion of cows to be on days 5 through 8 of the estrous cycle at the initiation of the timed artificial insemination (AI; Ovsynch) program for first postpartum AI. Anovulatory cows (those that have not initiated estrous cycles before the presynchronization) can respond to the presynchronization GnRH injections to initiate their first estrous cycle and later become pregnant if they ovulate in response to (GnRH-2). TAI, timed artificial insemination.

first AI services. For example, Double-Ovsynch decreased the percentage of cows with low circulating progesterone concentrations (<0.50 ng/mL) at GnRH-1 (12.0% vs 30.1%) and increased the percentage of cows with medium progesterone concentrations (0.50 < progesterone ≤ 3.0 ng/mL) at GnRH-1 (80.0% vs 57.0%), and with a CL at GnRH-1 (94.0% vs 67.8%). Double-Ovsynch also increased the percentage of cows with high progesterone (>3.0 ng/mL) at $PGF_{2\alpha}$ (88.0% vs 76.3%) and tended to increase average circulating progesterone at $PGF_{2\alpha}$ (3.52 ± 0.17 vs 3.09 ± 0.21 ng/mL).[18]

Similar progesterone and CL responses were reported for PG-3-G,[19] in addition to both programs tending to or increasing the percentage of cows ovulating to GnRH-1 and GnRH-2.[18,19] Thus, Presynch options that included GnRH administration induced ovulation in noncycling cows and seemed to improve most aspects of synchronization before or during the Ovsynch protocol. Cows that lack a CL at the first GnRH administration of the timed AI program, which includes anovular or cycling cows treated during proestrus, estrus, and metestrus, have reduced concentrations of progesterone compared with cows with a CL. These groups of cows may represent approximately 30% to 40% of cows subjected to timed AI and are those that have the poorest pregnancy outcomes to timed AI.

Presynchronization Five-day Programs

Ovulation to the first GnRH injection improves synchronization of the estrous cycle and reduces the period of follicular dominance, both factors are associated with improved pregnancy outcomes.[6,20] As a result, studies comparing 5- versus 7-day Ovsynch -programs in dairy cows[20] (see **Fig. 1**) reported greater percentages of cows to be pregnant when inseminated following the 5- than the 7-day programs because proestrus is prolonged and follicular dominance is reduced in more cows exposed to the 5-day Ovsynch program. Recent unpublished studies in which cows exposed to either the 5- or 7-day program, pregnancy risk did not differ when both groups of cows received a standard dose of PGF on days 5 and 6 in the 5-day program or on days 7 and 8 in the 7-day program.

One limitation to the 5-day program is the inability of a single dose of $PGF_{2\alpha}$ to induce complete CL regression in all cows (particularly a "new" CL that resulted from GnRH-induced ovulation). Therefore, 2 doses of $PGF_{2\alpha}$ are required (one on day 5 and another on day 6; see **Fig. 1**) to optimize luteal regression by either $PGF_{2\alpha}$ or by one of its analogs.[21] Even larger single doses administered on day 5 were less effective than 2 doses (**Table 2**).

Comparisons of various Presynch programs before the 5-day timed AI program showed that G-6-G produced pregnancy outcomes superior to Presynch 14 to 11 when Cosynch-72 was used.[22] When Presynch-12 was applied before timed AI, the percentage of cows pregnant was similar after both Cosynch-58 and Cosynch-72 programs (see **Table 2**).[23] Comparison of 2 Presynch programs and 2 times for administering the second GnRH injection and timed AI (58 vs 72 hours) produced no significant difference in pregnancy outcomes at day 30 after timed AI (**Table 3**).[23] At day 65 after timed AI, however, fewer cows treated with Presynch-10 and injected with GnRH and inseminated at 58 hours were pregnant compared with those injected with GnRH and inseminated at 72 hours. In contrast, no such differences were detected when cows were exposed to Double Ovsynch before the timed AI program.

Increasing doses (100 to 200 μL) of GnRH in 7-day Ovsynch programs have not increased the percentage of inseminated cows that are determined to be pregnant, although slightly more cows ovulated in response to GnRH-1. Applying 2 doses of $PGF_{2\alpha}$ 24 hours apart on days 7 and 8 in a 7-day program or increasing a single dose on day 7 by 50% also did not improve pregnancy risk (see **Table 3**), although slightly more CL regressed completely before timed AI. A recent report involving multiple herds, however, confirmed that pregnancy risk was increased by 3 percentage points when cows exposed to the 7-day program received a standard dose of $PGF_{2\alpha}$ on days 7 and 8 compared with only 1 dose on day 7.[24]

Programs Including Progesterone

A review of the literature (meta-analysis) indicates that use of a single progesterone intravaginal controlled internal drug release (CIDR) insert administered during the period between the first GnRH injection and the $PGF_{2\alpha}$ of the timed AI protocol increased the

Table 2
Pregnancy risk in dairy cows exposed to a 5-day timed AI program (Ovsynch) based on the number of doses of $PGF_{2\alpha}$

Program[a]	Pregnancy Risk 30–32 d After AI		No. of Studies
	Study Average, %	Study Weighted Average, %	
Doses of $PGF_{2\alpha}$			
1	31.8	32.7 (694)[c]	3
2	41.4	42.1 (691)	3
Two doses of $PGF_{2\alpha}$			
Cosynch-58[b]	52.9	50.7 (1144)	3
Cosynch-72[b]	52.4	52.4 (3094)	5

Abbreviations: AI, artificial insemination; GnRH, gonadotropin-releasing hormone; $PGF_{2\alpha}$, prostaglandin $F_{2\alpha}$.
[a] Labeled dose of $PGF_{2\alpha}$ on day 5 or one labeled dose on days 5 and 6 of a 5-day Ovsynch program (see **Fig. 1**).
[b] Cosynch-58 or Cosynch-72 = second GnRH injection and timed AI occur at 58 or 72 hours after the first $PGF_{2\alpha}$ injection, respectively.
[c] No. of cows.

Table 3
Pregnancy risk in dairy cows exposed to a 7-day timed AI program (Ovsynch) based on the number of doses of PGF$_{2\alpha}$

Doses of PGF$_{2\alpha}$[a]	Pregnancy Risk 39–65 d After AI		
	Study Average, %	Study Weighted Average, %	No. of Studies
Labeled dose	46.6	43.8 (506)[b]	2
50% increase or 2 doses 24 h apart	48.1	47.5 (643)	2

Abbreviations: AI, artificial insemination; PGF$_{2\alpha}$, prostaglandin F$_{2\alpha}$.
[a] Labeled dose of PGF$_{2\alpha}$ on day 7; 50% increase in labeled dose, or labeled dose on day 7 and 8 of a 7-day Ovsynch program (see Fig. 1).
[b] No. of cows.

percentage of pregnant cows at day 60 after AI compared with untreated controls (34.2% vs 29.6%), and the benefit from progesterone supplementation was similar for cows with and without a CL.[25] In general, therefore, pregnancy risk was greater for cows treated with progesterone than for controls (Table 4). Nevertheless, pregnancy risk for cows without CL treated with a single insert was 10.5% less than that of untreated cows that had a CL at the initiation of the timed AI program (29% vs 32%).

Cows benefitting the most from supplemental progesterone are those that are anovular or not in diestrus at the onset of the timed AI program. Incorporating a single progesterone insert as part of a timed AI program increased fertility in cows that lacked a CL at the first GnRH injection, but did not restore fertility to the same level as those cows starting the timed AI program in diestrus. This difference is likely related to the difference in amount of progesterone released by a CL during diestrus and a single progesterone insert.

Several recent studies targeted potential problem cows for supplemental progesterone administration as part of timed AI programs. Ovaries were examined for the presence of a CL by ultrasound at the beginning of Ovsynch after earlier treatment with 2 injections of PGF$_{2\alpha}$ 14 days apart.[26] Cows without a CL were treated with Ovsynch with or without progesterone via a CIDR insert. Cows with a CL served as a control. Percentage of cows without a CL diagnosed pregnant at 33 days after timed AI increased from 24.3% to 32.3% when treated with progesterone; 38% of control cows with a CL became pregnant. In another study,[27] cows without a CL at the onset of a 5-day Ovsynch program were treated with 2 CIDR inserts concurrently and pregnancy risk was compared with contemporary no-CL cows and cows in diestrus (bearing a CL). Pregnancy outcome at 32 days after timed AI did not differ between

Table 4
Pregnancy risk of dairy cows exposed to a 7-day timed AI program (Ovsynch) before first postpartum AI with or without progesterone

Program[a]	Pregnancy Risk 27–40 d After AI		
	Study Average, %	Study Weighted Average, %	No. of Studies
Control	34.6	33.2 (3459)[b]	11
Progesterone (CIDR)[a]	39.4	37.6 (3562)	11

Abbreviations: AI, artificial insemination; PGF$_{2\alpha}$, prostaglandin F$_{2\alpha}$.
[a] Cows were treated with various ovulation synchronization programs, eight of which also included presynchronization programs. Progesterone-releasing intravaginal controlled internal drug release (CIDR) inserts were applied during 7 days beginning at GnRH-1 and removed when PGF$_{2\alpha}$ was administered (see Fig. 1).
[b] No. of cows.

cows with a CL and those treated with 2 CIDR inserts (49.9% and 46.8%, respectively), but were greater than untreated, no-CL cows (30.8%).

The same design used in a 7-day Ovsynch program produced similar results.[28] Cows without a CL and treated with 2 CIDR inserts had greater pregnancy risk at first service than no-CL control cows (42.2% vs 31.1%), and pregnancy risk in the 2-CIDR no-CL cows did not differ from that in control cows starting treatment in diestrus (42.2% vs 38.4%), respectively.

REPEAT SERVICE (RESYNCHRONIZATION) PROGRAMS FOR LACTATING DAIRY COWS
Early Not Pregnancy Diagnosis

Increased efficiency of reproduction occurs when not pregnant status in previously inseminated cows is determined as soon as possible.[29] Means to detect not pregnant status relatively soon after insemination includes the following.

- Monitoring of blood concentrations of progesterone or commercially available kits to measure blood or milk pregnancy-associated glycoproteins (ie, PAGs);
- Presence of estrus determined by visual heat detection, heat detection aids, or by using other electronic methods (pressure-sensitive, rump-mounted transmitters or physical activity monitors); and
- Absence of uterine fluid, CL, and embryo via transrectal ultrasonography.

Early detection of not pregnant status facilitates earlier reinsemination of nonpregnant (open) cows. Although detection of pregnancy status earlier is associated with improved overall herd fertility measures, more embryo loss is observed than if pregnancy status was detected later. Methods to facilitate reinsemination of open cows are described hereafter.

Original studies reporting timed AI programs initiated in cows diagnosed not pregnant (NPD) involved starting either a 5- or 7-day Ovsynch program in cows on the day of NPD. When using transrectal ultrasonography to diagnose pregnancy on a weekly basis, it is common that one evaluates cows that were inseminated 30 to 36 days before the NPD. If the NPD falls on a Monday, then most cows that received a timed AI on Thursday would be day 32 of pregnancy. If transrectal palpation were used for pregnancy diagnosis, then a common interval for days because last AI would fall between days 37 and 43, with most cows receiving a timed AI falling on day 39. Starting cows in a timed AI Resynch-Ovsynch program at NPD often falls on either day 32 or 39 for most of the cows, depending on the method of pregnancy diagnosis.

Presynchronization Before Resynchronization

In some herds, cows NPD are started on a timed AI program on the day of NPD. In other herds, to reinseminate cows sooner after an NPD, the first GnRH injection of the timed AI is administered to all cows eligible for the next pregnancy diagnosis (unknown pregnancy status) either 5 or 7 days before NPD depending on which timed AI program is used (ie, 5 vs 7 day).

Applying a presynchronization treatment such as GnRH or human chorionic gonadotropin to ovulate a follicle and initiate a new follicular wave in cows with unknown pregnancy status has been tested for its profertility effects. Simple Resynch-Ovsynch programs initiated at day 32 or 39 after previous AI were compared with treatments that included a presynchronization GnRH or human chorionic gonadotropin injection administered 7 days before Ovsynch. At both initiation times, the pre-GnRH or pre-human chorionic gonadotropin injection increased pregnancy risk by 4% to 5% units (**Table 5**).

Table 5
Pregnancy risk of nonpregnant dairy cows exposed to a 7-day Resynch-Ovsynch timed AI program initiated at a not pregnant diagnosis at either 32 or 39 days after previous AI with or without presynchronization injections of either GnRH or hCG

	Pregnancy Risk 32–39 d After AI		
Program	Study Average, %	Study Weighted Average, %	No. of Studies
Control Resynch	29.3	29.0 (3657)[b]	11
Pre-GnRH or pre-hCG + Resynch[a]	34.2	33.5 (2996)	8

Abbreviations: AI, artificial insemination; GnRH, gonadotropin-releasing hormone; hCG, human chorionic gonadotropin; $PGF_{2\alpha}$, prostaglandin $F_{2\alpha}$.
[a] GnRH or hCG injection administered 7 days before Ovsynch-56.
[b] No. of cows.

Addition of progesterone in the form of a CIDR to nonpregnant cows in designed studies in 7-day Resynch-Ovsynch programs initiated at the NPD failed to increase pregnancy risk of cows, whereas when tested in a 5-day Ovsynch program initiated at day 32, progesterone increased pregnancy outcome.[30] As previously noted, the greatest pregnancy advantage accrues from applying progesterone to cows without a CL rather than those with a CL.

In the previously cited summary (see **Table 5**), detection of estrus was not applied and all cows received only the timed AI. In herds in which cows are housed in dry lots or free stall barns with or without turn-out dry lots, detection of estrus is often applied to cows in addition to using timed AI programs for cows not detected in estrus. In subsequent studies, a pre-GnRH injection was applied as a presynchronization treatment and cows were inseminated when detected in estrus. The timed AI program was discontinued when cows were reinseminated at estrus, or in the absence of estrus, the complete timed AI program was carried out.

In 2 such studies (**Table 6**), fewer cows were detected in estrus and inseminated before the timed AI program was initiated when the pre-GnRH injection was applied compared with the control Resynch (37.4% vs 50.3%; calculated from **Table 7** data), even though resulting pregnancy risks were not different. In the face of similar pregnancy risk after insemination, cows detected in estrus and inseminated became pregnant earlier than timed AI cows.

Table 6
Pregnancy risk of nonpregnant cows exposed to a 7-day Resynch-Ovsynch timed AI program initiated at not pregnant diagnosis at either 32 or 39 days after previous AI: Insemination at estrus or at appointment (timed AI)

	Pregnancy Risk 32–39 d After AI		
Program	Study Average, %	Study Weighted Average, %	No. of Studies
Control Resynch	32.3	32.3 (1501)[b]	—
Estrus	39.2	39.1 (756)	2
Timed AI	25.5	25.4 (745)	2
Pre-GnRH + Resynch[a]	35.6	33.9 (1398)	
Estrus	41.7	41.2 (523)	2
Timed AI	29.5	29.6 (875)	2

Abbreviations: AI, artificial insemination; GnRH, gonadotropin-releasing hormone.
[a] GnRH injection administered 7 days before Ovsynch-56.
[b] No. of cows.

Table 7
Pregnancy risk of nonpregnant cows exposed to presynchronization programs before a 7-day Resynch-Ovsynch timed AI program including GnRH or $PGF_{2\alpha}$ after a not pregnant diagnosis

Program[a]	Pregnancy Risk 29–32 d After AI		No. of Studies
	Study Average, %	Study Weighted Average, %	
Pre-GnRH Resynch	34.7	38.2 (642)[b]	2
Estrus	33.3	34.3 (115)	—
Timed AI	36.1	39.1 (527)	—
Pre-$PGF_{2\alpha}$ + Resynch	31.8	34.4 (1505)	4
Estrus	34.8	34.8 (846)	—
Timed AI	29.6	34.0 (659)	—

Abbreviations: AI, artificial insemination; Pre-GnRH, gonadotropin-releasing hormone; ND, not pregnant diagnosis; $PGF_{2\alpha}$, prostaglandin $F_{2\alpha}$.

[a] Control = Ovsynch-56 initiated at day 32 (NPD); Pre-GnRH = GnRH injection given 7 days before NPDs (at which time Ovsynch-56 was initiated); $PGF_{2\alpha}$ = injection of $PGF_{2\alpha}$ at 7, 11, or 12 days before initiating Ovsynch.

[b] No of cows.

Subsequent studies endeavored to presynchronize estrous cycles with $PGF_{2\alpha}$ to facilitate estrus expression and earlier reinsemination after an NPD (see **Table 7**). In some cases, when $PGF_{2\alpha}$ was administered on and shortly after the NPD, pregnancy risk was improved.[31] In most cases fertility was not improved,[14] but more cows detected in estrus were inseminated earlier than cows assigned to a timed AI program. In general, when applying Resynch programs to dairy cows at NPD, using presynchronization $PGF_{2\alpha}$ facilitates estrus expression, whereas using a pre-GnRH injection suppresses estrus expression.

TIMING OF SECOND GONADOTROPIN-RELEASING HORMONE ADMINISTRATION AND TIMED ARTIFICIAL INSEMINATION

Success of timed AI programs depends on adequate duration of proestrus and proper timing of insemination relative to ovulation. For the standard Ovsynch program, with 7 days between the initial GnRH and $PGF_{2\alpha}$ injections, administering the final GnRH 56 hours after $PGF_{2\alpha}$ and performing AI 16 hours later seems to optimize pregnancy risk in dairy cows.[32] Conversely, extending the proestrus longer than 56 hours and inseminating cows concurrently with the final GnRH injection may reduce fertility in dairy cows.[33,34] Allowing 56 hours of proestrus provides additional growth of the ovulatory follicle and increased exposure to estradiol,[35] which is thought to be needed to avoid short estrous cycles after induced ovulation. For 7-day Ovsynch programs, optimal timing of the second (or breeding) injection of GnRH is approximately 56 hours after $PGF_{2\alpha}$ (Ovsynch-56) with AI occurring approximately 16 hours later (or 72 hours after $PGF_{2\alpha}$) compared with timed AI at either 48 or 72 hours, concurrent with the second GnRH injection (**Table 8**).

In contrast, for cows subjected to the 5-day Ovsynch program, which results in smaller ovulatory follicles and reduced concentrations of estradiol in the plasma around the time of AI compared with the 7-day Ovsynch protocol,[20] the duration of proestrus should be extended to 72 hours.[25,30] Therefore, a careful balance involving follicle and oocyte maturation and timing between sperm and oocyte availability must be considered so that optimal fertility can be achieved. Extending the duration of the proestrus to 72 hours when applying the 5-day timed AI program compensated for a

Table 8
Pregnancy risk of dairy cows exposed to a 7-day Ovsynch timed AI program and various times of GnRH injection relative to PGF$_{2\alpha}$

Program	Pregnancy Risk 28–40 d After AI		No. of Studies
	Study Average, %	Study Weighted Average, %	
Cosynch-48[a]	29.5	28.4 (1640)[d]	6
Cosynch-72[b]	28.7	29.0 (1582)	7
Ovsynch-56[c]	36.0	33.7 (1729)	5

Abbreviations: AI, artificial insemination; GnRH, gonadotropin-releasing hormone; PGF$_{2\alpha}$, prostaglandin F$_{2\alpha}$.
[a] Cosynch 48 = GnRH and AI at 48 hours after PGF$_{2\alpha}$.
[b] Cosynch72 = GnRH and AI at 72 hours after PGF$_{2\alpha}$.
[c] Ovsynch-56 = GnRH at 56 hours after PGF$_{2\alpha}$ and AI 16 hours later.
[d] No. of cows.

less optimal interval between induced ovulation and insemination, which allowed for the administration of the final GnRH concurrently with AI at 72 hours after PGF$_{2\alpha}$ without decreasing pregnancy risk.[30]

ARTIFICIAL INSEMINATION PROGRAMS FOR REPLACEMENT DAIRY HEIFERS

When heifers are inseminated after detected estrus without any hormone synchronization, it is not uncommon for conception risk to exceed 60%. Even when inseminations were performed after PGF$_{2\alpha}$ injections (and the majority of heifers express estrus on days 2–5 after injection) and inseminations were made after detected estrus, conception risk is commonly greater than 60%. These are traditional and proven ways to inseminate heifers, but they require time and skilled labor for heat detection. In large pens of heifers, such as found in heifer grower operations who contract to raise heifers for dairy producers, inseminations are often based on both estrus and timed AI programs, followed by cleanup bulls.

Gender-biased or sexed semen is often used when inseminating replacement heifers because of their better fertility than lactating cows. Conception risk is limited to approximately 70% to 80% of what is achieved with conventional semen.

Seven-day Programs

When applying timed AI in heifers, pregnancy risk will be slightly reduced to the mid 50% range compared with insemination after detected estrus. The benefit of not needing estrus detection expertise, however, makes timed AI of heifers attractive for many heifer developers. A 7-day timed AI program in heifers includes a progesterone insert (eg, CIDR) used for 7 days and PGF$_{2\alpha}$ injected upon its removal, in addition to a GnRH injection at CIDR insertion and a second GnRH injection between the PGF$_{2\alpha}$ injection and timed AI (see **Fig. 1**). These results also hold true for the 7-day CIDR programs when heifers were inseminated after detected estrus up until 72 hours after PGF$_{2\alpha}$ and then the remaining heifers were injected with GnRH and inseminated at 72 hours in the absence of estrus.

Five-day Programs

The most consistent results for timed AI in heifers are found using the 5-day programs (see **Fig. 1**). A series of recent studies were conducted in a large number of dairy heifers to examine some variations of the 5-day timed AI program. In study 1 (**Fig. 5**), ovulation in dairy heifers was synchronized and 2 injections of PGF$_{2\alpha}$

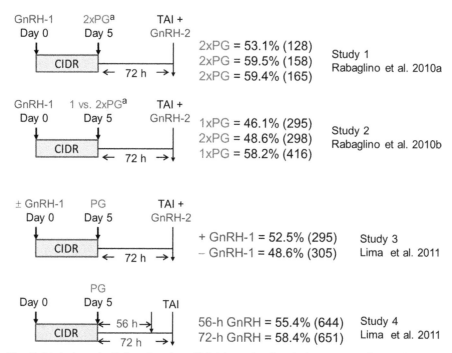

Fig. 5. Variations in 5-day timed artificial insemination (AI) programs for replacement heifers are discussed in the text. GnRH, gonadotropin-releasing hormone; PG, prostaglandin $F_{2\alpha}$; TAI, timed artificial insemination. [a] Two injections 12 h apart.

were administered on day 5 (one when the CIDR insert was removed and another 12 hours later). Pregnancy risk did not differ in 2 separate experiments, but ranged from 53% to 59%.[36]

In study 2 (see **Fig. 5**), a comparison was made between using one or 2 $PGF_{2\alpha}$ injections at the time of CIDR insert removal. No differences in pregnancy risk was detected in 2 experiments.[37]

In study 3 (see **Fig. 5**), only 1 $PGF_{2\alpha}$ injection was used and the researchers addressed the need for the GnRH-1 injection. Results from study 3 showed no advantage for using the GnRH-1 injection when 1 $PGF_{2\alpha}$ injection was administered because pregnancy risks ranged from 48% to 52%.[38]

In study 4 (see **Fig. 5**), no GnRH-1 injection was used with only 1 $PGF_{2\alpha}$ injection and the proper timing of GnRH-2 was tested. Results showed that the inconvenience of handling the heifers an extra time to administer GnRH-2 at 56 hours (16 hours before the timed AI) was not necessary to maximize pregnancy risk. In contrast, for those heifers that did not show estrus during the 72 hours after $PGF_{2\alpha}$ and CIDR removal, extending the time to the GnRH injection to 72 hours (coincident with the timed AI) improved their pregnancy outcome from 44.7% to 53%.[38]

One further study demonstrated that when GnRH-1 was administered at the time of CIDR insertion in a 5-day program, administering 2 $PGF_{2\alpha}$ injections (24 hours apart; one with CIDR insert removal and one 24 hours later) was advantageous to improve pregnancy risk compared with not using GnRH-1 and using only 1 $PGF_{2\alpha}$ injection (59.4% vs 53.5%, respectively).

Synchronization of ovulation in dairy heifers using a progesterone insert with administrations of GnRH and PGF$_{2\alpha}$ in 5-day programs can successfully occur. Several options are successful. The results indicated that the 5-day program is effective and the GnRH-1 injection is not necessary when using only one PGF$_{2\alpha}$ injection. Extending the timing of the GnRH-2 to 72 hours (coincident with the timed AI) benefitted heifers that did not show estrus during the 72 hours after CIDR insert removal.

REFERENCES

1. Butler WR, Smith RD. Interrelationships between energy balance and postpartum reproductive function in dairy cattle. J Dairy Sci 1989;72:767–83.
2. Royal MD, Darwash AO, Webb R, et al. Declining fertility in dairy cattle: changes in traditional and endocrine parameters of fertility. Anim Sci 2000;70:487–501.
3. Crowe MA, Diskin MG, Williams EJ. Parturition to resumption of ovarian cyclicity: comparative aspects of beef and dairy cows. Animal 2014;8:40–53.
4. Wiltbank MC, Pursley JR. The cow as an induced ovulator: timed AI after synchronization of ovulation. Theriogenology 2014;81:170–85.
5. Bisinotto RS, Ribeiro ES, Santos JEP. Synchronisation of ovulation for management of reproduction in dairy cows. Animal 2014;8:151–9.
6. Vasconcelos JLM, Silcox RW, Rosa GJM, et al. Synchronization rate, size of the ovulatory follicle, and pregnancy rate after synchronization of ovulation beginning on different days of the cycle in lactating dairy cows. Theriogenology 1999;52:1067–78.
7. Moreira F, Orlandi C, Risco CA, et al. Effects of presynchronization and bovine somatotropin on pregnancy rates to a timed artificial insemination protocol in lactating dairy cows. J Dairy Sci 2001;84:1646–59.
8. El-Zarkouny SZ, Cartmill JA, Hensley BA, et al. Pregnancy in dairy cows after synchronized ovulation regimens with or without presynchronization and progesterone. J Dairy Sci 2004;87:1024–37.
9. Navanukraw C, Redmer DA, Reynolds LP, et al. A modified presynchronization protocol improves fertility to timed artificial insemination in lactating dairy cows. J Dairy Sci 2004;87:1551–7.
10. Galvao KN, Sa Filho MF, Santos JEP. Reducing the interval from presynchronization to initiation of timed artificial insemination improves fertility in dairy cows. J Dairy Sci 2007;90:4212–8.
11. Colazo MG, Ponce-Barajas P, Ambrose DJ. Pregnancy per artificial insemination in lactating dairy cows subjected to 2 different intervals from presynchronization to initiation of Ovsynch protocol. J Dairy Sci 2013;96:7640–8.
12. Melendez P, Gonzalez G, Aguilar E, et al. Comparison of two estrus-synchronization protocols and timed artificial insemination in dairy cattle. J Dairy Sci 2006;89:4567–72.
13. Chebel RC, Santos JEP. Effect of inseminating cows in estrus following a presynchronization protocol on reproductive and lactation performances. J Dairy Sci 2010;93:4632–43.
14. Chebel RC, Scanavez AA, Silva PRB, et al. Evaluation of presynchronized resynchronization protocols for lactating dairy cows. J Dairy Sci 2010;96:1009–20.
15. Souza AH, Ayres H, Ferreira RM, et al. A new presynchronization system (Double-Ovsynch) increases fertility at first postpartum timed AI in lactating dairy cows. Theriogenology 2008;70:208–15.

16. Herlihy MM, Giordano JO, Souza AH, et al. Presynchronization with Double-Ovsynch improves fertility at first postpartum artificial insemination in lactating dairy cows. J Dairy Sci 2012;95:7003–14.

17. Stevenson JS, Pulley SL. Pregnancy per artificial insemination after presynchronizing estrous cycles with the Presynch-10 protocol or prostaglandin F2a injection followed by gonadotropin-releasing hormone before Ovsynch-56 in 4 dairy herds of lactating dairy cows. J Dairy Sci 2012;95:6513–22.

18. Ayres H, Ferreira RM, Cunha AP, et al. Double-Ovsynch in high-producing dairy cows: effects on progesterone concentrations and ovulation to GnRH treatments. Theriogenology 2013;79:159–64.

19. Stevenson JS, Pulley SL, Mellieon HI Jr. Prostaglandin F2a and gonadotropin-releasing hormone administration improve progesterone status, luteal number, and proportion of ovular and anovular dairy cows with corpora lutea before a timed artificial insemination program. J Dairy Sci 2012;95:1831–44.

20. Santos JEP, Narciso CD, Rivera F, et al. Effect of reducing the period of follicle dominance in a timed artificial insemination protocol on reproduction of dairy cows. J Dairy Sci 2010;93:2976–88.

21. Ribeiro ES, Bisinotto RS, Favoreto MG, et al. Fertility in dairy cows following pre-synchronization and administering twice the luteolytic dose of prostaglandin F2a as one or two injections in the 5-day timed artificial insemination protocol. Theriogenology 2012;78:273–84.

22. Ribeiro ES, Cerri RLA, Bisinotto RS, et al. Reproductive performance of grazing dairy cows following presynchronization and resynchronization protocols. J Dairy Sci 2011;94:4984–96.

23. Ribeiro ES, Monteiro APA, Lima FS, et al. Effects of presynchronization and length of proestrus on fertility of grazing dairy cows subjected to a 5-day timed artificial insemination protocol. J Dairy Sci 2012;95:2513–22.

24. Wiltbank MC, Baez GM, Cochrane F, et al. Effect of a second treatment with pros-taglandin $F_{2\alpha}$ during the Ovsynch protocol on luteolysis and pregnancy in dairy cows. J Dairy Sci 2015;98:8644–54.

25. Bisinotto RS, Martinez N, Sinedino LDP, et al. Meta-analysis of progesterone sup-plementation during timed artificial insemination programs in dairy cows. J Dairy Sci 2014;98:2472–87.

26. Stevenson JS, Tenhouse DE, Krisher RL, et al. Detection of anovulation by heat-mount detectors and transrectal ultrasonography before treatment with proges-terone in a timed insemination protocol. J Dairy Sci 2008;91:2901–15.

27. Bisinotto RS, Ribeiro ES, Lima FS, et al. Targeted progesterone supplementation improves fertility in lactating dairy cows without a corpus luteum at the initiation of the timed artificial insemination protocol. J Dairy Sci 2013;96:2214–25.

28. Bisinotto RS, Castro LO, Pansani MB, et al. Progesterone supplementation to lactating dairy cows without a corpus luteum at initiation of the Ovsynch protocol. J Dairy Sci 2015;98:2515–28.

29. Fricke PM. Scanning the future–ultrasonography as a reproductive management tool for dairy cattle. J Dairy Sci 2002;85:1918–26.

30. Bisinotto RS, Ribeiro ES, Martins LT, et al. Effect of interval between induction of ovulation and artificial insemination (AI) and supplemental progesterone for resynchronization on fertility of dairy cows subjected to a 5-d timed AI program. J Dairy Sci 2010;93:5798–808.

31. Silva E, Sterry RA, Kolb D, et al. Effect of pretreatment with prostaglandin F2alpha before resynchronization of ovulation on fertility of lactating dairy cows. J Dairy Sci 2007;90:5509–17.

32. Pursley JR, Silcox RW, Wiltbank MC. Effect of time of artificial insemination on pregnancy rates, calving rates, pregnancy loss, and gender ratio after synchronization od ovulation in lactating dairy cows. J Dairy Sci 1998;81:2139–44.

33. Brusveen DJ, Cunha AP, Silva CD, et al. Altering the time of the second gonadotropin-releasing hormone injection and artificial insemination (AI) during Ovsynch affects pregnancies per AI in lactating dairy cows. J Dairy Sci 2008; 91:1044–52.

34. Sterry RA, Welle ML, Fricke PM. Treatment with gonadotropin-releasing hormone after first timed artificial insemination improves fertility in noncycling lactating dairy cows. J Dairy Sci 2006;89:4237–45.

35. Peters MW, Pursley JR. Timing of final GnRH of the Ovsynch protocol affects ovulatory follicle size, subsequent luteal function, and fertility in dairy cows. Theriogenology 2003;60:1197–204.

36. Rabaglino MB, Risco CA, Thatcher MJ, et al. Application of one injection of prostaglandin F(2alpha) in the five-day Co-Synch+CIDR protocol for estrous synchronization and resynchronization of dairy heifers. J Dairy Sci 2010;93:1050–8.

37. Rabaglino MB, Risco CA, Thatcher MJ, et al. Use of a five-day progesterone-based timed AI protocol to determine if flunixin meglumine improves pregnancy per timed AI in dairy heifers. Theriogenology 2010;73:1311–8.

38. Lima FS, Ayres H, Favoreto MG, et al. Effects of gonadotropin-releasing hormone at initiation of the 5-d timed artificial insemination (AI) program and timing of induction of ovulation relative to AI on ovarian dynamics and fertility of dairy heifers. J Dairy Sci 2011;94:4997–5004.

Embryo Transfer (Techniques, Donors, and Recipients)

Patrick E. Phillips, DVM[a],*, Marianna M. Jahnke, MS[b]

KEYWORDS

- Bovine • Embryo transfer • Donor • Recipient • MOET
- In vitro maturation/ In vitro fertilization

KEY POINTS

- Donor and recipient management are critically important in the success of in vivo embryo transfer (ET).
- Experience through training and mentorship is critical to development of skill sets required for a successful ET program.
- Guidance by the International Embryo Transfer Society and the American Embryo Transfer Association provides excellent references for the novice ET practitioner.
- Advanced reproductive technologies, such as ovum pickup, in vitro processes, and cloning, are rapidly changing the face of ET today.

HISTORY

The eternal attempt to control the reproductive parameters of domestic animals and man can be traced back 5000 years to Egypt, where Pharaohs tried to create Apis bulls by positioning cows in open fields during storms in an attempt to have them struck by lightning.[1] In more recent times, it was shown that Walter Heape is credited with the first mammalian embryo transfer (ET) when he took the embryos from a rabbit and transferred them to a surrogate doe in 1890.[2] The first recorded successful transfer and live birth from an embryo derived from cattle was in 1951 by Willett and colleagues[3] at the University of Wisconsin. It was not until the late 1960s and early 1970s that commercialization of in vivo ET technology in cattle began to

The authors have nothing to disclose.
[a] Veterinary Diagnostic and Production Animal Medicine, Iowa State University College of Veterinary Medicine, 2434 LVMC, Ames, IA 50011, USA; [b] Veterinary Diagnostic and Production Animal Medicine, Iowa State University College of Veterinary Medicine, 2428 LVMC, Ames, IA 50011, USA
* Corresponding author.
E-mail address: ovadoc@iastate.edu

flourish, and significant research inroads regarding collection and transfer of bovine embryos began. Pioneers, such as Peter Elsden, Tim Rawson, George Seidel, Bob Baker, and John Hasler, showed that initial work involving surgical recovery of bovine embryos was possible, but work on nonsurgical techniques had to be developed for this technology to expand and grow. By the late 1970s, nonsurgical recoveries were widely used, which opened the door for dairy cattle, especially Holsteins, to be used as donors.[4] It was not until the early to mid-1980s that nonsurgical transfer of bovine embryos became prevalent. The transition from surgical to nonsurgical transfers was slowed by 2 main problems. The first is that the pregnancy rate using surgical transfer techniques was significantly higher initially than nonsurgical in certain operations. The second impediment to this transition was the lack of useful tools to accomplish the transfer. IMV Technologies developed the initial nonsurgical ET gun that was introduced in North America in 1984 to 1985.[4] Overcoming these 2 challenges quickly led to nonsurgical transfer becoming adopted universally in the ET profession.

A major development in the ET world was the ability to cryopreserve bovine embryos at $-196°C$ and keep them indefinitely. In 1973, Wilmut and Rowson[5] were the first to cryopreserve bovine blastocysts, using dimethyl sulfoxide (DMSO), and subsequently establishing a day 42 pregnancy in a recipient cow after thaw. The remainder of this article describes how knowledge and technology have been expanded to find better effectiveness in production and preservation of bovine embryos.

DONOR MANAGEMENT

Selection of superior genetic or phenotypic animals has been the basis of donor selection since ET's inception. The addition of indices and genomics has further refined the selection process of animals destined to become donors. The donors today can be selected by the marketplace, industry ranking, or simply the owner's desire to produce more offspring from a particular animal. Additional criteria, from a reproductive management viewpoint, include age, tract development, nutrition, body condition score (BCS), lactation, parity, days open, environment, and endocrine factors to name a few.[6]

Shull[7] looked at donor management from a problematic viewpoint. When expected outcomes are not realized in commercial ET, it can be into 1 of 3 categories: the owner, the practitioner, or the animal herself. The owner is the first category to analyze. Misconceptions as to response, fertility, and recovered embryos have to be met with facts. The average number of viable embryos recovered per flush in 2013 was 6.8.[8] Another issue to confront is the use of frozen semen from poor fertility bulls or using sexed semen. In 2013, embryo recoveries from sexed semen produced viable embryos 25.1% of the time, whereas embryo recoveries from nonsorted semen produced viable embryos 55.95% of the time.[8] The above issues can be confronted with education of the owner about the industry and averages for each category.[7]

The second category of management concerns involves the practitioner. This area involves inexperience, substandard donor hormone protocols, poor equipment, facilities, and inexperienced staff. Again, repetitive training and help formulating a battery of tested protocols will aid in the management problem.[7] In addition, enhanced record keeping by the practitioner will allow the individual donor cow's history to aid in management changes being made, using fact and not conjecture.

The third category is the animal herself. Less than average embryo production can be related to many factors that were stated above. For example, understanding the difference in how *Bos taurus* and *Bos indicus* respond, or the difference between heifers and cows, or the difference between dairy and beef breeds, is essential to capitalizing on the embryo produced. Manipulation of the estrous cycle to enhance estrus, correcting physical abnormalities of the reproductive tract, and nutritional counseling with the owner of that BCS 2.0 cow with a calf at her side will not only enhance the owner's own education but also prevent wasting a great deal of time and increase the practitioners success rate.[6]

SUPEROVULATION

Early efforts to superovulate cattle in the early 1970s used equine chorionic gonadotropin (eCG) until follicle-stimulating hormone (FSH) became available.[9] eCG had numerous drawbacks, including a long half-life, being highly antigenic, and having post-eCG reproductive quiescence. As FSH emerged on the market, it was originally porcine in origin. The pituitary extract of FSH today is contaminated with luteinizing hormone (LH) to varying levels. It has been found that increased levels of LH in FSH products actually decrease the superovulatory and viable embryo response in cattle. It is thought that endogenous LH levels are adequate for successful superovulation.[10] Another viewpoint has shown that FSH with varying levels of LH at the end of the superovulation protocol enhances ovulatory rates in cattle.

Donor animals are typically started on a superovulatory schedule no sooner than 45 days after calving. Initial work depended on the initiation of cyclicity and ovulation in the donor with formation of a prostaglandin-sensitive corpora lutea 9 to 13 days after ovulation during the superovulation protocol. Because porcine follicle-stimulating hormone has a very short half-life, about 5 hours, it requires administration twice daily during the superovulation protocol.[11] Many protocols have been developed over time, but commonly, a decreasing dose protocol with administration of a prostaglandin F2α concurrently with FSH at the end of the protocol has been used. This type of protocol is wholly dependent on the cow or heifer cycling normally at the time of superovulation.

More recently, protocols have been developed that were designed to increase the success rate of embryo recovery and quality through the use of exogenous progestogens, such as the controlled internal drug release (CIDR) and dominant follicle removal. The use of the CIDR has allowed practitioners the flexibility to start a superovulatory schedule anytime during the estrous cycle. Removal of the dominant follicle allows for a new cohort of antral follicles to begin developing and respond to the FSH therapy in greater numbers.[12] Removal of the dominant follicle has been accomplished by numerous methods, including ultrasound-guided aspiration, estradiol-17β, and gonadotropin-releasing hormone (GnRH).[13] Although estradiol-17β is illegal for use in cattle in the United States, it is used extensively around the world, including Canada. Dominant follicle ovulation, with subsequent follicular wave recruitment using GnRH, is widely used in the United States today. Studies have shown that this method is effective only 50% to 60% of the time in timed artificial insemination programs.[14] It has also been shown that GnRH in combination with a CIDR is as effective in removal of the dominant follicle and subsequent follicular wave recruitment as estradiol 17β when used in superovulation.[15] Removal of the dominant follicle reduces the effect of inhibin, produced by this follicle, which allows for FSH responsive small follicles to be recruited and grow with the use of a superovulation scheme. Superovulation protocols are continually being refined and simplified for ease of use by the producer and veterinarian and to reduce stress on the donor animal.

Fig. 1 shows a common schedule using CIDRs and GnRH. In no way is this advocated as the only program available, but is used only to show the timeframes involved in a typical superovulatory program.

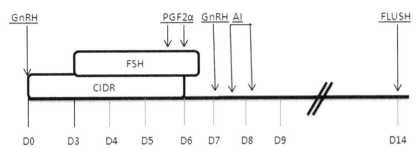

Fig. 1. Example of a superovulation schedule using CIDRs and GnRH. PGF2α, prostaglandin F2α.

EMBRYO RECOVERY

The industry has moved to nonsurgical recovery of embryos since the 1970s. Today, silicone catheters have been specifically produced that have the proper diameter and length for all types of cattle. Unlike the Foley catheter that was originally used in the 1970s, today's catheters are reusable and autoclavable. With the advent of a strong export market for US genetics, the recovery systems have been adapted to be totally closed during the recovery process. The process is performed in 1 of 2 ways generally. The first is a gravity system, wherein 1 to 2 L of a specialized media such as Dulbecco's phosphate-buffered saline (DPBS) is gently lavaged into each uterine horn in aliquots of 50 to 200 mL at a time and recovered into a specialized filter for trapping the embryos. The second form of recovery is the syringe technique, whereby the media are syringed into each horn and recovered via the syringe into an embryo filter.

It is imperative to the successful recovery of embryos and subsequent establishment of pregnancies to insure that all surfaces and products that may come in contact with the embryo or media are nontoxic and sterile. The industry encountered a major setback in the 1980s when a syringe manufacturer changed the sterilization process used for its syringes without notification of end-users. The new γ-irradiation procedure used affected the lubricant used on the plunger of the syringe, and it became toxic. As practitioners and ET companies found out, the new syringes had a toxic lubricant, which decreased their pregnancies to zero.[4] Today, products from media, catheters, syringes, tubing, and filters are manufactured and tested to ensure sterility and safety.

The media used today, such as DPBS, originally used Fraction V bovine serum albumin (BSA) as a protein additive that acted as a surfactant to aid in the removal of the embryo from the endometrium and help keep it in suspension during the recovery process. As global export markets expanded in the 1980s and 1990s, concerns about the biosecurity of the BSA and possible contamination with bovine viral diarrhea virus (BVD) emerged. This problem necessitated the development of surfactants that were not of animal origin. Many have been developed, but the most common used today is polyvinyl alcohol. However, tested and sterilized BSA is still used by many practitioners today in both their flush and their holding media.

One of the major improvements in the recovery process for bovine embryos was the development of the embryo filter. Originally, recovered lavage fluid from the uterus would be collected in a glass flask or graduated cylinder and allowed to sit, undisturbed, for 30 to 60 minutes, allowing the embryos to drop to the bottom. The supernatant would be decanted off carefully, and the remaining fluid would be placed in a gridded search dish to find the embryos. Today, the many embryo filters on the market do fundamentally the same thing. They trap the 150- to 200-μm embryos on a 50- to

70-μm stainless steel or plastic filter. The filter allows the fluid to escape, but captures the embryos on the filter for searching and processing.

One of the final aspects of the recovery process is the skill of the practitioner. ET training is available commercially and in sponsored wet laboratories at scientific meetings American Association of Bovine Practitioners (AABP) as well at numerous Colleges of Veterinary Medicine in the United States. Although this training can range from 3 to 7 days, the training teaches the technical side of embryo recovery, cryopreservation, and transfer. From this point, it may take years to become proficient as an ET specialist that not only understands the technical aspect of ET but also fully grasps the "art" of ET.

EMBRYO MORPHOLOGY

Embryos are routinely evaluated after collection, before transfer or freezing for storage. Embryo morphologic evaluation is important to differentiate unfertilized oocytes from embryos, determine embryo quality and identify abnormalities, and determine if the stage of development is consistent with the embryo age.[16]

According to the International Embryo Transfer Society (IETS), embryos should be morphologically evaluated under a microscope using at least ×50 magnification to identify any abnormalities such as cracked zona pellucida. The overall diameter of a bovine embryo is 150 to 190 μm, which is unchanged from a 1-cell zygote until the blastocyst stage of development. The embryo is composed of a glycoprotein layer surrounding the plasma membrane of the embryo (zona pellucida) and cells (blastomeres) that eventually differentiates into inner cell mass (ICM) and trophoblast cells as the embryo develops. The zona pellucida, present from 1 cell until the expanded blastocyst stage, is a protective shell surrounding the embryo that acts as a physical barrier against pathogens. It also contains sperm receptors to assist during fertilization, blocking the penetration of accessory sperm. The ICM will give rise to the fetus while the trophoblast cells will eventually form the outer layer of the placenta. During the differentiation event (blastulation), a fluid-filled cavity (blastocoel cavity) is formed between the ICM and trophoblast cells (**Fig. 2**). During development, the blastocoel cavity grows progressively larger, causing the thinning and the subsequent hatching of the zona pellucida.[17]

Embryos recovered on days 6 to 8 after the onset of estrus should be classified into groups based on their stage of development and quality grade using the IETS classification system (**Table 1**). This classification system consists of a 2-digit code for stage of development and quality grade, respectively.

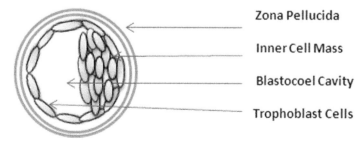

Zona Pellucida

Inner Cell Mass

Blastocoel Cavity

Trophoblast Cells

Fig. 2. Illustration of a blastocyst stage bovine embryo. (*Adapted from* Jahnke MJ, West JK, Youngs CR. Evaluation of in vivo derived embryos. In: Hopper RM, editor. Bovine reproduction. Hoboken (NJ): Wiley and Sons; 2014. p. 735; with permission.)

Table 1
Bovine embryo stage and quality description

Stage of Development		Quality of Embryos	
Code	Stage	Code	Quality Description
1	Unfertilized	1	Excellent or good
2	Two- to 12-cell	2	Fair
3	Early morula	3	Poor
4	Morula	4	Dead or degenerating
5	Early blastocyst		
6	Blastocyst		
7	Expanded blastocyst		
8	Hatched blastocyst		
9	Expanded hatched blastocyst		

From Stringfellow D, Givens M. Manual of the International Embryo Transfer Society. 4th edition. Champaign (IL): International Embryo Transfer Society; 2010; with permission.

The specific code for stage of development is numeric, ranging from (1, unfertilized oocyte, to 9, expanding hatched blastocyst) (**Fig. 3**). The blastomeres multiply through cleavage divisions from a single cell. As blastomere number increases and compacts to a tight-cluster of cells, a morula forms around day 6 postestrus.

One-Cell or Unfertilized (Stage 1)

An oocyte collected around day 7 is called an unfertilized ovum (UFO). A UFO usually has a perfectly spherical oolemma or vitelline membrane; the cytoplasm appears granular, and it contains a reasonable amount of space between the zona and the cell called perivitelline space (**Fig. 4**). However, UFOs may be degenerating by day 7 and show a more fragmented appearance that can be confusing to the untrained eye.

Two-Cell to 12-Cell (Stage 2)

Embryos that are recovered around day 7 containing 2 to 12 cells are severely delayed in their stage of development and should considered dead or degenerate (**Figs. 5 and 6**).

Early Morula (Stage 3)

Embryos in this stage have divided into 16 or more cells, and individual blastomeres are difficult to distinguish from one another (**Fig. 7**).

Morula (Stage 4)

Individual blastomeres have formed a tight cell mass through compaction, but cells have not yet differentiated (**Fig. 8**).

Early Blastocyst (Stage 5)

A fluid-filled cavity called a blastocoel cavity starts forming inside the cell mass. The blastocoel cavity allows blastomeres to differentiate into the outer trophoblast cells and ICM (**Fig. 9**).

Blastocyst (Stage 6)

The blastocyst (stage 6) is a stage of development whereby the embryo has a defined outer trophoblast layer, blastocoel cavity, and ICM (**Fig. 10**). At this stage, the embryo occupies most of the perivitelline space, and the zona pellucida is still the same thickness.

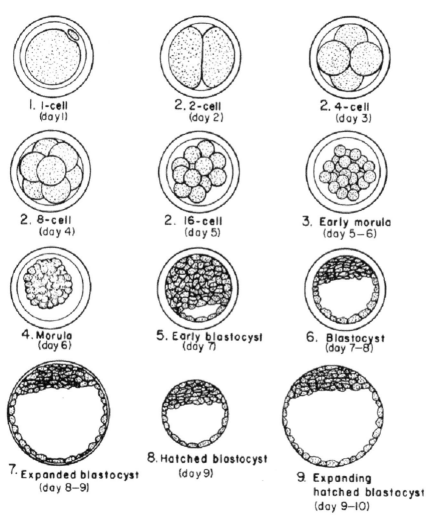

Fig. 3. Illustration of normal bovine embryonic development. (*From* Stringfellow DA, Seidel SM. Manual of the International Embryo Transfer Society, 4th edition. Champaign (IL): International Embryo Transfer Society; 2010; with permission.)

Expanded Blastocyst (Stage 7)

The most distinguished feature of this stage is an increase in the overall diameter of the embryo in addition to thinning of the zona pellucida (**Fig. 11**).

Hatched Blastocyst (Stage 8)

At this stage of embryonic development, the embryo is beginning to hatch or has completely escaped through a crack in the zona pellucida (**Fig. 12**). Embryos in this phase can also be collapsed, creating a different appearance (**Fig. 13**).

Hatched Expanded Blastocyst (Stage 9)

Embryos at this stage will be hatched from the zona pellucida and re-expanded (**Fig. 14**).

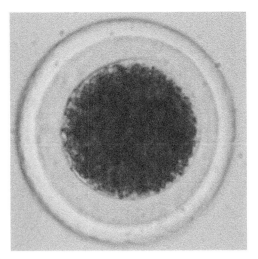

Fig. 4. Unfertilized ovum.

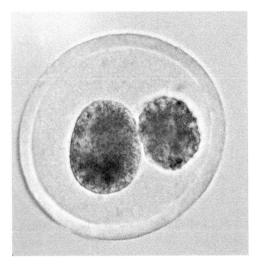

Fig. 5. Two cell.

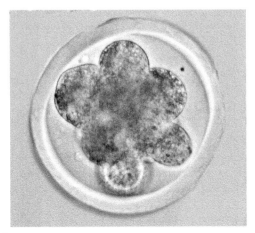

Fig. 6. Four to 8 cell.

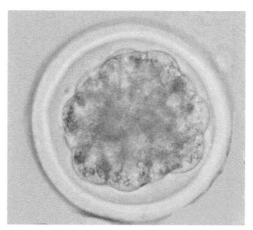

Fig. 7. Early morula.

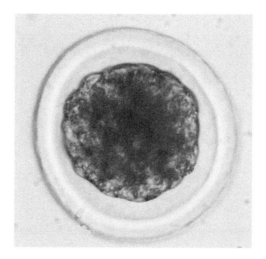

Fig. 8. Morula.

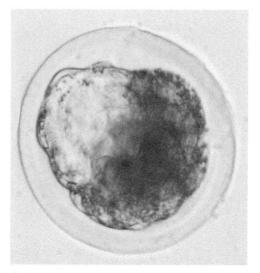

Fig. 9. Early blastocyst.

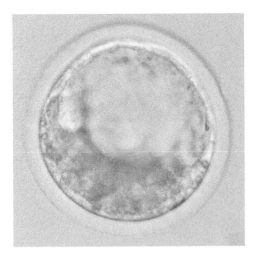

Fig. 10. Blastocyst.

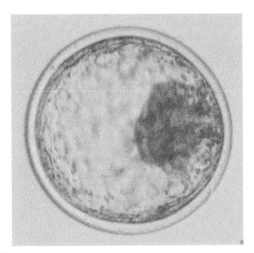

Fig. 11. Expanded blastocyst.

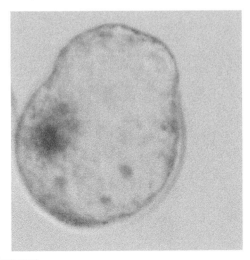

Fig. 12. Hatched blastocyst.

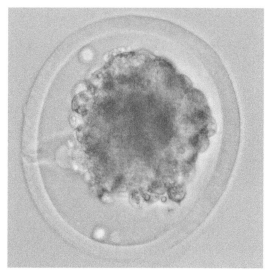

Fig. 13. Collapsed blastocyst.

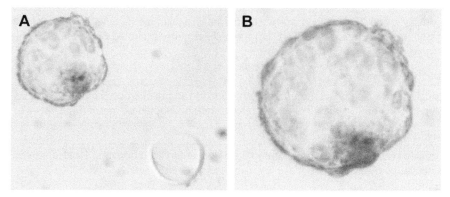

Fig. 14. (*A, B*) Hatched expanded blastocyst.

EMBRYO QUALITY CODES RECOMMENDED BY THE INTERNATIONAL EMBRYO TRANSFER SOCIETY

Embryo quality grade is determined by visual assessment of an embryo's morphologic characteristics. This visual assessment is a subjective evaluation. The best predictor of an embryo's viability is its stage of development relative to the given day after fertilization.[18] Some of the characteristics that can affect the quality of an embryo are uniform size and color of the blastomeres, presence or absence of vacuoles among the cells, presence or absence of extruded cells, and shape of the zona pellucida. Embryos of excellent, good, or fair quality grade yield the highest pregnancy rates. Quality codes 1 and 2 tolerate the freezing procedure without any diminish pregnancy rate. Poor quality embryos should only be transferred fresh. Generally, unless otherwise specified, only code 1 embryos should be exported. From a superovulated cow undergoing an embryo recovery on day 7, a wide variation of embryo stage and quality is expected. The codes for embryo quality range numerically from 1 to 4 as follows.

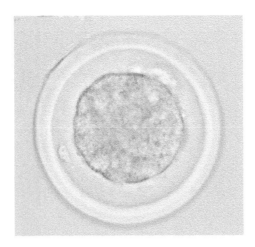

Fig. 15. 4-1.

Quality Code 1: Excellent or Good

Irregularities are relatively minor in quality 1 code embryo. At least 85% of the cellular material should be an intact, viable embryo mass (**Figs. 15–17**).

Quality Code 2: Fair

A quality code 2 embryo presents moderate irregularities in overall shape of the embryo mass or size. At least 50% of the cellular material should be an intact, viable embryo mass (**Figs. 18–20**).

Quality Code 3: Poor

A quality code 3 contains major irregularities in the shape of embryo mass or size, color, and density. At least 25% of the cellular material should be intact (**Figs. 21–23**).

Quality Code 4: Dead or Degenerate

A quality code 4 includes degenerated embryos, unfertilized oocytes, 1-cell embryos, or nonviable (**Figs. 24–26**).

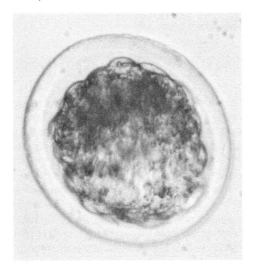

Fig. 16. 5-1.

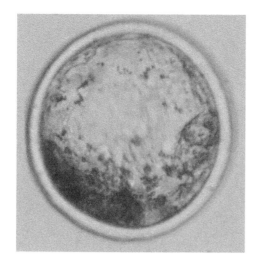

Fig. 17. 6-1.

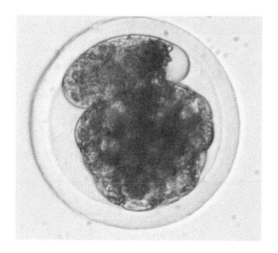

Fig. 18. 4-2.

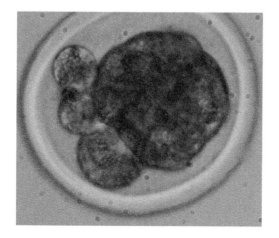

Fig. 19. 4-2.

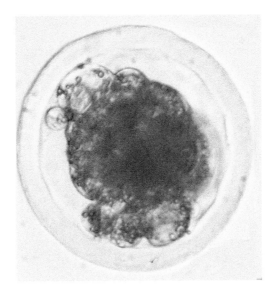

Fig. 20. 4-2.

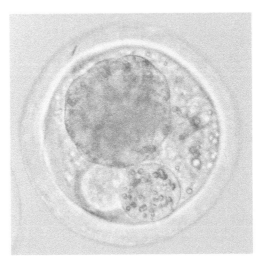

Fig. 21. 4-3.

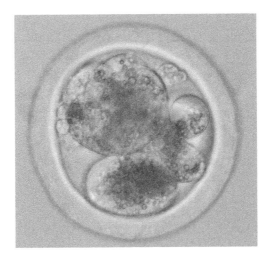

Fig. 22. 4-3.

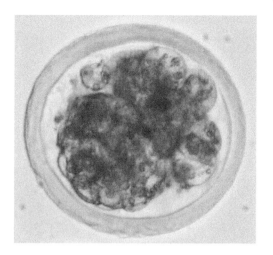

Fig. 23. 4-3.

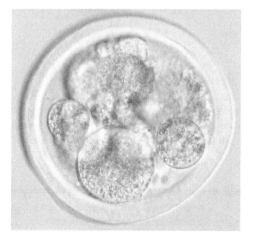

Fig. 24. Degenerate (2–4).

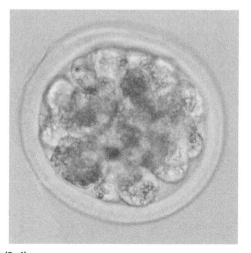

Fig. 25. Degenerate (2–4).

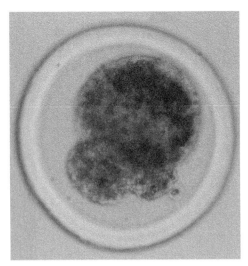

Fig. 26. Unfertilized (1–4).

EMBRYO MANIPULATION
Embryo Splitting

Embryo splitting is a safe and efficient way to create monozygotic twins. During this procedure, the embryo is divided into 2 halves using a micromanipulator and a micro-blade (**Fig. 27**). Each half produced via embryo splitting is called a demi-embryo.

Embryo Biopsying

This procedure consists of removing a small group of cells from the embryo using a microblade attached to a micromanipulator (**Figs. 28** and **29**). Embryo biopsy is used to evaluate the genetic material for diagnosis of specific genetic defects or for determination of embryo sex. In addition, embryo biopsy can garner material for genomic testing.

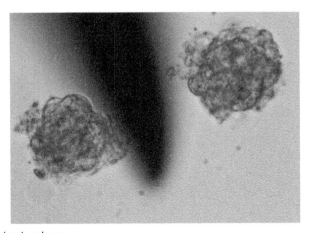

Fig. 27. Two demi-embryos.

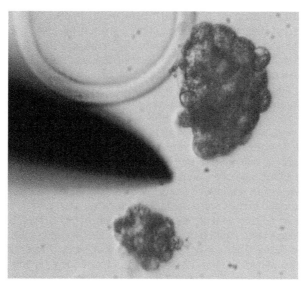

Fig. 28. Embryo and biopsy.

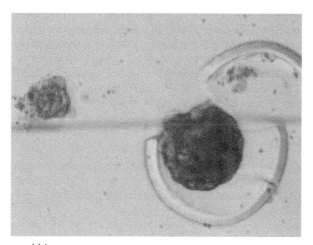

Fig. 29. Embryo and biopsy.

Embryo Gender Determination

This procedure uses amplified DNA from biopsied cells with a procedure called polymerase chain reaction, which identifies the presence or absence of the male chromosome Y and determines the gender of the embryo.

CRYOPRESERVATION

The indefinite stasis of biological life at supercooled temperatures has been discussed since the early 20th century.[19] It was not until the accidental discovery by Sir Christopher Polge and colleagues in 1949 that one could successfully slow-freeze rooster spermatozoa using glycerol as a cryoprotectant.[20]

Today, cryopreservation of biological tissue and gametes is found in 2 basic categories. The first is vitrification, or "glassing," which is the use of high cryoprotectant concentrations and very rapid temperature decrease to $-196°C$. Typical cryoprotectants used for this include DMSO, polyethylene glycol, and even glycerol. The effect is to freeze gametes in the absence of ice crystal formation, thus preserving the intracellular architecture and membranes. Until recently, it has not been a commercial option for the practitioner due to very stringent variables used in the process.[21]

The second procedure used widely today for embryo freezing is the slow-freezing process using lower molar concentration of cryoprotectant such as glycerol or ethylene glycol. This procedure, with or without the use of sugars such as sucrose or arabinogalactan, is designed to slowly replace the intracellular water with cryoprotectant with the added help of the sugars to provide additional osmotic pressure extracellularly to help insure minimal ice crystal formation during the freezing process. Embryos are exposed to the cryoprotectant, held at stable temperature to allow equilibration for a short amount of time, then slowly cooled ($-0.5°C$/min) to $-32.0°C$, and then directly plunged into liquid nitrogen at $-196.0°C$. Two different cryoprotectants are mainly used today. The first one used is 1.0 M glycerol. This cryoprotectant requires a stepwise dehydration and rehydration of the embryo, which requires additional equipment for the thaw process. This technique is known as the "long-thaw" process. The second slow-freeze process used is 1.5M ethylene glycol. This cryoprotectant allows for the rapid thaw of the embryo in 25°C water and then is directly transferred to the recipient using the straw it was frozen in.[22] This type of slow-freeze process is called Direct Transfer and is the most common process used today in the bovine ET industry. Commercial freezing units are available today for the practitioner and researcher that are economical and exacting in time and temperature control. **Table 2** is a subset from the American Embryo Transfer Association (AETA) and shows the volume of commercial in vivo bovine embryos recovered, frozen or transferred in the United States currently by AETA members.

RECIPIENT MANAGEMENT

Probably one of the most important yet underappreciated aspects of a successful ET program is the recipient.[23] Management of this herd requires fundamental understanding of recipient selection, nutrition, estrus synchronization, disease management, and marketing.

Recipient selection is one of the first objectives for an ET program to achieve. Depending on whether one is dealing with an assembled herd or a closed herd, there are a few criteria that need to be addressed. Although heifers used as recipients are a common practice in many places, it does come with its own perils. These animals

Table 2
Historical production, freezing, and transfer of in vivo produced embryos in the United States

Year	Total Viable Embryos	Average Viable/ Flush	Total Embryo Frozen	Total Fresh Embryos Transferred	Total Frozen Embryos Transferred
2002	172,118	7.46	110,715	59,682	69,978
2007	332,846	5.69	216,697	110,223	137,772
2013	301,671	6.80	215,525	85,876	215,699

Courtesy of American Embryo Transfer Association Annual Survey of Members; with permission.

typically will give higher pregnancy rates than cows, ranging from 10% to 23%.[4] The downside is that this animal is used to carry genetics that typically are not selected for calving ease. Calving management has to be a primary concern when using heifers as recipients. An additional downside to heifer usage in the beef world is milk production. Will she be able to maximize weaning weights of her ET offspring as compared with an advanced parity cow in the herd? Advanced parity cows from 3 to 8 years of age are the optimum recipient with better milk production, better reproductive history, and better colostrum and can be selected for disposition.[23]

Nutrition can be a critical factor in a successful recipient pool. Ideally, beef recipients should have a BCS between 2.5 and 3.5, and dairy recipients should be in the range of 5.5 to 6.5. Extremely thin or overweight animals tend to have lower pregnancy rates than a properly fitted cow or heifer. Nutritional factors that need to be addressed not only include higher starch and fat diets before implantation, but also additives, such as organic trace minerals, mold and mycotoxin abatement programs, bunk management, bunk space, and feeding practices.[24]

Successful outcomes in an ET program depend on proper estrus synchronization. Although developed timed synchronization protocols are strived for for recipients, it is apparent that embryo quality plays a more significant role in successful outcome than degree of synchrony.[23] Visual estrus detection has for many years been considered the gold standard for defining estrus synchronization. Ideally, it should be performed twice daily for 30 minutes in the early AM and later PM and not be associated with outside distractions such as feeding. Newer strategies for estrus synchronization are being developed using timed ovulation programs that are seen in the artificial insemination industry. These pharmacologic programs using progestogens and gonadotropins have been shown to be successful as visual heat detection, and in many places, are replacing visual estrus detection.[25]

Recipient health is a major part of the management strategy for an ET program. Its application and implementation must be done well before the animals are used as a recipient. Specific disease conditions that must be ruled out before the animals are used as a recipient include BVD, enzootic bovine leukosis, neospora, Johnes, and Brucellosis. Testing of the recipient pool ensures that these conditions do not become a limiting factor in the overall success rate of the program or yield affected high value calves.

ADVANCED REPRODUCTIVE TECHNOLOGIES

In vitro produced (IVP) embryos and embryo cloning are on the verge of changing bovine ET, as it is known, very soon. The rapid advancement in this technology has allowed for the numerous advantages in commercial ET today. Donors in an IVP program can have ovum pickup (OPU) performed every 12 to 18 days up to 100 plus days pregnant using an ultrasound-guided follicular aspiration unit. Oocytes recovered in the field are sent to laboratories where maturation and fertilization (IVF) are performed. The use of sex-sorted semen is common in these programs and yield better results than its use in conventional ET programs. After 6 days in the laboratory, the IVF embryos are transported back to the farm using a temperature-controlled incubator designed for transit via conventional carriers, where they are transferred into synchronized recipients.

Cryopreservation of IVP embryos has made significant advances in recent years. Frozen IVP embryos have similar pregnancy rates as conventional ET embryos when using grade I embryos. These embryos are being cryopreserved using the Direct Transfer method, allowing minimal handling on the farm. **Table 3** shows how IVP embryo technology has expanded over the last 10 years.

Table 3
Historical production, transfer, and freezing of in vitro produced embryos in the United States

Year	OPU Recoveries	Viable Oocytes	Transferred IVP Embryos	Frozen IVP Embryos	Transferred Frozen IVP Embryos
2003	2781	12,063	1558	908	344
2006	2328	10,984	3472	1243	545
2010	6876	109,615	24,452	3955	2290
2013	22,046	416,612	101,502	34,652	12,310

Courtesy of American Embryo Transfer Association Annual Survey of Members; with permission.

SUMMARY

ET technology in cattle has had an impressive history that has garnered much attention and research over the last 50 years. Innovation in techniques and knowledge concerning bovine ET is preparing the profession to move into a new era of Advanced Reproductive Technologies, such as IVF and cloned embryos, on a very wide and global scale. Traditional multiple ovulation embryo transfer practices will still exist for many practitioners for years to come. An important part of the future of ET is the ability to train and mentor new veterinarians in the field. Organizations such as the AETA and the IETS can provide the fundamental basis for this education, but the industry in the field will be the trainer to hone the skills of the next generation of ET Practitioners.

REFERENCES

1. Breasted James H. Ancient Records of Egypt. Vol. 4: The 20th to the 26th Dynasties. Chicago, IL: University of Chicago; 1906. p. 348–57.
2. Heape W. Preliminary note on the transplantation and growth of mammalian ova within a uterine foster-mother. Proceedings of the Royal Society of London 1890; 48:457–8.
3. Willett EL, Black WG, Casida LE, et al. Successful transplantation of a fertilized bovine ovum. Science 1951;113:247.
4. Hasler JF. Forty years of embryo transfer in cattle: a review focusing on the journal Theriogenology, the growth of the industry in North America, and personal reminisces. Theriogenology 2014;81:152–69.
5. Wilmut I, Rowson LEA. The successful low-temperature preservation of mouse and cow embryos. J Reprod Fertil 1973;33:352–3.
6. Santos JEP, Cerri RLA, Sartori R. Nutritional management of the donor cow. Theriogenology 2008;69:88–97.
7. Shull JW. Managing the problem beef embryo donor. In: Proceedings. Society For Theriogenology. Montgomery, AL; 2009. p. 283–8.
8. American Embryo Transfer Association website. AETA Annual Surveys. Available at: www.aeta.org/survey.asp. Accessed July 15, 2014.
9. Betteridge KJ. Techniques and results in cattle superovulation. In: Betteridge KJ, editor. Embryo transfer in farm animals. Ottawa (ON): Canada Department of Agriculture; 1977. p. 1–9. Monograph 16.
10. Looney C, Bondioli K, Hill K, et al. Superovulation of donor cows with bovine follicle-stimulating hormone (bFSH) produced by recombinant DNA technology. Theriogenology 1988;29:271.

11. Laster D. Disappearance of and uptake of I125 FSH in the rat, rabbit, ewe and cow. J Reprod Fertil 1972;30:407–15.
12. Shaw DW, Good TE. Recovery rates and embryo quality following dominant follicle ablation in superovulated cattle. Theriogenology 2000;8(53):1521–8.
13. Bó GA, Mapletoft RJ. Historical perspectives and recent research on superovulation in cattle. Theriogenology 2014;81:38–48.
14. Small JA, Colazo MG, Kastelic JP, et al. Effects of progesterone presynchronization and eCG on pregnancy rates to GnRH-based, timed-AI in beef cattle. Theriogenology 2009;71:698–706.
15. Wock JM, Lyle LM, Hockett ME. Effect of gonadotropin-releasing hormone compared with estradiol-17β at the beginning of a superstimulation protocol on superovulatory response and embryo quality. Reprod Fertil Dev 2007;1(20):228–9.
16. Jahnke MJ, West JK, Youngs CR. Evaluation of in vivo derived embryos. In: Hopper RM, editor. Bovine reproduction. Hoboken (NJ): Wiley and Sons; 2014. p. 733–48.
17. Stringfellow DA, Seidel SM. Manual of the International Embryo Transfer Society. 3rd edition. Champaign (IL): International Embryo Transfer Society; 1998. p. 1–79.
18. Mapletoft RJ, Hasler JF. Embryo Transfer 101 with a Technical Slant. In: Proceedings CETA/AETA Joint Convention. Champaign IL; 2006. p. 3–20.
19. Luyet BJ. The vitrification of organic colloids and of protoplasm. Biodynamics 1937;1:1–14.
20. Polge C, Smith AU, Parker AS. Revival of spermatozoa after vitrification and dehydration at low temperatures. Nature 1949;164:666.
21. Arav A. Cryopreservation of oocytes and embryos. Theriogenology 2014;81:96–102.
22. Leibo SP, Pool TB. The principal variables of cryopreservation: solutions, temperatures, and rate changes. Fertil Steril 2011;2(96):269–76.
23. Schmidt J. Thriving, surviving, and nose-diving in beef recipient management. In: Proceedings of American Embryo Transfer Association, Champaign, IL; 2010; p. 35-42.
24. Oetzel GR. The effect of nutrition on reproduction: applications for ET donors and recipients. In: Proceedings American Embryo Transfer Association, Champaign, IL; 2012. p. 50–9.
25. Bó GA, Mapletoft RJ. Strategies for donor and recipient selection, treatment, and management. In: Proceedings American Embryo Transfer Association, Champaign, IL; 2013. p. 16–24.

Management of Reproductive Disease in Dairy Cows

Robert O. Gilbert, BVSc, MMedVet, MRCVS

KEYWORDS

- Retained fetal membranes • Metritis • Cervicitis • Endometritis • Anovulation
- Cystic ovarian disease

KEY POINTS

- Retained fetal membranes increase risk of metritis but treatment of uncomplicated cases is not usually justified. Supplementation of vitamin E, selenium or beta carotene in deficient herds can reduce incidence.
- Incidence of puerperal metritis is higher in primipara and in cows with obstetrical complications. Affected cows should be treated with antibiotics.
- Endometritis is associated with postpartum negative energy balance. Affected cows have reduced fertility and increased embryonic loss.
- Cervicitis and purulent vaginal discharge are associated with obstetrical complications, reduce fertility and increase embryonic loss. Where permissible (not in the USA) intrauterine cefapirin is an effective treatment.
- Anovulation is most common in cows in poor body condition and negative energy balance, but also has a genetic basis. Cows respond to inclusion of progesterone in synchronization protocols. Anovulation is associated with increased risk of embryonic and fetal loss.

INTRODUCTION

Postpartum diseases are common in dairy cows, and their incidence contributes to reduced fertility and increased risk of culling, making their prevention and management extremely important. Reproductive efficiency has a major impact on economic success of any dairy production unit. Optimizing reproductive efficiency contributes to overall efficiency of production units, minimizing environmental impacts and contributing to sustainability of food production. Additionally, control of reproductive diseases is important for maintenance of health and welfare of dairy cows; for minimizing use of antibiotics; and ensuring a wholesome, safe, and nutritious product.

Disclosure: The author is coinventor of a vaccine to prevent metritis (US patent W02014084964-A1).
Department of Clinical Sciences, College of Veterinary Medicine, Cornell University, Tower Road, Ithaca, NY 14853-6401, USA
E-mail address: rob.gilbert@cornell.edu

THE PERIPARTURIENT COW

Many of the important disorders of the postpartum period are attributable to metabolic and immune changes that occur, sometimes inevitably, as the cow makes the transition from late pregnancy to early lactation. In the last weeks of pregnancy metabolic demands of the fetus reach a maximum while at the same time voluntary dry matter intake decreases some 20%.[1] Cows also have to contend with major changes in diet after parturition to diets supporting lactation, and with the metabolic demands of lactation.[1-3] Inevitably, feed intake fails to meet the initial demands of lactation, and cows experience a period of negative energy balance, requiring mobilization of tissue reserves.[4] The combined effects of onset of lactation and physiologic events of parturition result in transient deficiencies in several vitamins and minerals and changes in immune function.[2,3,5-7] These, in turn, play a role in pathogenesis of important postpartum uterine disorders, including retained fetal membranes (RFM), metritis, and endometritis, and ovarian disorders, such as anovulation and ovarian follicular cysts. Mobilization of fat reserves results in increased circulating concentrations of nonesterified fatty acids. Liver capacity for metabolizing lipids can be overwhelmed leading to export of β-hydroxybutyrate, which accumulates in blood. Periparturient concentrations of nonesterified fatty acids and β-hydroxybutyrate can predict cows at risk of uterine disease.[8-10] Altered blood mineral status has also been linked to impaired immune function[11-16] and subsequent uterine disease.[17] The transition is also a period of oxidative stress and antioxidant capacity is diminished.[18]

In conjunction with the metabolic changes outlined previously, early lactation cows develop insulin resistance. This may be a mechanism to preferentially allocate energy reserves to milk production.[1,19] Additionally, growth hormone receptors in the liver are reduced, leading to lower insulinlike growth factor 1 concentrations, which are related to susceptibility to uterine disease.[20,21] Insulin restores growth hormone responsiveness[22] and increases follicular secretion of estradiol.[23] Obstetric complications add to the vulnerable status of the postpartum cow. Dystocia, birth of twins, or birth of stillborn calves all increase the risk of metritis and endometritis.[24-28]

RETAINED FETAL MEMBRANES

Although bovine fetal membranes are normally expelled within 3 to 8 hours after delivery of the calf[29] RFM is usually defined as failure of expulsion by 24 hours. The incidence in dairy cows is about 5% to 15% and is higher for older cows than for primipara.[30,31] The incidence of RFM is increased by abortion, stillbirth, multiple birth, dystocia, uterine torsion, heat stress, hydrops allantois, and periparturient hypocalcemia.[31] Cows induced to calve by pharmacologic means, such as exogenous corticosteroid administration, frequently have RFM. A high incidence of RFM is associated with many infectious conditions, including brucellosis, campylobacteriosis, and aspergillosis. Nutritional causes, such as overconditioning of dry cows and deficiencies of carotene, selenium, and vitamin E, have been incriminated. Low birth weight and premature parturition are significant risk factors for RFM.[31] Cattle that have RFM once may be at greater risk of the condition after subsequent parturition[31] and cows with RFM have a higher incidence of metabolic diseases, mastitis, metritis, and even subsequent abortion.[32]

Placental maturation is accompanied by structural and functional changes, some of which fail in cows with RFM. Numbers of placental binucleate cells, which secrete prostaglandin (PG) E_2, normally decline in late pregnancy but fail to do so in cows with RFM, leading to increased ratios of $PGE_2/PGF_{2\alpha}$.[33] Cows with RFM typically have lower circulating estradiol concentration in the immediate prepartum period than unaffected herdmates[34] (**Fig. 1**) and reduced aromatase (CYP19) gene

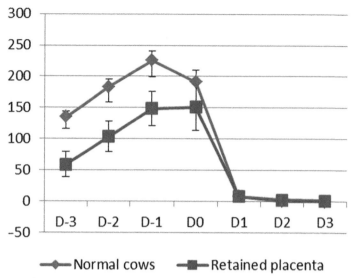

Fig. 1. Cows with RFM have lower circulating estradiol concentration (picogram per milliliter) during the prepartum period. D0, day of parturition. (*Courtesy of* S.H. Cheong, W.R. Butler and R.O. Gilbert, BVSc, MMedVet, Cornell University, Ithaca, NY.)

expression has been reported in retained membranes.[35] RFM is mediated by impaired neutrophil function beginning in late pregnancy. Reduced neutrophil migration toward tissue extracts of placentomes can be detected 2 weeks before calving in cows that go on to develop RFM.[36,37] Other neutrophil functions are also impaired. Expression of proinflammatory mediators is reduced in the prepartum period in cows with RFM.[38] Impaired neutrophil function has also been recorded in hypocalcemic cows. Indeed, many of the etiologic factors associated with RFM have also been correlated to impairment of neutrophil function, including vitamin and mineral deficiencies, heat stress, or exogenous corticosteroid administration. The poor neutrophil function in affected cows extends into the postpartum period, and probably mediates most of the complications usually associated with RFM.[39] Major histocompatibility complex compatibility of dam and calf results in increased risk of RFM.[40–43] RFM is not associated with decreased uterine muscular contraction; cows with RFM have increased frequency and amplitude of uterine contractions.[44,45]

Clinical signs of RFM are usually obvious unless the membranes are retained within the uterus or only project into the cervix or vagina and require a vaginal examination to be detected.

Cows with RFM produce less milk in the affected lactation. This is especially true for affected first lactation cows.[46] Cows with RFM are at increased risk of developing metritis, endometritis, ovarian cysts,[30] or mastitis.[47,48] Increased risk of mastitis reinforces the importance of impaired immune function in the pathogenesis of RFM. Cows with RFM tend to experience more days to first insemination, more days from first insemination to conception, and more days open than cows without RFM.[49]

Manual removal of the retained membranes provides no benefit and may do harm, particularly when future reproductive potential is used as the outcome.[50–52] Risco and colleagues,[53] however, observed that cows with RFM, dystocia, or both that were left untreated had similar reproductive outcomes to untreated cows, which had not suffered from these disorders.

Treatment of cows with RFM with gonadotropin-releasing hormone (GnRH), F2α, or oxytocin is not beneficial in terms of placental release or future reproductive performance.[53] Similarly, oral administration of calcium chloride gel had no effect of subsequent metritis, days to first insemination, or pregnancy to first insemination.[54]

Many practitioners in different parts of the world still rely on intrauterine infusion of antibiotics as a treatment of RFM, despite a lack of evidence for its efficacy. Intrauterine infusion of oxytetracycline may reduce the incidence of subsequent fever[55] but has no effect on subsequent reproductive performance.[56] Intrauterine infusion of oxytetracycline is associated with detectable milk residues in all treated cows, which can persist for 144 hours (mean, 52 hours) after the last infusion.[57] Intrauterine infusion of 1 g of ceftiofur (an extralabel use of the compound, illegal in some jurisdictions) between 14 and 20 days after RFM was not associated with significantly improved reproductive performance, but treated cows were less likely to be culled from the herd (and correspondingly more likely to calve again).[58,59] Note that antibiotic therapy, especially with tetracyclines, which has the ability to inhibit matrix metalloproteinases (zinc-dependent extracellular proteinases), may actually prolong RFM. Benign neglect, without attempts at manual removal, and systemic administration of antibiotics to cows showing fever or other signs of metritis is at least as effective as more invasive treatment (**Box 1**).[60–62]

The most effective strategy for prevention of RFM is to ensure that cows have continued access to feed during the prepartum period, to avoid regrouping and other forms of social stress during this period, and to ensure that dietary selenium and vitamin E are adequate. Nutritional strategies to prevent milk fever are likely to be beneficial in limiting incidence of RFM. Routine treatment of cows at calving with either

---

Box 1
Retained fetal membranes

Definition
- Retention of membranes for more than 24 hours

Risk factors
- Abortion, stillbirth, twins, dystocia
- Hypocalcemia
- Deficiency of betacarotene, vitamin A, vitamin E, selenium
- Infectious disease
- Induced parturition

Treatment
- Benign neglect

Consequences
- Increased risk of metritis, mastitis
- Reduced milk yield

Prevention
- Maintain dry matter intake in dry period
- Supplement vitamin E, selenium, betacarotene if necessary
- Monensin supplementation

PGF$_{2\alpha}$ or oxytocin is not effective in preventing RFM.[63] Feeding of monensin has been reported to decrease incidence of RFM in multiparous cows,[64] although this effect was not noticed in another (smaller) trial.[65] Supplementation with betacarotene may reduce incidence of RFM in multiparous cows.[66]

PUERPERAL METRITIS

Acute puerperal metritis usually occurs in the first 10 days postpartum and is characterized by an enlarged, flaccid uterus; a fetid, watery red-brown discharge; and usually fever[67,68] and other signs of systemic illness, such as depression or decreased milk yield and feed intake. Fever may follow development of other signs by 1 or 2 days[69] and is sometimes not detected.[24,69] Risk of metritis is increased by RFM, obstetric complications, and twin birth. It is more common in cows that are overconditioned or underconditioned. Feeding urea to dry cows has been implicated as a cause of postpartum uterine infection.[70] The condition is more prevalent in dairy cows than in beef animals and occurs with higher frequency in primiparous cows. The lactation incidence rate of metritis is about 15% to 20%, but may be much higher in some herds. Milk yield of affected cows is reduced.[71–74] Metritis contributes to delayed conception and increased risk of culling.[72,74] Costs of acute metritis are associated with treatment costs, increased culling, and impaired fertility. Cows with metritis are at increased risk for other postpartum complications, such as displaced abomasum, and for endometritis.

Cows that have diminished food intake during the late dry period have increased risk of puerperal metritis[75]; these cows frequently show elevated β-hydroxybutyrate or nonesterified fatty acid concentrations in peripheral blood. They have impaired immune function, partially mediated by low intracellular glycogen content of neutrophils. Circulating cortisol and estradiol concentrations tend to be increased immediately postpartum in affected cows.[71] Milk yield is depressed, particularly in affected first lactation animals.[71]

Bacteria commonly involved in puerperal metritis are *Escherichia coli*, and the gram-negative anaerobes *Prevatella melaninogenica* and *Fusobacterium necrophorum*.[76–78] Specific strains of *E coli* expressing specific virulence factors seem to be implicated; *E coli* are the earliest invaders and their presence increases the risk for subsequent invasion of the uterus by other pathogens.[79,80] Of several virulence factors expressed by metritis-causing *E coli*, the most important seems to be FimH, a pili adhesive protein enabling the bacteria to adhere to and colonize epithelial surfaces.[81] FimH adhesion is mediated by mannose, and in vitro mannose is capable of preventing adhesion to cultured uterine epithelial cells.[80] However, intrauterine administration of mannose was ineffective in preventing metritis.[82] Cows with FimH-expressing *E coli* in the uterus during the first 2 days postpartum have impaired reproductive performance[77,83] and are more likely to be infected with *F necrophorum* at 8 to 10 days postpartum.[83] *F necrophorum* expresses several virulence factors, but a leukotoxin known to be highly toxic to bovine neutrophils seems to be of most importance. Adhesion to bovine endothelial cells is mediated by virulence factor FomA.[84] *F necrophorum* is synergistic with *Trueperella pyogenes* in etiology of several conditions including abscesses, footrot, summer mastitis, and calf diphtheria[85] and this synergy also contributes to uterine disease.[77,83,86] *T pyogenes* seems to be more prominent in uterine disease later in the postpartum period (endometritis, cervicitis and purulent vaginal discharge).

Diagnosis of metritis is usually uncomplicated but affected cows should be examined thoroughly to exclude peracute mastitis, abomasal displacement, pneumonia, peritonitis, or other systemic disease. Traditionally, fever has been regarded as an essential component of acute puerperal metritis but it may not be prominent.[24]

Acute puerperal metritis usually responds favorably to systemic administration of antimicrobial drugs. If necessary, more aggressive supportive therapy, including fluid therapy, should be instituted. Many of the *E coli* involved in pathogenesis of acute puerperal metritis are antibiotic resistant, but cephalosporin antibiotics remain the best choice based on microbial sensitivity and for uterine distribution.[87] Although drainage of the fetid uterine contents is intuitively appealing, the uterus is friable and may be penetrated easily by a siphon tube at this stage. Manipulation of the uterus can result in bacteremia, and any attempt at drainage should be avoided or at least delayed until after beginning antimicrobial treatment.[67] Many antimicrobial drugs have been found to be useful in the treatment of cows with acute puerperal metritis. Several studies have found systemic administration of ceftiofur to be effective in advancing resolution of clinical signs[88,89] but not in improving fertility.[90] The same is true for systemic ampicillin treatment.[69] Given concerns over antibiotic resistance and residues, some have advocated waiting 2 days before instituting antibiotic treatment, given a self-cure rate of approximately 30%.[90] There is no evidence that other forms of treatment, such as estrogens[91] or oral calcium gels,[54] improve clinical condition or reproductive response of cows with metritis. Intrauterine administration of antibiotics has generally not been found to be beneficial; in one exception, high doses of oxytetracycline were used for a protracted period.[56] Many bacteria isolated from cows with metritis are resistant to tetracycline.[92]

Most cows recover promptly from toxic puerperal metritis with timely treatment, or sometimes, spontaneously.[93] In rare instances, fatal liver failure[94] or amyloidosis[95] may be complications of puerperal metritis. Acute puerperal metritis increases the risk of subsequent infertility.[96–98] Cows with acute puerperal metritis are at increased risk of later purulent vaginal exudate or endometritis (**Box 2**).[69]

Effective means of preventing metritis would be extremely valuable to dairy producers. Although reduced dry matter intake in the dry period is a major contributor to the pathogenesis, it is not clear how to avoid a reduction in voluntary intake, which occurs in some cows even in the absence of any social stressors, such as group changes and by eliminating competition for bunk space by feeding cows individually (Cheong SH, Butler WR, Gilbert RO, unpublished data, 2015). Although overcrowding affects feeding behavior,[99,100] there is no evidence that stocking rate affects metritis incidence.[101] Nevertheless, it seems prudent to avoid overcrowding dry cows, frequent group changes, and mixing heifers and older cows. Hygiene plays a role in metritis prevalence, and attention should be paid to hygiene in calving pens.[102] Herds using straw bedding in calving pens have lower incidence of metritis than those using other forms of bedding.[103] Recently, a multivalent vaccine has been reported to reduce risk of metritis in dairy cows[104] and is currently in clinical trials.

There is some prospect of genetic selection for reduction of metritis incidence. Some investigators have reported heritability of metritis to be 0.19 and 0.26 for primiparous and second lactation cows, respectively.[105] Others have reported more modest heritability, ranging from 0.02 to 0.07.[106–108] We have observed large differences in metritis incidence in first lactation daughters of different bulls calving in the same year in one large herd (**Table 1**). Polymorphisms in genes encoding toll-like receptors and the leptin receptor gene have been linked to metritis incidence.[109,110] Because this is currently an area of active research more concrete guidelines are likely to emerge.

Box 2
Puerperal metritis

Definition

- First 10 days postpartum
- Enlarged, atonic uterus
- Fetid, watery, red-brown discharge
- Signs of systemic disease
- Fever (inconsistent)

Risk factors

- RFM
- Obstetric complications
- Twin birth

Treatment

- Systemic ceftiofur
- Ampicillin
- Supportive therapy if required

Consequences

- Reduced milk yield
- Delayed conception
- Increased risk of endometritis
- Increased risk of culling

Prevention

- Maintain dry matter intake
- Calving pen hygiene
- Future possibilities
  - Vaccination
  - Genetic selection

Table 1
Incidence of metritis in half sib groups during 1 year in a single dairy farm

Sire	Number of Daughters	Proportion with Metritis (%)
A	138	39.1
B	213	23.5
C	191	21.5
D	296	10.1

Proportion differs significantly by sire ($P < .0001$). Note that these data have not been corrected for age, season, obstetric intervention, or other factors that may influence incidence of metritis.
(*Courtesy of* K.N. Galvão, DVM, PhD and R.O. Gilbert, BVSc, MMedVet, Cornell University, Ithaca, NY.)

PYOMETRA

Pyometra occurs as a specific postpartum condition in postpartum cows. It is characterized by the accumulation of purulent or mucopurulent exudates in the uterus in the presence of an active corpus luteum in acyclic cows. It affects about 4% of dairy cows each lactation,[111] but its incidence may be increased by routine use of GnRH in the early postpartum period.[112] In general, ovulation is delayed in cows with significant uterine pathogen load[113] but if cows do ovulate in the face of ongoing uterine contamination they risk development of pyometra, because the endometrial damage may impair endogenous release of $PGF_{2\alpha}$. Traditionally *T pyogenes* have been the most common bacteria isolated from cases of pyometra[114] but metagenomic methods demonstrate prevalence of *Fusobacterium pyogenes* in affected animals.[115] A specific form of pyometra is also seen in cows infected with *Tritrichomonas fetus*[116] and is not considered further here.

The treatment of choice for pyometra is $PGF_{2\alpha}$ or its analogues.[51,117–120] Treatment results in luteolysis, behavioral estrus, expulsion of accumulated exudate, and bacteriologic clearance of the uterus in about 90% of treated cases. Recurrence of pyometra after a single treatment occurs in 9% to 13% of cases.[117,118] First service conception rate of approximately 30% or more follows treatment, but 80% of animals may be expected to conceive within three to four inseminations.[117,119]

Estrogens, in the form of estradiol cypionate of diethylstilbestrol, have also been used for the treatment of pyometra (such use is now illegal in many countries). It should be remembered that estrogens are luteolytic in cows. The clinical response to estrogen therapy is poorer than that expected after treatment with $PGF_{2\alpha}$,[118] and posttreatment conception results are poorer. Both a higher[117] and a lower[118] incidence of cystic ovarian disease after treatment of pyometra with estrogens relative to PGs has been reported (**Box 3**). In one study,[118] nitrofurazone infusion into the uterus was combined with either estradiol or prostaglandin treatment. In both cases, the use of nitrofurazone significantly depressed posttreatment conception rates. These data provide additional evidence against intrauterine infusion as a modality of treatment of bovine uterine disorders.

ENDOMETRITIS

Endometritis (sometimes referred to as subclinical endometritis) is defined as inflammation of the endometrium. It is a local disease and is not accompanied by systemic

---

Box 3
Pyometra

Definition
- Intrauterine accumulation of pus in presence of a corpus luteum
- Usually in early postpartum period

Diagnosis
- Transrectal palpation or ultrasonography (distinguish from pregnancy)

Treatment
- $PGF_{2\alpha}$ or analogues
- May need to be repeated

Prognosis
- Usually good

signs. It typically occurs in clinically relevant form after 4 weeks postpartum. Endometritis requires endometrial cytology[39,121–123] or biopsy[124] for convincing diagnosis, but its presence can be inferred from the pH, protein, or leukocyte esterase concentration of recovered uterine lavage fluid,[125,126] or more simply the appearance or optical density[127] of this fluid. Transrectal ultrasonography is also useful for diagnosis, but with moderate sensitivity and specificity.[128] The prevalence of endometritis in the immediate prebreeding period (approximately 40–60 days postpartum) is high in dairy cows and exerts a substantial negative effect on subsequent reproductive performance,[26,122,129] reducing conception to insemination and increasing pregnancy loss between 28 and 60 days after insemination.

The major risk factor for development of endometritis seems to be periparturient negative energy balance.[26,123,130] Acute puerperal metritis in the early postpartum period increases risk of subsequent endometritis.[26,69] The major bacteria associated with endometritis are the same as those implicated in the pathogenesis of puerperal metritis: E coli, T pyogenes, and the gram-negative anaerobes P melaninogenica and F pyogenes. E coli seems to be an early invader and has largely disappeared by the time endometritis is diagnosed. T pyogenes is more often isolated contemporaneously with the diagnosis.[77,78,83]

Virtually all cows show evidence of mild uterine inflammation at 2 weeks postpartum. By 4 to 6 weeks postpartum, up to half of cows still have cytologic endometritis. Attempts to diagnose endometritis before about 4 weeks postpartum are confounded by physiologic inflammation associated with endometrial remodeling. Overall prevalence of endometritis at about 40 to 60 days postpartum is about 26%, but herd prevalence ranges widely (5% to more than 50%).[26,129]

Endometritis reduces pregnancy to first artificial insemination and overall risk of pregnancy in the affected lactation.[26,122,131] The consequences of subclinical endometritis were less severe in first lactation animals; although first service conception rate was diminished by endometritis in both age groups, overall time to pregnancy was not affected in primiparous cows with subclinical endometritis (**Box 4**).[26]

Routine diagnosis of endometritis is seldom practical for all cows in a herd. However, it may be useful to examine a cohort of cows (eg, 20 cows) by endometrial cytology to obtain insight into the prevalence of the condition on a specific farm. Then, if prevalence is high, steps are initiated to better manage transition cows to minimize periparturient negative energy balance.

Because individual cows are seldom diagnosed with endometritis, treatment is usually moot. Kasimanickam and coworkers[131] show that intrauterine infusion of a specific formulation of cefapirin (Metricure) has beneficial effects on subsequent reproductive performance of affected cows. This product is not available in the United States. Several studies have examined PG administration for treatment or prevention of endometritis, without any evidence of efficacy, either for reducing incidence or improving reproduction.[132–134]

Prevention of endometritis rests largely on management of dietary intake and periparturient energy balance. Reduction of metritis incidence reduces endometritis risk. Calving and postpartum hygiene are important.

CERVICITIS AND PURULENT VAGINAL DISCHARGE

Although visible purulent vaginal exudate may accompany more severe forms of endometritis, it has become clear that cows may have visible reproductive tract exudate but be free of endometritis. It is assumed by most investigators that primary cervicitis is the major cause of a vaginal exudate in the absence of endometrial

---

Box 4
Endometritis

Definition and diagnosis

- Demonstration of endometrial inflammation (cytology, biopsy, or indirect methods)
- Vaginal exudate may be attributable to endometritis or other reproductive tract disorders

Risk factors

- Metritis
- Negative energy balance in early postpartum period

Treatment

- Intrauterine infusion of cefapirin where permitted
- Prostaglandin not effective

Consequences

- Reduced conception per insemination
- More days open
- Increased pregnancy loss

Prevention

- Manage transition cows for minimal negative energy balance
- Hygiene in calving pens

---

inflammation. Several lines of evidence support this conclusion. In pioneering work on identifying clinical findings associated with reduced fertility, LeBlanc and colleagues[135] found that increased cervical diameter after 3 weeks postpartum was one factor (along with purulent vaginal discharge) predicting reduced likelihood of pregnancy. Indeed, identification of an enlarged cervix was recognized as a harbinger of poor fertility much earlier.[136] It now seems likely that these cows have cervical damage, sustained during parturition and independent of endometritis, although the two conditions can coexist. Dubuc and colleagues[123] found that endometritis and purulent vaginal discharge had independent and additive detrimental effects on reproduction and that they had largely separate risk factors. Endometritis was predisposed to mainly by negative energy balance, whereas cervicitis/purulent vaginal discharge was most commonly a consequence of obstetric complications, including RFM. Both conditions occur with higher frequency in cows that have suffered from acute puerperal metritis.[71] Direct evidence for the presence of cervicitis, diagnosed by cytology, has recently been presented by Deguillaume and colleagues.[137] They found that cervicitis existed independently of endometritis. Prevalence of endometritis alone in their study was 13%, cervicitis only was 11%, and 32% of cows had both conditions. Both contributed to reduced hazard of pregnancy, and cows with both conditions fared worse than those with either one. Identification of cervicitis as a common postpartum disorder does not completely clarify the question of origin of purulent exudate in the vagina. Approximately half of cows with cervicitis have purulent vaginal discharge, and vice versa.[137,138] In some cases, purulent vaginal discharge may reflect more severe endometritis. However, the source of exudate in some cases remains unresolved, and may indicate primary vaginitis in some animals (**Box 5**).

Box 5
Cervicitis/purulent vaginal discharge

Definition/diagnosis

- Demonstrable vaginal exudate (may require vaginoscopy or Metricheck examination
- Exudate may be attributable to severe endometritis, but may occur in absence of endometrial inflammation
- Primary cervicitis is the cause in at least some cases

Risk factors

- Obstetric complications
- Puerperal metritis

Treatment

- Cefapirin where permissible

Consequences

- Reduced conception
- Prolonged days open
- Increased pregnancy loss

Prevention

- Prevention of metritis
- Management of obstetric problems

Whatever the source, presence of purulent vaginal exudate is associated with reduced reproductive performance. Presence of purulent material in the vagina may be conveniently detected by use of a dedicated instrument, the Metricheck (Simcro, New Zealand). This device scoops mucus or exudate from the cranial vagina for examination. Depending only on visible exudate or palpation findings can result in missing up to 40% of cases of purulent vaginal exudate.[135]

There are few effective treatment options for purulent vaginal exudate. A formulation of cephapirin specially fabricated for intrauterine administration (Metricure) has been shown convincingly to improve reproductive performance in treated cows when administered to affected cows after 4 weeks postpartum. Metricure is not available in the United States. There is no evidence in favor of intrauterine infusions other than cephapirin, and they should be avoided. Although $PGF_{2\alpha}$ is often used for treating purulent vaginal discharge, evidence for its efficacy is equivocal,[133,138] although it may have beneficial effects on reproduction independent of endometritis/cervicitis. Despite the weak evidence in its favor, $PGF_{2\alpha}$ may be the best treatment option, especially in the United States; it avoids additional antibiotic use, is inexpensive, and has other beneficial effects on reproduction (including presynchronization for controlled breeding programs).

ANOVULATION

In the United States approximately 20% of postpartum cows fail to ovulate by the end of the postpartum voluntary waiting period (60–65 d). These cows have lower pregnancy rates than ovulatory cows, and are at higher risk of embryonic loss. Galvão and colleagues[139] reported that cows ovulating before 21 days postpartum had greater hazard of pregnancy than those ovulating for the first time between 21 and 49 days postpartum, which in turn performed better than those ovulating for the first time after 49 days postpartum. Dubuc and colleagues[140] reported that in their study population of high-producing dairy cows 28% of cows ovulated by 21 days postpartum, 56% by 35 days, 74% by 49 days, and 21 remained anovulatory by 63 days postpartum. Major risk factors for anovulation or delayed first ovulation are negative energy balance before and after parturition, inflammation indicated by the acute-phase protein haptoglobin in the first week postpartum, and the presence of cytologic endometritis. Body condition score at calving and at the onset of the breeding period and especially body condition loss over this period are predictive, as is any disease condition during the postpartum period. There is little effect of milk yield on anovulation. Low circulating concentrations of betacarotene in the prepartum period may contribute to anovulation (**Fig. 2**).[141]

Importantly, the time to first postpartum ovulation and the risk of anovulation persisting up to or beyond 60 days in milk are much more highly heritable than most reproductive traits (approximately 17%–23%), providing a potential selection tool for enhanced fertility.[142] Although endometritis and anovulation exert a detrimental effect on reproduction, these effects seem to be independent and additive (see **Fig. 2**).[143]

The first priority in management of anovulatory cows is prevention of the condition. Careful management of body condition score can help minimize the proportion of

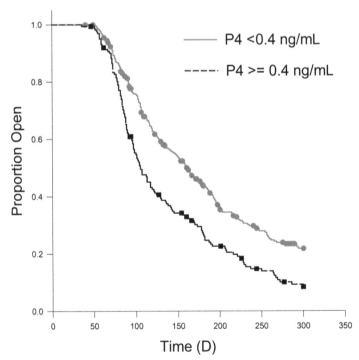

Fig. 2. Effect of progesterone concentration at 3 weeks on subsequent reproduction. Cows with increased progesterone concentration (ovulation) by 21 days postpartum had superior reproductive performance to those ovulating for the first time later in lactation. (*Courtesy of R.O. Gilbert, BVSc, MMedVet, Cornell University, Ithaca, NY.*)

cows remaining anovulatory at the end of the voluntary waiting period. Virtually all diseases of the postpartum period add to the risk of anovulation, so efforts directed at minimizing uterine and other disorders also reduce the incidence of anovulation. One advantage of programs that synchronize ovulation is that they provoke ovulation in previously anovulatory cows, allowing some measure of reproductive success. However, previously anovulatory cows achieve results inferior to those of previously cycling cows. One strategy for improving fertility in anovulatory cows is to augment ovulation synchronization protocols with progesterone (CIDR-Synch protocols). Alternatively, two consecutive OvSynch protocols (Double OvSynch) may achieve the desired result of having a corpus luteum at the onset of the breeding OvSynch program. Another problem in previously anovulatory cows is that they often do not undergo complete luteolysis in response to the second $PGF_{2\alpha}$ injection of OvSynch. In these cases, giving two $PGF_{2\alpha}$ injections ensures complete luteolysis and improves pregnancy to AI (two injections seem to give better results than a single injection of a larger dose).

CYSTIC OVARIAN FOLLICLES

Ovarian follicular cysts may be regarded as a special form of anovulation (**Box 6**). In this case follicles develop up to and beyond the normal ovulatory size (usually 15–18 mm). They may become partially luteinized. Older definitions of cystic ovarian follicles require modification. Typically, these defined cystic follicles as being greater than 25 mm in diameter. In fact, follicles become functionally cystic at the point when they fail to ovulate, which may be at a much smaller size. Older definitions also stipulated that the cystic structure needed to persist for at least 10 days. Modern investigations using serial ultrasonography indicate that cysts are dynamic, with one replacing the previous one as follicular waves emerge and grow and successive

---

Box 6
Anovulation

Definition

- Failure to ovulate and return to cyclicity by end of voluntary waiting period

Diagnosis

- Progesterone profile
- Serial examination (palpation/ultrasonography)

Risk factors

- Periparturient negative energy balance
- Body condition score (at calving, at onset of breeding, loss in early lactation)
- Endometritis
- Genetic factors

Treatment

- Incorporation of progesterone into synchronization protocols
- Ensure complete luteolysis before insemination (two injections of $PGF_{2\alpha}$)

Prevention

- Manage negative energy balance and body condition score
- Genetic selection in future

dominant follicles fail to ovulate.[144] These follicles may produce physiologic amounts of estradiol but fail to induce a preovulatory luteinizing hormone (LH) surge, despite normal pituitary LH concentrations. Pathogenesis of cystic ovaries is not fully understood, but there is evidence that once an LH surge has been generated, the hypothalamus is not able to generate a subsequent ovulatory LH surge if it is not exposed to progesterone in the interim. Evidence in support of this hypothesis comes from experiments in which preovulatory follicles were aspirated after the LH surge, but before ovulation. In some cases a functional corpus luteum formed, and these cows had normal cycles. In others, in which a corpus luteum did not form, subsequent dominant follicles grew beyond normal ovulatory size (cysts) until placement of a progesterone-releasing intravaginal device, which restored normal ovulatory function.[145] Surgical removal of the corpus hemorrhagicum has the same effect.[146] In a similar experiment, cows were given daily luteolytic doses of $PGF_{2\alpha}$ beginning at ovulation. Cows that developed normal corpora lutea had normal cycles. Those in which progesterone concentrations remained low developed ovarian follicular cysts.[147] Normal hypothalamic response to estradiol, with ability to drive an ovulatory LH surge, is restored by progesterone treatment, using a CIDR for a minimum of 3 days.[148] Spontaneous development of ovarian follicular cysts may be mediated by uterine infection or negative energy balance, which is also known to alter GnRH/LH pulsatility.[149] Cystic ovarian follicles are usually encountered in high-producing dairy cows and in early lactation (**Box 7**).

Treatment of ovarian follicular cysts depends on restoring or inducing an ovulatory surge of LH. Because cystic cows have adequate stores of pituitary LH and are responsive to GnRH, exogenous administration of GnRH usually induces ovulation or luteinization of a functional follicle (not ovulation of the cystic follicle). Treatment with progesterone (eg, by administration of a CIDR for 3 or more days[148]) may restore the hypothalamic ability to induce an ovulatory surge of LH by appropriate GnRH release. Therefore, GnRH, LH analogues (eg, human chorionic gonadotropin), or progesterone are suitable treatments for cows with ovarian follicular cysts. Because current protocols for synchronization of ovulation incorporate GnRH, they are usually effective for treating cystic follicles.

PREGNANCY LOSS

There is increasing awareness that several cows identified as pregnant at 28 or 35 days after insemination are no longer pregnant at 60 or more days after

---

Box 7
Ovarian follicular cysts

Definition
- Anovulatory follicle larger than normal ovulatory size

Risk factors
- Negative energy balance
- Uterine infection

Treatment
- GnRH
- Human chorionic gonadotropin
- Progesterone

insemination. These losses are important because they delay establishment of successful pregnancy and because cows that are mistakenly assumed still to be pregnant are no longer intensively observed or managed to be reinseminated. Summarizing 14 separate studies, Santos and colleagues[150] reported an average pregnancy loss of 12.8%, equal to 0.85% per day in the period from about 28 to 45 days after insemination (depending on the study). Pregnancy loss between 28 and 60 days after insemination can be 9% in cows that have had no other postpartum disease, and increases to 14% with a single diagnosis of disease and up to 16% with diagnosis of two or more postpartum diseases before insemination.[151] Diseases associated with pregnancy loss in dairy cows include obstetric complications, endometritis, postpartum fever, mastitis, and lameness.[151] Endometritis has a strong association with pregnancy loss; cows previously diagnosed with endometritis, but in which the condition has resolved, have increased risk of pregnancy loss compared with cows that never had endometritis. Cows in which endometritis remains unresolved at time of insemination had three-fold higher loss (over 40%).[152] In grazing cows in Florida, embryonic loss between Days 30 and 65 was significantly increased by calving problems, metritis, or purulent vaginal exudate (cows were not examined for cytologic evidence of endometritis).[153] Pregnancy losses are much higher in lactating dairy cows than in heifers or beef cows.[150] Anovular cows experience a rate of pregnancy loss almost twice that of cyclic control animals.[150] High milk yield does not seem to mediate increased embryonic loss.[150] Cows carrying twins are at increased risk of pregnancy failure (**Box 8**).[154]

Several interventions have been associated with improved embryo survival in dairy cows. These include treatment with recombinant bovine somatotropin, perhaps because bovine somatotropin accelerates embryo development.[150] Nutritional interventions are also feasible. Feeding high-starch diets in the postpartum period increases the number of cows that are cyclic at the end of the voluntary waiting period, which alone has a positive effect on pregnancy per insemination and risk of pregnancy loss. Several fatty acids have been found to have a beneficial effect on embryo quality. Cows fed diets incorporating fats after 30 days postpartum had reduced risk of pregnancy loss between 30 and 60 days after insemination.[150] It seems likely that sequential diets (high starch followed by lipid supplementation) to

---

Box 8
Pregnancy loss

Definition

- Death of embryo or early fetus after positive diagnosis of pregnancy

Risk factors

- Postpartum disease, especially endometritis
- Anovulation before breeding

Consequence

- Prolonged days open

Prevention

- Prevention of postpartum disease
- Dietary intervention to increase early ovulation and enhance embryo quality
- Positive effect of bovine somatotropin

stimulate cyclicity and then to enhance embryo quality and survival have promise for success.

REFERENCES

1. Bell AW. Regulation of organic nutrient metabolism during transition from late pregnancy to early lactation. J Anim Sci 1995;73(9):2804–19.
2. Kimura K, Goff JP, Kehrli ME Jr, et al. Effects of mastectomy on composition of peripheral blood mononuclear cell populations in periparturient dairy cows. J Dairy Sci 2002;85(6):1437–44.
3. Goff JP, Kimura K, Horst RL. Effect of mastectomy on milk fever, energy, and vitamins A, E, and beta-carotene status at parturition. J Dairy Sci 2002;85(6): 1427–36.
4. Roche JR, Friggens NC, Kay JK, et al. Invited review: body condition score and its association with dairy cow productivity, health, and welfare. J Dairy Sci 2009; 92(12):5769–801.
5. Goff JP, Horst RL. Physiological changes at parturition and their relationship to metabolic disorders. J Dairy Sci 1997;80(7):1260–8.
6. Kimura K, Goff JP, Kehrli ME Jr, et al. Phenotype analysis of peripheral blood mononuclear cells in periparturient dairy cows. J Dairy Sci 1999;82(2):315–9.
7. Nonnecke BJ, Kimura K, Goff JP, et al. Effects of the mammary gland on functional capacities of blood mononuclear leukocyte populations from periparturient cows. J Dairy Sci 2003;86(7):2359–68.
8. Ospina PA, Nydam DV, Stokol T, et al. Association between the proportion of sampled transition cows with increased nonesterified fatty acids and beta-hydroxybutyrate and disease incidence, pregnancy rate, and milk production at the herd level. J Dairy Sci 2010;93(8):3595–601.
9. Ospina PA, Nydam DV, Stokol T, et al. Associations of elevated nonesterified fatty acids and beta-hydroxybutyrate concentrations with early lactation reproductive performance and milk production in transition dairy cattle in the northeastern United States. J Dairy Sci 2010;93(4):1596–603.
10. Ospina PA, Nydam DV, Stokol T, et al. Evaluation of nonesterified fatty acids and beta-hydroxybutyrate in transition dairy cattle in the northeastern United States: critical thresholds for prediction of clinical diseases. J Dairy Sci 2010;93(2): 546–54.
11. Martinez N, Risco CA, Lima FS, et al. Evaluation of peripartal calcium status, energetic profile, and neutrophil function in dairy cows at low or high risk of developing uterine disease. J Dairy Sci 2012;95(12):7158–72.
12. Martinez N, Sinedino LD, Bisinotto RS, et al. Effect of induced subclinical hypocalcemia on physiological responses and neutrophil function in dairy cows. J Dairy Sci 2014;97(2):874–87.
13. Cebra CK, Heidel JR, Crisman RO, et al. The relationship between endogenous cortisol, blood micronutrients, and neutrophil function in postparturient Holstein cows. J Vet Intern Med 2003;17(6):902–7.
14. Shankar AH, Prasad AS. Zinc and immune function: the biological basis of altered resistance to infection. Am J Clin Nutr 1998;68(2 Suppl):447S–63S.
15. Dang AK, Prasad S, De K, et al. Effect of supplementation of vitamin E, copper and zinc on the in vitro phagocytic activity and lymphocyte proliferation index of peripartum Sahiwal (Bos indicus) cows. J Anim Physiol Anim Nutr (Berl) 2012; 97(2):315–21.

16. Spears JW, Weiss WP. Role of antioxidants and trace elements in health and immunity of transition dairy cows. Vet J 2008;176(1):70–6.
17. Bicalho ML, Lima FS, Ganda EK, et al. Effect of trace mineral supplementation on selected minerals, energy metabolites, oxidative stress, and immune parameters and its association with uterine diseases in dairy cattle. J Dairy Sci 2014; 97(7):4281–95.
18. Abuelo A, Hernandez J, Benedito JL, et al. Oxidative stress index (OSi) as a new tool to assess redox status in dairy cattle during the transition period. Animal 2013;7(8):1374–8.
19. Bell AW, Bauman DE. Adaptations of glucose metabolism during pregnancy and lactation. J Mammary Gland Biol Neoplasia 1997;2(3):265–78.
20. Wathes DC, Cheng Z, Fenwick MA, et al. Influence of energy balance on the somatotrophic axis and matrix metalloproteinase expression in the endometrium of the postpartum dairy cow. Reproduction 2011;141(2):269–81.
21. Wathes DC, Cheng Z, Chowdhury W, et al. Negative energy balance alters global gene expression and immune responses in the uterus of postpartum dairy cows. Physiol Genomics 2009;39(1):1–13.
22. Butler ST, Marr AL, Pelton SH, et al. Insulin restores GH responsiveness during lactation-induced negative energy balance in dairy cattle: effects on expression of IGF-I and GH receptor 1A. J Endocrinol 2003;176(2):205–17.
23. Butler ST, Pelton SH, Butler WR. Insulin increases 17 beta-estradiol production by the dominant follicle of the first postpartum follicle wave in dairy cows. Reproduction 2004;127(5):537–45.
24. Benzaquen ME, Risco CA, Archbald LF, et al. Rectal temperature, calving-related factors, and the incidence of puerperal metritis in postpartum dairy cows. J Dairy Sci 2007;90(6):2804–14.
25. Potter TJ, Guitian J, Fishwick J, et al. Risk factors for clinical endometritis in postpartum dairy cattle. Theriogenology 2010;74(1):127–34.
26. Cheong SH, Nydam DV, Galvão KN, et al. Cow-level and herd-level risk factors for subclinical endometritis in lactating Holstein cows. J Dairy Sci 2011;94(2): 762–70.
27. Bicalho RC, Cheong SH, Galvão KN, et al. Effect of twin birth calvings on milk production, reproductive performance, and survival of lactating cows. J Am Vet Med Assoc 2007;231(9):1390–7.
28. Bicalho RC, Galvão KN, Cheong SH, et al. Effect of stillbirths on dam survival and reproduction performance in Holstein dairy cows. J Dairy Sci 2007;90(6): 2797–803.
29. Wehrend A, Hofmann E, Bostedt H. The duration of expulsion and the separation of the afterbirth in breeding cows: a contribution to the improvement of parturition monitoring. Dtsch Tierarztl Wochenschr 2005;112(1):19–24 [in German].
30. Grohn YT, Rajala-Schultz PJ. Epidemiology of reproductive performance in dairy cows. Anim Reprod Sci 2000;60-61:605–14.
31. Joosten I, Van Eldik P, Elving L, et al. Factors related to the etiology of retained placenta in dairy cattle. Anim Reprod Sci 1987;14:251–62.
32. Gröhn YT, Erb HN, McCulloch CE, et al. Epidemiology of reproductive disorders in dairy cattle: associations among host characteristics, disease and production. Prev Vet Med 1990;8(1):25–39.
33. Slama H, Vaillancourt D, Goff AK. Control of in vitro prostaglandin F2 alpha and E2 synthesis by caruncular and allantochorionic tissues from cows that calved normally and those with retained fetal membranes. Domest Anim Endocrinol 1994;11(2):175–85.

34. Wischral A, Verreschi IT, Lima SB, et al. Pre-parturition profile of steroids and prostaglandin in cows with or without foetal membrane retention. Anim Reprod Sci 2001;67(3–4):181–8.

35. Ghai S, Monga R, Mohanty TK, et al. Term placenta shows methylation independent down regulation of Cyp19 gene in animals with retained fetal membranes. Res Vet Sci 2012;92(1):53–9.

36. Kimura K, Goff JP, Kehrli ME Jr, et al. Decreased neutrophil function as a cause of retained placenta in dairy cattle. J Dairy Sci 2002;85(3):544–50.

37. Benedictus L, Jorritsma R, Knijn HM, et al. Chemotactic activity of cotyledons for mononuclear leukocytes related to occurrence of retained placenta in dexamethasone induced parturition in cattle. Theriogenology 2011;76(5):802–9.

38. Boro P, Kumaresan A, Pathak R, et al. Alteration in peripheral blood concentration of certain pro-inflammatory cytokines in cows developing retention of fetal membranes. Anim Reprod Sci 2015;157:11–6.

39. Gilbert RO, Grohn YT, Guard CL, et al. Impaired post partum neutrophil function in cows which retain fetal membranes. Res Vet Sci 1993;55(1):15–9.

40. Joosten I, Sanders MF, Hensen EJ. Involvement of major histocompatibility complex class I compatibility between dam and calf in the aetiology of bovine retained placenta. Anim Genet 1991;22(6):455–63.

41. Joosten I, Van Eldik P, Elving L, et al. Factors affecting occurrence of retained placenta in cattle. Effect of sire on incidence. Anim Reprod Sci 1991;25:11–22.

42. Joosten I, Hensen EJ. Retained placenta: an immunological approach. Anim Reprod Sci 1992;28:451–61.

43. Davies CJ, Hill JR, Edwards JL, et al. Major histocompatibility antigen expression on the bovine placenta: its relationship to abnormal pregnancies and retained placenta. Anim Reprod Sci 2004;82-83:267–80.

44. Martin LR, Williams WF, Russek E, et al. Postpartum uterine motility measurements in dairy cows retaining their fetal membranes. Theriogenology 1981;15(5):513–24.

45. Burton MJ. Uterine motility in periparturient dairy cattle. St Paul (MN): University of Minnesota; 1986 [Dissertation/Thesis].

46. Rajala PJ, Grohn YT. Effects of dystocia, retained placenta, and metritis on milk yield in dairy cows. J Dairy Sci 1998;81(12):3172–81.

47. Schukken YH. Retained placenta and mastitis. Cornell Vet 1989;79(2):129–31.

48. Schukken YH, Erb HN, Scarlett JM. A hospital-based study of the relationship between retained placenta and mastitis in dairy cows. Cornell Vet 1989;79(4):319–26.

49. Maizon DO, Oltenacu PA, Grohn YT, et al. Effects of diseases on reproductive performance in Swedish Red and White dairy cattle. Prev Vet Med 2004;66(1–4):113–26.

50. Palmer CC. Clinical studies on retained placenta in the cow. J Am Vet Med Assoc 1932;80(1):59.

51. Paisley LG, Mickelsen WD, Anderson PB. Mechanisms and therapy for retained fetal membranes and uterine infections of cows: a review. Theriogenology 1986;25(3):353–81.

52. Bolinder A, Seguin B, Kindahl H, et al. Retained fetal membranes in cows: manual removal versus nonremoval and its effect on reproductive performance. Theriogenology 1988;30(1):45–56.

53. Risco CA, Archbald LF, Elliott J, et al. Effect of hormonal treatment on fertility in dairy cows with dystocia or retained fetal membranes at parturition. J Dairy Sci 1994;77:2562–9.

54. Hernandez J, Risco CA, Elliott JB. Effect of oral administration of a calcium chloride gel on blood mineral concentrations, parturient disorders, reproductive performance, and milk produciton of dairy cows with retained fetal membranes. J Am Vet Med Assoc 1999;215(1):72–6.

55. Stevens RD, Dinsmore RP, Cattell MB. Evaluation of the use of intrauterine infusions of oxytetracycline, subcutaneous injections of fenprostalene, or a combination of both, for the treatment of retained fetal membranes in dairy cows. J Am Vet Med Assoc 1995;15(12):1612–5.

56. Goshen T, Shpigel NY. Evaluation of intrauterine antibiotic treatment of clinical metritis and retained fetal membranes in dairy cows. Theriogenology 2006; 66(9):2210–8.

57. Dinsmore RP, Stevens RD, Cattell MB, et al. Oxytetracycline residues in milk after intrauterine treatment of cows with retained fetal membranes. J Am Vet Med Assoc 1996;209(10):1753–5.

58. Eiler H, Hopkins FM. Successful treatment of retained placenta with umbilical cord injections of collagenase in cows. J Am Vet Med Association 1993; 203(3):436–43.

59. Guerin P, Thiebault JJ, Delignette-Muller ML, et al. Effect of injecting collagenase into the uterine artery during a caesarean section on the placental separation of cows induced to calve with dexamethasone. Vet Rec 2004;154(11):326–8.

60. Drillich M, Pfutzner A, Sabin HJ, et al. Comparison of two protocols for the treatment of retained fetal membranes in dairy cattle. Theriogenology 2003;59(3–4): 951–60.

61. Drillich M, Mahlstedt M, Reichert U, et al. Strategies to improve the therapy of retained fetal membranes in dairy cows. J Dairy Sci 2006;89(2):627–35.

62. Drillich M, Reichert U, Mahlstedt M, et al. Comparison of two strategies for systemic antibiotic treatment of dairy cows with retained fetal membranes: preventive vs. selective treatment. J Dairy Sci 2006;89(5):1502–8.

63. Stevens RD, Dinsmore RP. Treatment of dairy cows at parturition with prostaglandin F2 alpha or oxytocin for prevention of retained fetal membranes. J Am Vet Med Association 1997;211(10):1280–4.

64. Melendez P, Gonzalez G, Benzaquen M, et al. The effect of monensin controlled-release capsule on the incidence of retained fetal membranes, milk yield and reproductive responses in Holstein cows. Theriogenology 2006;66: 234–41.

65. Beckett S, Lean I, Dyson R, et al. Effects of monensin on the reproduction, health, and milk production of dairy cows. J Dairy Sci 1998;81(6):1563–73.

66. Oliveira RC, Guerreiro BM, Morais Junior NN, et al. Supplementation of prepartum dairy cows with beta-carotene. J Dairy Sci 2015;98(9):6304–14.

67. Gilbert RO, Schwark WS. Pharmacologic considerations in the management of peripartum conditions in the cow. Vet Clin North Am Food Anim Pract 1992;8(1): 29–56.

68. Sheldon IM, Lewis GS, LeBlanc S, et al. Defining postpartum uterine disease in cattle. Theriogenology 2006;65(8):1516–30.

69. Lima FS, Vieira-Neto A, Vasconcellos GS, et al. Efficacy of ampicillin trihydrate or ceftiofur hydrochloride for treatment of metritis and subsequent fertility in dairy cows. J Dairy Sci 2014;97(9):5401–14.

70. Barnouin J, Chacomac JP. A nutritional risk factor for early metritis in dairy farms in France. Prev Vet Med 1992;13:27.

71. Galvão KN, Flaminio MJ, Brittin SB, et al. Association between uterine disease and indicators of neutrophil and systemic energy status in lactating Holstein cows. J Dairy Sci 2010;93(7):2926–37.
72. Giuliodori MJ, Magnasco RP, Becu-Villalobos D, et al. Metritis in dairy cows: risk factors and reproductive performance. J Dairy Sci 2013;96(6):3621–31.
73. Dubuc J, Duffield TF, Leslie KE, et al. Effects of postpartum uterine diseases on milk production and culling in dairy cows. J Dairy Sci 2011;94(3):1339–46.
74. Wittrock JM, Proudfoot KL, Weary DM, et al. Short communication: metritis affects milk production and cull rate of Holstein multiparous and primiparous dairy cows differently. J Dairy Sci 2011;94(5):2408–12.
75. Huzzey JM, Veira DM, Weary DM, et al. Prepartum behavior and dry matter intake identify dairy cows at risk for metritis. J Dairy Sci 2007;90(7):3220–33.
76. Santos TM, Gilbert RO, Bicalho RC. Metagenomic analysis of the uterine bacterial microbiota in healthy and metritic postpartum dairy cows. J Dairy Sci 2011; 94(1):291–302.
77. Machado VS, Oikonomou G, Bicalho ML, et al. Investigation of postpartum dairy cows' uterine microbial diversity using metagenomic pyrosequencing of the 16S rRNA gene. Vet Microbiol 2012;159(3–4):460–9.
78. Santos TM, Bicalho RC. Diversity and succession of bacterial communities in the uterine fluid of postpartum metritic, endometritic and healthy dairy cows. PLoS One 2012;7(12):e53048.
79. Santos NR, Galvão KN, Brittin SB, et al. The significance of uterine *E. coli* infection in the early postpartum period of dairy cows. Reprod Domest Anim 2008;43:63.
80. Sheldon IM, Rycroft AN, Dogan B, et al. Specific strains of *Escherichia coli* are pathogenic for the endometrium of cattle and cause pelvic inflammatory disease in cattle and mice. PLoS One 2010;5(2):e9192.
81. Bicalho RC, Machado VS, Bicalho ML, et al. Molecular and epidemiological characterization of bovine intrauterine *Escherichia coli*. J Dairy Sci 2010; 93(12):5818–30.
82. Machado VS, Bicalho ML, Pereira RV, et al. The effect of intrauterine administration of mannose or bacteriophage on uterine health and fertility of dairy cows with special focus on *Escherichia coli* and *Arcanobacterium pyogenes*. J Dairy Sci 2012;95(6):3100–9.
83. Bicalho ML, Machado VS, Oikonomou G, et al. Association between virulence factors of *Escherichia coli*, *Fusobacterium necrophorum*, and *Arcanobacterium pyogenes* and uterine diseases of dairy cows. Vet Microbiol 2012;157(1–2): 125–31.
84. Kumar A, Menon S, Nagaraja TG, et al. Identification of an outer membrane protein of *Fusobacterium necrophorum* subsp. necrophorum that binds with high affinity to bovine endothelial cells. Vet Microbiol 2015;176(1–2):196–201.
85. Nagaraja TG, Narayanan SK, Stewart GC, et al. *Fusobacterium necrophorum* infections in animals: pathogenesis and pathogenic mechanisms. Anaerobe 2005;11(4):239–46.
86. Dohmen MJ, Joop K, Sturk A, et al. Relationship between intra-uterine bacterial contamination, endotoxin levels and the development of endometritis in postpartum cows with dystocia or retained placenta. Theriogenology 2000;54(7): 1019–32.
87. Bicalho RC, Santos TM, Gilbert RO, et al. Susceptibility of *Escherichia coli* isolated from uteri of postpartum dairy cows to antibiotic and environmental bacteriophages. Part I: isolation and lytic activity estimation of bacteriophages. J Dairy Sci 2010;93(1):93–104.

88. Drillich M, Beetz O, Pfutzner A, et al. Evaluation of a systemic antibiotic treatment of toxic puerperal metritis in dairy cows. J Dairy Sci 2001;84(9):2010–7.

89. Zhou C, Boucher JF, Dame KJ, et al. Multilocation trial of ceftiofur for treatment of postpartum cows with fever. J Am Vet Med Assoc 2001;219(6):805–8.

90. Haimerl P, Heuwieser W. Invited review: antibiotic treatment of metritis in dairy cows: a systematic approach. J Dairy Sci 2014;97(11):6649–61.

91. Risco CA, Hernandez J. Comparison of ceftiofur hydrochloride and estradiol cypionate for metritis prevention and reproductive performance in dairy cows affected with retained fetal membranes. Theriogenology 2003;60(1):47–58.

92. Santos TM, Gilbert RO, Caixeta LS, et al. Susceptibility of *Escherichia coli* isolated from uteri of postpartum dairy cows to antibiotic and environmental bacteriophages. Part II: in vitro antimicrobial activity evaluation of a bacteriophage cocktail and several antibiotics. J Dairy Sci 2010;93(1):105–14.

93. McLaughlin CL, Stanisiewski E, Lucas MJ, et al. Evaluation of two doses of ceftiofur crystalline free acid sterile suspension for treatment of metritis in lactating dairy cows. J Dairy Sci 2012;95(8):4363–71.

94. Sweeney RW, Divers TJ, Whitlock RH, et al. Hepatic failure in dairy cattle following mastitis or metritis. J Vet Intern Med 1988;2(2):80–4.

95. Johnson R, Jamison K. Amyloidosis in six dairy cows. J Am Vet Med Assoc 1984;185(12):1538–43.

96. Moss N, Lean IJ, Reid SW, et al. Risk factors for repeat-breeder syndrome in New South Wales dairy cows. Prev Vet Med 2002;54(2):91–103.

97. Toni F, Vincenti L, Ricci A, et al. Postpartum uterine diseases and their impacts on conception and days open in dairy herds in Italy. Theriogenology 2015;84(7): 1206–14.

98. Elkjaer K, Labouriau R, Ancker ML, et al. Short communication: large-scale study on effects of metritis on reproduction in Danish Holstein cows. J Dairy Sci 2013;96(1):372–7.

99. Olofsson J. Competition for total mixed diets fed for ad libitum intake using one or four cows per feeding station. J Dairy Sci 1999;82(1):69–79.

100. Proudfoot KL, Veira DM, Weary DM, et al. Competition at the feed bunk changes the feeding, standing, and social behavior of transition dairy cows. J Dairy Sci 2009;92(7):3116–23.

101. Silva PR, Dresch AR, Machado KS, et al. Prepartum stocking density: effects on metabolic, health, reproductive, and productive responses. J Dairy Sci 2014; 97(9):5521–32.

102. Schuenemann GM, Nieto I, Bas S, et al. Dairy calving management: effect of perineal hygiene scores on metritis. J Dairy Sci 2011;94(E-Suppl 1):744.

103. Kaneene JB, Miller R. Epidemiological study of metritis in Michigan dairy cattle. Vet Res 1994;25(2–3):253–7.

104. Machado VS, Bicalho ML, Meira Junior EB, et al. Subcutaneous immunization with inactivated bacterial components and purified protein of *Escherichia coli*, *Fusobacterium Necrophorum* and *Trueperella pyogenes* prevents puerperal metritis in Holstein dairy cows. PLoS One 2014;9(3):e91734.

105. Lin HK, Oltenacu PA, Van Vleck LD, et al. Heritabilities of and genetic correlations among six health problems in Holstein cows. J Dairy Sci 1989;72(1):180–6.

106. Zwald NR, Weigel KA, Chang YM, et al. Genetic selection for health traits using producer-recorded data. II. Genetic correlations, disease probabilities, and relationships with existing traits. J Dairy Sci 2004;87(12):4295–302.

107. Zwald NR, Weigel KA, Chang YM, et al. Genetic selection for health traits using producer-recorded data. I. Incidence rates, heritability estimates, and sire breeding values. J Dairy Sci 2004;87(12):4287–94.

108. Lyons DT, Freeman AE, Kuck AL. Genetics of health traits in Holstein cattle. J Dairy Sci 1991;74(3):1092–100.

109. Oikonomou G, Angelopoulou K, Arsenos G, et al. The effects of polymorphisms in the DGAT1, leptin and growth hormone receptor gene loci on body energy, blood metabolic and reproductive traits of Holstein cows. Anim Genet 2009; 40(1):10–7.

110. Pinedo PJ, Galvao KN, Seabury CM. Innate immune gene variation and differential susceptibility to uterine diseases in Holstein cows. Theriogenology 2013; 80(4):384–90.

111. Akordor FY, Stone JB, Walton JS, et al. Reproductive performance of lactating Holstein cows fed supplemental beta-carotene. J Dairy Sci 1986;69(8):2173–8.

112. Etherington WG, Bosu WT, Martin SW, et al. Reproductive performance in dairy cows following postpartum treatment with gonadotrophin releasing hormone and/or prostaglandin: a field trial. Can J Comp Med 1984;48(3):245–50.

113. Sheldon IM, Noakes DE, Rycroft AN, et al. Influence of uterine bacterial contamination after parturition on ovarian dominant follicle selection and follicle growth and function in cattle. Reproduction 2002;123(6):837–45.

114. Ribeiro MG, Risseti RM, Bolanos CA, et al. Trueperella pyogenes multispecies infections in domestic animals: a retrospective study of 144 cases (2002 to 2012). Vet Q 2015;35(2):82–7.

115. Knudsen LR, Karstrup CC, Pedersen HG, et al. Revisiting bovine pyometra: new insights into the disease using a culture-independent deep sequencing approach. Vet Microbiol 2015;175(2–4):319–24.

116. BonDurant RH. Pathogenesis, diagnosis, and management of trichomoniasis in cattle. Vet Clin North Am Food Anim Pract 1997;13(2):345–61.

117. de Kruif A, van der Wielen NJ, Brand A, et al. Oestrogens and prostaglandins in the treatment of cattle affected with pyometra (author's transl). Tijdschr Diergeneeskd 1977;102(15):851–6 [in Dutch].

118. Fazeli M, Ball L, Olson JD. Comparison of treatment of pyometra with estradiol cypionate or cloprostenol followed by infusion or non-infusion with nitrofurazone. Theriogenology 1980;14(5):339–47.

119. Ott RS, Gustafsson BK. Use of prostaglandins for treatment of bovine pyometra and postpartum infections: a review. Compendium of Continuing Education for Practicing Veterinarians 1981;3:S184.

120. el-Tahawy Ael G, Fahmy MM. Partial budgeting assessment of the treatment of pyometra, follicular cysts and ovarian inactivity causing postpartum anoestrus in dairy cattle. Res Vet Sci 2011;90(1):44–50.

121. Gilbert RO, Shin ST, Guard CL, et al. Incidence of endometritis and effects on reproductive performance of dairy cows. Theriogenology 1998;49(1):251.

122. Gilbert RO, Shin ST, Guard CL, et al. Prevalence of endometritis and its effects on reproductive performance of dairy cows. Theriogenology 2005;64(9): 1879–88.

123. Dubuc J, Duffield TF, Leslie KE, et al. Risk factors for postpartum uterine diseases in dairy cows. J Dairy Sci 2010;93(12):5764–71.

124. Bonnett BN, Martin SW, Meek AH. Associations of clinical findings, bacteriological and histological results of endometrial biopsy with reproductive performance of postpartum dairy cows. Prev Vet Med 1993;15:205–20.

125. Cheong SH, Nydam DV, Galvao KN, et al. Use of reagent test strips for diagnosis of endometritis in dairy cows. Theriogenology 2012;77(5):858–64.
126. Denis-Robichaud J, Dubuc J. Determination of optimal diagnostic criteria for purulent vaginal discharge and cytological endometritis in dairy cows. J Dairy Sci 2015;98(10):6848–55.
127. Machado VS, Knauer WA, Bicalho ML, et al. A novel diagnostic technique to determine uterine health of Holstein cows at 35 days postpartum. J Dairy Sci 2012;95(3):1349–57.
128. Barlund CS, Carruthers TD, Waldner CL, et al. A comparison of diagnostic techniques for postpartum endometritis in dairy cattle. Theriogenology 2008;69(6): 714–23.
129. Dubuc J, Duffield TF, Leslie KE, et al. Definitions and diagnosis of postpartum endometritis in dairy cows. J Dairy Sci 2010;93(11):5225–33.
130. Hammon DS, Evjen IM, Dhiman TR, et al. Negative energy balance during the periparturient period is associated with uterine health disorders and fever in Holstein cows. J Dairy Sci 2004;87(Suppl.1):279.
131. Kasimanickam R, Duffield TF, Foster RA, et al. Endometrial cytology and ultrasonography for the detection of subclinical endometritis in postpartum dairy cows. Theriogenology 2004;62(1–2):9–23.
132. Galvão KN, Frajblat M, Brittin SB, et al. Effect of prostaglandin F-2 alpha on subclinical endometritis and fertility in dairy cows. J Dairy Sci 2009;92(10):4906–13.
133. Dubuc J, Duffield TF, Leslie KE, et al. Randomized clinical trial of antibiotic and prostaglandin treatments for uterine health and reproductive performance in dairy cows. J Dairy Sci 2011;94(3):1325–38.
134. Haimerl P, Arlt S, Heuwieser W. Evidence-based medicine: quality and comparability of clinical trials investigating the efficacy of prostaglandin F(2alpha) for the treatment of bovine endometritis. J Dairy Res 2012;79(3):287–96.
135. LeBlanc SJ, Duffield TF, Leslie KE, et al. Defining and diagnosing postpartum clinical endometritis and its impact on reproductive performance in dairy cows. J Dairy Sci 2002;85(9):2223–36.
136. Tennant B, Peddicord RG. The influence of delayed uterine involution and endometritis on bovine fertility. Cornell Vet 1968;58(2):185–92.
137. Deguillaume L, Geffre A, Desquilbet L, et al. Effect of endocervical inflammation on days to conception in dairy cows. J Dairy Sci 2012;95(4):1776–83.
138. LeBlanc SJ. Reproductive tract inflammatory disease in postpartum dairy cows. Animal 2014;8(Suppl 1):54–63.
139. Galvão K, Frajblat M, Butler W, et al. Effect of early postpartum ovulation on fertility in dairy cows. Reprod Domest Anim 2010;45:e207–11.
140. Dubuc J, Duffield TF, Leslie KE, et al. Risk factors and effects of postpartum anovulation in dairy cows. J Dairy Sci 2012;95(4):1845–54.
141. Kawashima C, Kida K, Schweigert FJ, et al. Relationship between plasma beta-carotene concentrations during the peripartum period and ovulation in the first follicular wave postpartum in dairy cows. Anim Reprod Sci 2009;111(1):105–11.
142. Bamber RL, Shook GE, Wiltbank MC, et al. Genetic parameters for anovulation and pregnancy loss in dairy cattle. J Dairy Sci 2009;92(11):5739–53.
143. Vieira-Neto A, Gilbert RO, Butler WR, et al. Individual and combined effects of anovulation and cytological endometritis on reproductive performance of dairy cows. J Dairy Sci 2014;97:1–11.
144. Cook DL, Smith CA, Parfet JR, et al. Fate and turnover rate of ovarian follicular cysts in dairy cattle. J Reprod Fertil 1990;90(1):37–46.

145. Gumen A, Sartori R, Costa FM, et al. A GnRH/LH surge without subsequent progesterone exposure can induce development of follicular cysts. J Dairy Sci 2002;85(1):43–50.
146. Gumen A, Wiltbank MC. Follicular cysts occur after a normal estradiol-induced GnRH/LH surge if the corpus hemorrhagicum is removed. Reproduction 2005; 129(6):737–45.
147. Kaneko K, Takagi N. Influence of repeated dinoprost treatment on ovarian activity in cycling dairy cows. Theriogenology 2014;81(3):454–8.
148. Gumen A, Wiltbank MC. Length of progesterone exposure needed to resolve large follicle anovular condition in dairy cows. Theriogenology 2005;63(1): 202–18.
149. Vanholder T, Opsomer G, de Kruif A. Aetiology and pathogenesis of cystic ovarian follicles in dairy cattle: a review. Reprod Nutr Dev 2006;46(2):105–19.
150. Santos JE, Thatcher WW, Chebel RC, et al. The effect of embryonic death rates in cattle on the efficacy of estrus synchronization programs. Anim Reprod Sci 2004;82-83:513–35.
151. Santos JE, Bisinotto RS, Ribeiro ES, et al. Applying nutrition and physiology to improve reproduction in dairy cattle. Soc Reprod Fertil Suppl 2010;67:387–403.
152. Lima FS, Bisinotto RS, Ribeiro ES, et al. Effects of 1 or 2 treatments with prostaglandin F(2)alpha on subclinical endometritis and fertility in lactating dairy cows inseminated by timed artificial insemination. J Dairy Sci 2013;96(10):6480–8.
153. Ribeiro ES, Lima FS, Greco LF, et al. Prevalence of periparturient diseases and effects on fertility of seasonally calving grazing dairy cows supplemented with concentrates. J Dairy Sci 2013;96(9):5682–97.
154. Lopez-Gatius F, Santolaria P, Yaniz J, et al. Factors affecting pregnancy loss from gestation Day 38 to 90 in lactating dairy cows from a single herd. Theriogenology 2002;57(4):1251–61.

Tritrichomonas foetus Prevention and Control in Cattle

Jeff D. Ondrak, DVM, MS

KEYWORDS

- Trichomoniasis • *Tritrichomonas foetus* • Venereal disease • Reproduction • Cattle

KEY POINTS

- *Tritrichomonas foetus* is an obligate parasite of the bovine reproductive tract causing a highly contagious venereal disease.
- Infection of cows with *T foetus* most often leads to pregnancy loss, but typically a return to normal fertility.
- Infection of older bulls with *T foetus* most often leads to unapparent, chronic infections and, if not detected, perpetuates the disease in the herd.
- Trichomoniasis control involves accurately identifying and removing infected bulls and managing cows appropriately.

INTRODUCTION

Bovine trichomoniasis, commonly referred to as trich, is a venereal disease of cattle caused by *Tritrichomonas foetus* that was first reported in the United States in a Pennsylvania dairy herd in 1932.[1] By the 1950s, it was reported in Western US beef herds[2] and it is now considered endemic in herds managed under range conditions with natural service breeding as found in the western United States, Florida, and worldwide. Trichomoniasis has been eliminated from many cattle populations around the world where management includes limited comingling of cattle and common use of artificial insemination for breeding.[3]

Although the management systems for cattle in areas where trichomoniasis has been eliminated differs from those used in endemic areas, it does suggest that control and potentially elimination of trichomoniasis is possible through the implementation of applicable management practices. The purpose of this article is to highlight basic information regarding trichomoniasis and suggest applications of this information in

The author has nothing to disclose.

Great Plains Veterinary Educational Center, University of Nebraska-Lincoln, P.O. Box 148, Clay Center, NE 68352, USA

E-mail address: jondrak@gpvec.unl.edu

Vet Clin Food Anim 32 (2016) 411–423

http://dx.doi.org/10.1016/j.cvfa.2016.01.010

0749-0720/16/$ – see front matter © 2016 Elsevier Inc. All rights reserved.

vetfood.theclinics.com

developing practical and effective herd-level control measures for beef cattle producers.

CLINICAL PRESENTATION
Individual Level

Bulls exhibit an absence of macroscopic and microscopic pathologic changes and a limited immunologic response to infection, which results in no visible clinical signs being exhibited by infected bulls[4] and the development of unapparent chronically infected bulls.[5] Although bulls do not demonstrate visible clinical signs of infection, the development of chronically infected bulls plays a significant role in the epidemiology of this disease and seems to be related to the age of the bull when it is exposed to T foetus.[6,7] The following studies highlight the difference in infection prevalence across age groups:

- In a survey of California beef herds, 2% of bulls 3 years of age and younger were infected with T foetus compared with 6.7% of bulls 4 years of age and older (P<.025).[8]
- An epidemiologic study in Florida found the mean age of infected bulls was 5.5 ± 1.6 years and mean age of uninfected bulls was 3.9 ± 2.3 years (P<.001).[9]
- Another study in Florida found bulls greater than 5 years of age were 2.2 (odds ratio, 2.2; 95% CI, 1.1–4.3; P = .022) times more likely to be infected than bulls 5 years of age or younger when all other factors were constant.[10]

One explanation for the relationship between age and chronically infected bulls may be the development of crypts, which are microscopic invaginations of the penile and preputial epithelium are are purported to increase in size and number as bulls age.[11–13] However, a more recent study brings into question the validity of the relationship of crypts to age-related chronic T foetus infections in bulls suggesting further work needs to be performed in this area.[14] Although older bulls seem to be more likely to become chronically infected with T foetus than young bulls, 2-year-old[15] and 3-year-old[16] bulls have been reported to be positive for T foetus.

Breed predisposition to T foetus infection has been proposed and several studies have reported T foetus infection prevalence by breed.[8–10,16,17] However, study bias in the form of uneven breed distribution across breeding groups and herds, which potentially affects risk of exposure leaves the validity of these findings in question.

Other unknown individual specific factors may also play a role in the development of chronic T foetus infections in bulls as suggested by this quote from an early trichomoniasis article, "The results indicate that there are distinct individual differences in natural resistance of bulls to infection with T foetus."[18]

T foetus can be isolated from the female bovine reproductive tract as soon as 4 days after introduction,[19] but does not seem to interfere with conception or maternal recognition of pregnancy[20] or express any macroscopic or microscopic lesions in the reproductive tract until after 50 days gestation.[21] As the infection progresses, mild inflammatory changes are noted with eventual fetal loss in a majority of the infected females up to 95 days after exposure.

Most fetal loss occurs within the first 5 months of gestation followed by a 2- to 6-month period of infertility as the immune system clears the parasite from the reproductive tract.[20] Complete clearance of T foetus from the female reproductive tract is expected in 5 to 20 weeks after infection, although some exceptions occur.[19]

Pyometras and cows with unusually long infections are the most notable exceptions to the usually limited infection. Pyometra may be one of the earliest clinical signs of

T foetus infection in the cow herd[22] and the purulent debris in the uterine lumen frequently contains abundant numbers of *T foetus*.[1] Chronically infected cows have been reported to carry infections for as long as 300 days[23] and 22 months after breeding.[24] Carrier cows have been reported to remain infected through normal pregnancy with *T foetus* being isolated up to 9 weeks[25] and 63 to 97 days[26] after delivering an apparently normal calf.

A summary of probable outcomes of *T foetus* infection in bovine females and their expected incidence rate based on expert opinion and clinical experience applied to a computer model are shown below[27]:

- Early embryonic death: 13.1% to 50.2%;
- Abortions: 3.1% to 14.1%;
- Fetal macerations: 0.6% to 2.4%;
- Pyometras: 2.1% to 8.0%;
- Pregnant carrier state: 0.2% to 0.7%; and
- Infertile, *T foetus* infection cleared: 9.4% to 35.4%.

These values are merely estimates, but serve as a reference for the level of common and less common outcomes that might be expected during a natural trichomoniasis outbreak investigation. Early embryonic death, abortion, and temporary infertility after *T foetus* infection clearance are expressed as early termination of pregnancy and an early return to estrus, which is the most common clinical sign of *T foetus* infection in the bovine female.[28]

The immune response in cows seems to result in an amnestic response to repeated *T foetus* infections, causing subsequent infections to be significantly shorter in duration.[29,30] However, this amnestic response seems to be short lived with an estimated length of partially protective immunity of less than 15 months.[31]

Herd Level

Clinical signs on a herd basis are the summation of clinical signs exhibited by individuals within the herd associated with the parasite's impact on female reproductive performance. Observant livestock owners may detect the early return to estrus as the first clinical sign of *T foetus* infection during the breeding season. Early estrus may lead to an infected cow found not pregnant at the end of the breeding season if a limited length breeding season is used. Reports from trichomoniasis affected herds indicate the percentage of nonpregnant cows at the end of the breeding season may reach as high as 45.3%[32] and 57%.[33]

If an extended breeding season is used, then early return to estrus may lead to cows found pregnant at the end of the breeding season, but bred much later in the breeding season than normally expected. In 1 report, cows exposed to *T foetus*–infected bulls experienced calving intervals of 96.5 and 98.9 days longer than nonexposed cows during the first and second year of herd infection, respectively.[31]

Although not visible, pyometra and fetal maceration can be detected through transrectal palpation of the reproductive tract by a skilled palpator and may be an early indicator of the presence of *T foetus* infection in a herd.[34,35]

MAGNITUDE OF EFFECT

Trichomoniasis exerts its most prominent impact on a cattle operation through its negative effect on the herd's reproductive performance, resulting in fewer pregnant cows and subsequently fewer calves to sell for income. Additional factors related to trichomoniasis that exert a negative influence on the profitability of a beef cattle operation include feed and other maintenance costs for nonproductive cows, replacement costs of *T foetus*–infected bulls and nonproductive females, testing costs to control *T foetus* in the herd, and reduced weaning weights owing to late born calves.

A computer spreadsheet simulation model was used to assess the impact of trichomoniais on individual cattle operations.[27] The model made the following predictions:

- A 14% to 50% reduction in calf crop;
- A 12% to 30 day longer breeding season;
- A 5% to 12% reduction in the suckling period;
- A reduction of 4% to 10% in monetary return per calf born; and
- A 5% to 35% reduction in the return per cow confined with a fertile bull.

Because production costs vary greatly between cattle operations, a single dollar value cannot be placed on overall reduction in the return per cow. However, a 5% to 35% reduction in return is significant in light of the typically small profit margins found on most cattle operations.

Another computer spreadsheet simulation model was used to evaluate the effect of trichomoniasis vaccination on reproductive efficiency in beef herds.[36] The model estimated a reduced income of up to 23% for a 300 cow herd when *T foetus* was left uncontrolled in the herd, which closely agrees the previous studies findings.

Studies have shown the prevalence of *T foetus*–infected bulls varies greatly between infected herds with prevalence ranges of 4.0% to 38.5%[8] and 1.8% to 27.0%[10] being reported, which may account for the variability of the impact of this disease on different cattle operations.

The prevalence of *T foetus*–infected bulls in different management groups within a single ranch or farm may also play a significant role in the magnitude of effect of trichomoniasis. An outbreak investigation into reproductive failure on a large Florida ranch found a *T foetus*–positive bull prevalence range of 0.9% to 35.9% across 11 distinct units of the ranch.[9] However, no direct relationship between the prevalence of infected bulls and nonpregnant cows could be determined. A more recent outbreak investigation in Nebraska found a *T foetus*–positive bull prevalence range of 0.0% to 40.0% and a positive correlation between the prevalence of infected bulls in a management group and the proportion of nonpregnant cows in that group ($r^2 = 0.97$).[37]

RISK FACTORS AND EPIDEMIOLOGY
Risk Factors

The leading risk factors for trichomoniasis have been well-defined and include use of natural service for breeding,[17] extensive range management,[17,38] no defined breeding season,[38] neighboring a *T foetus*–positive herd,[39] and commingling of cattle.[40] The common thread to these risk factors is their relationship to the transmission of *T foetus*.

Transmission of *T foetus* is considered to be strictly venereal under natural conditions and occurs during coitus between infected and uninfected cattle.[28] The rate of natural transmission is high, with up to 95% of naïve females becoming infected after a single exposure through coitus with an infected bull.[21] Uninfected bulls have also been shown to be capable transferring the organism from infected to uninfected females. However, the rate of transmission was low and required a time lapse of less than 20 minutes between coitus with the infected and noninfected cows.[41]

Although *T foetus* is considered an obligate parasite of the bovine reproductive tract, it is capable of surviving temperatures used to preserve semen for artificial insemination, which suggests that semen contaminated with this organism at the time of cryopreservation could lead to transmission of the organism through this non-venereal mode of transmission.[42]

Other less common methods of transmission have been described, including experimentally transferring the organism from infected to noninfected cows using a glass rod[19] and transfer through the use of an improperly sanitized vaginal speculum.[26] These nonvenereal means of transmission are rare in practice, but are mentioned as a reminder that care must be taken to avoid iatrogenic transfer of *T foetus* from infected to noninfected animals.

Prevalence

A variety of prevalence estimates for multiple US geographic regions have been reported in the literature. However, many prevalence estimates are based on single bull specimen culture results (vs repeated sampling) and the protocols for obtaining, maintaining, and examining these cultured specimens (if reported at all) leave the accuracy of many estimates in question.

Two studies that seem to provide reliable estimates of prevalence of *T foetus*–infected herds in specific US geographic locations were conducted at the state-wide level in California and Florida. In 1988 and 1989, investigators found 9 of 57 sampled herds (15.8%) in California with at least 1 *T foetus*–positive bull and a prevalence of *T foetus*–positive bulls of 4.1% across all bulls sampled.[8] A survey of Florida cattle operations from 1997 through 1999 found 17 of 59 (28.8%) herds with at least one infected bull and a prevalence of *T foetus*–positive bulls across all bulls tested of 6.0%.[10]

Both of these prevalence estimates were considerable higher than a study conducted in Colorado and Nebraska abattoirs which found only 0.172% of bulls *T foetus*–positive by a culture.[43] The lower prevalence in this study may represent a regional difference in *T foetus* prevalence owing to differences in herd management between regions, varying levels of regulatory trichomoniasis control programs, and fluctuations in *T foetus* prevalence related to the cyclic nature of the disease. It is important to note all of these studies relied on single bull samples which may lead to under detection of *T foetus*–positive bulls.[15]

More recently, the prevalence of *T foetus*–positive bulls in various states has been assessed and investigators found 1 of 374 (0.27%) Alabama bulls positive,[44] 2 of 1118 (0.18%) Tennessee bulls positive,[45] and between 2007 and 2010 an average herd prevalence of 2.17% in Wyoming.[46]

SAMPLE COLLECTION

Testing bulls to determine their *T foetus* status is a basic component of trichomoniasis control programs, and it seems to be straightforward process. However, there are 3 phases of any diagnostic testing process that must be completed successfully to arrive at a correct diagnosis, and the preanalytical phase (the portion of the testing process involving collection and handling of samples before performing an analysis of the specimen) is reported to account for approximately 62% of the total diagnostic errors.[47]

This supports the suggestion by other authors[48] that optimizing the diagnostic test itself is helpful, but more attention to preanalytical factors will be necessary for increasingly accurate determination the infection status of individual animals. The remainder of this section will focus on the preanalytical factors associated with *T foetus* testing.

Sexual rest of at least 1 to 2 weeks is recommended before specimen collection to allow the number of organisms to increase and therefore improve the likelihood of accurately identifying *T foetus*–positive bulls.[49] Situations may arise during the breeding season when testing is warranted but sexual rest cannot be ensured. Under these circumstances, it is critical to be aware that known *T foetus*–infected bulls have been found to be intermittently test negative when tested during the breeding season, which means that multiple tests are required to ensure an accurate diagnosis.[31]

Various specimen collection techniques have been used for bull *T foetus* testing, including artificial vagina washing,[50] preputial swabbing with a cotton swab,[51] preputial scraping with a specially designed instrument similar to the commercially available Tricamper device (Queensland Department of Primary Industries and Fisheries, Brisbane QLD),[52] preputial lavage,[51] and preputial specimen aspiration via pipette.[18]

Multiple studies have examined the differences between these techniques with equivocal results.[48,51–56] Because of the lack of evidence supporting 1 collection technique for *T foetus* recovery over another and the convenience of the pipette aspiration technique under field conditions typically encountered in the United States, pipette aspiration has become the method of choice for *T foetus* preputial specimen collection in the United States.[49]

Recently, a new preputial sample collection device, TRICHIT (Morris Livestock Products, Delavan, WI), has become available. The device is similar to a standard uterine infusion pipette with a small plastic cup attached to one end that purportedly increases the specimen collection volume while reducing blood contamination. To the author's knowledge, no studies have been published to compare the performance of the TRICHIT with other collection devices or techniques.

Regardless of the device used to collect the preputial sample, the location within the prepuce from which the sample is collected may play a role in being able to consistently identify *T foetus*–infected bulls. A study found the highest number of *T foetus* at the midshaft and caudal sections of the free portion of the penis followed by the prepuce adjacent to the free portion of the penis and then the remainder of the penile and preputial locations.[57] This result suggests that preputial sampling should involve scraping the penis as long as care is taken to avoid excessive trauma to the penis.

The appropriate specimen for *T foetus* testing has been described as "cloudy and blood tinged."[12] The presence of turbidity and blood in the specimen presumably indicates the collection process was vigorous enough to dislodge the organisms from the epithelial crypts. No substantiating data were given by the authors to support this idea and no other references were found containing documentation to confirm or dispute this suggestion. Excessive blood in the specimen should be avoided especially for samples tested by polymerase chain reaction (PCR) because blood is reported to be potentially inhibitory to the PCR.[48]

It is not uncommon for the prepuce of bulls, and especially young bulls, to be contaminated with feces or other debris, which may affect the accuracy of test results. Non–*T foetus* trichomonads, typically of fecal origin, complicate culture-based testing, but can be overcome through the use of *T foetus*–specific PCR testing.[58] A recent study found that bacteria that is not inhibited by the growth media may interfere with *T foetus* identification by culture and PCR and adversely affect the diagnostic sensitivity of these tests.[59] Because of this finding, samples with gross contamination should be discarded and a second sample collected and submitted for testing.

Specimen volume would also seem to be a consideration when assessing the quality of a preputial sample. A single study addressing this issue found an average volume of specimen collected by the pipette method to be 0.52 mL and the investigators found no relationship between specimen volume and the number of *T foetus* present in the specimen.[56]

From this information, it would seem that a quality sample collected from the preputial cavity of a bull for *T foetus* testing would be turbid, slightly blood tinged, approximately 0.5 mL or greater in volume, and free of gross contamination. Once collected and inoculated into the diagnostic laboratory recommended transport media, the sample should be protected from extremely cold or hot temperatures until delivered to the laboratory.[60–63]

TESTING STRATEGIES FOR CONTROL

The standard testing protocol for controlling trichomoniasis in an infected herd has been to subject all bulls in the herd to 3 culture-based tests at 1 week or greater intervals.[15] PCR testing seems to have greater sensitivity and specificity than culture leading to the suggestion by some that fewer sampling events may be adequate to identify all *T foetus*–positive bulls in the herd. However, studies[37,61] have shown this is not the case and 3 individual samples collected at weekly intervals from all bulls should be tested to provide a high level of confidence that all infected bulls in the herd have been identified, regardless of the test used.

TESTING STRATEGIES FOR SURVEILLANCE

Routine, systematic testing of bulls for *T foetus* can provide early detection of a disease incursion and is a key component of a trichomoniasis prevention program for herds in trichomoniasis-endemic areas, herds neighboring *T foetus*–positive herds, or herds recovering from a recent outbreak. The decision to test and what testing protocol to use should be guided by the local prevalence of trichomoniasis, the herd owner's aversion to the risk of a disease incursion, and balancing the cost and benefits of testing.

In general, surveillance testing occurs sometime between the end of 1 breeding season and the beginning of the next, and includes a single test of all bulls in the herd. The advantage of surveillance testing closely after the breeding season is early detection of infection, which allows time to develop and implement a complete trichomoniasis control program before the next breeding season. Bulls tested under this program must not be exposed to cows before the next breeding season. Alternatively, all bulls may be tested immediately before the breeding season, which has the advantage of timing the test to coincide with an annual breeding soundness examination, thereby reducing the number of times the bulls must be handled. However, this may not allow sufficient time for appropriate management of the disease before the start of the breeding season.

In multiunit operations surveillance, testing may be focused on specific management groups that have a greater risk for infection rather than testing the entire bull population[37] to decrease the cost of testing. This strategy requires well-kept herd records and a willingness to accept the risk of undetected infected bulls.

Another option to decrease the cost of surveillance testing is pooling of samples. Evidence in the literature suggests pooling of samples provides a significant cost savings without a significant reduction in the ability to detect *T foetus*–positive herds.[64,65] In this scenario, all bulls in the herd are sampled a single time and samples are placed in individual media containers for shipment, and all pooling is performed at the diagnostic laboratory.

Before any surveillance testing is undertaken, the issue of false positives should be fully explored. In populations of bulls with a very low prevalence of trichomoniasis — virgin, yearling bulls for example, occasional positive test results will unexpectedly occur[66] and owners and veterinarians should be prepared to interpret these results in a way that minimizes the impact of these false-positive tests.

STRATEGIES TO ELIMINATE FROM INFECTED HERD

The distinctive epidemiologic features of *T foetus*, specifically venereal transmission, typically transient infection in females, and a predilection for the prepuce in chronically infected older bulls, seem to offer the opportunity for rapid control and elimination of the organism from an infected herd. With this in mind and based on the information provided in the previous sections, suggested strategies to eliminate *T foetus* from an infected herd include the following:

- Sample and test all herd bulls 3 times regardless of the test used and cull all test positive bulls, or
- Cull all herd bulls to eliminate the time and money spent on testing while eliminating any risk of misclassifying a bull as *T foetus*–negative, which would allow the organism to remain in the herd. However, this option carries a financial burden that may be unacceptable to the herd owner.
- Cull all nonproductive cows (ie, cows not pregnant at the end of the breeding season or that fail to deliver a live calf before the next breeding season), or
- Establish 2 distinct female management groups based on their potential for *T foetus* infection with virgin heifers and cows delivering live calves in 1 group and nonproductive cows in the other. This option involves risk of maintaining *T foetus* in the herd through the nonproductive cows and requires fastidious management, including absolute isolation of the nonproductive cows from all other cattle and use of artificial insemination or bulls exclusive to this group.
- Consider vaccinating all females with an approved trichomoniasis vaccine, which will not prevent infection, but seems to reduce fetal loss associated with infection and the duration of infection.[67,68]
- Implement prevention strategies for high-risk herds as described in Strategies for Prevention in Uninfected Herds.

STRATEGIES FOR PREVENTION IN UNINFECTED HERDS
Low-Risk Herds

These herds are low risk for the introduction of *T foetus* based on a low local prevalence of the disease and the use of management practices that reduce the risk of the introduction of trichonomiasis into the herd. With this in mind and based on the information provided in the previous sections, suggested strategies for prevention of *T foetus* in low-risk herds include the following.

- Develop communication networks with neighbors to ensure rapid notification if trichomoniasis is diagnosed in a neighboring herd.
- Monitor fences and cattle to rapidly identify when unplanned commingling with another herd has occurred so immediate steps can be taken to address the problem and reduce the risk of introducing trichomoniasis.
- Maintain herd records to monitor herd reproductive performance and identify animals within management groups for early detection of a potential trichomoniasis incursion and efficient management of the outbreak.
- Observe interstate and intrastate animal health regulations regarding trichomoniasis and other diseases. Although regulations are in place to protect the livestock industries of each state, they should be considered a barrier to trichomoniasis introduction and not a complete prevention program at the herd level.

- Purchase replacement animals, preferably virgin bulls and heifers, from a reputable source. The purchase of nonvirgin bulls and cows, especially from herds with unknown reproductive performance, increases the risk of trichomoniasis introduction. The risk accepted when purchasing nonvirgin replacements may be greatly reduced by verifying the source herd has excellent reproductive performance, testing the bulls to ensure their negative status, and purchasing pregnant cows.

High-Risk Herds

Herds are considered high risk for the introduction of *T foetus* based on a relatively high local prevalence of the disease and the use of management practices that increase the risk of the introduction of trichomoniasis into the herd, as describe. With this in mind and based on the information provided in the previous sections, suggested strategies for prevention of *T foetus* in high risk herds include the following.

- Implement prevention strategies for low-risk herds as described in Low-risk Herds.
- Plan a pasture use program to minimize contact with neighboring cattle.
- Use proper artificial insemination protocols with semen from a reputable source in specific management groups or the entire herd to greatly reduce the risk of *T foetus* transmission.
- Maintain a young bull battery to reduce the rate of transmission and the potential development for chronic carrier bulls.
- Isolate and/or test cattle if unplanned commingling with neighboring herds has occurred. Females should be isolated from the rest of the herd until after the breeding season and their pregnancy status can be confirmed. Bulls should be isolated and tested to ensure they are *T foetus*-negative, which may require 3 tests at weekly intervals.
- Restrict the duration of the breeding season to less than 120 days to reduce the opportunity for transmission of the disease within the herd and to more easily monitor reproductive performance.
- Institute a surveillance testing program as described in Testing Strategies for Surveillance.

TRICH COLLABORATIVE, ONLINE, NOVEL, SCIENCE-BASED, USER-FRIENDLY, LEARNING, TOOL

Creating an effective herd management program for trichomoniasis that is customized to the herd and considers the many factors related to *T foetus* control can seem overwhelming especially in light of the variation between herds regarding *T foetus* status, risk of exposure, herd owner willingness to accept risk, and ability to implement appropriate management practices. To assist producers and veterinarians in this endeavor Trich CONSULT (Collaborative, Online, Novel, Science-based, User-friendly, Learning, Tool) was developed as a web-based trichomoniasis assessment tool that incorporates science-based recommendations into an interactive format that mimics a conversation with an expert.

Trich CONSULT uses a series of questions to assess the *T foetus* status and management practices of a herd and based on the responses to the questions provides feedback to allow the individual to evaluate the importance of implementing the suggested trichomoniasis control strategies. Each question also includes a link to additional information and references to aid the individual in making informed decisions. After all the questions have been answered a customized 3- to 4-page report may be generated that summarizes the questions and responses with positive reaction for good decisions and warnings for poor decisions. Trich CONSULT is currently available for use free of charge at www.trichconsult.org.

SUMMARY AND DISCUSSION

Trichomoniasis has been long recognized as a venereal disease of cattle that can have a significant impact on the reproductive performance of infected herds through pregnancy losses and decreased pounds of calf at weaning. Characteristics of this disease such as strictly venereal transmission and typically transient female infections lend itself to control. However, unapparent, chronic infections in older bulls have been an obstacle to eliminating trichomoniasis from many extensively managed cattle populations around the world. Strict adherence to trichomoniasis prevention and control strategies related to the management of nonproductive females and nonvirgin bulls is the key to effectively controlling this disease.

REFERENCES

1. Emmerson MA. Trichomoniasis in cattle. J Am Vet Med Assoc 1932;81:636–40.
2. Fitzgerald PR, Johnson AE, Thorne J, et al. Trichomoniasis in range cattle. Vet Med 1958;53:249–52.
3. Skirrow SZ, BonDurant RH. Bovine trichomoniasis. Vet Bull 1988;58:591–603.
4. Parsonson IM, Clark BL, Dufty J. The pathogenesis of Tri*trichomonas foetus* infection in the bull. Aust Vet J 1974;50:421–3.
5. Rhyan JC, Wilson KL, Wagner B, et al. Demonstration of *Tritrichomonas foetus* in the external genitalia and of specific antibodies in preputial secretions of naturally infected bulls. Vet Pathol 1999;36:406–11.
6. Christensen HR, Clark BL, Parsonson IM. Incidence of *Tritrichomonas foetus* in young replacement bulls following introduction into an infected herd. Aust Vet J 1977;53:132–4.
7. Christensen HR, Clark BL. Spread of *Tritrichomonas foetus* in beef bulls in an infected herd. Aust Vet J 1979;55:205.
8. BonDurant RH, Anderson ML, Blanchard P, et al. Prevalence of trichomoniasis among California beef herds. J Am Vet Med Assoc 1990;196:1590–3.
9. Rae DO, Chenoweth PJ, Genho PC, et al. Prevalence of Tritrichomonas fetus in a bull population and effect on production in a large cow-calf enterprise. J Am Vet Med Assoc 1999;214:1051–5.
10. Rae DO, Crews JE, Greiner EC, et al. Epidemiology of *Tritrichomonas foetus* in beef bull populations in Florida. Theriogenology 2004;61:605–18.
11. Samuelson JD, Winter AJ. Bovine vibriosis: the nature of the carrier state in the bull. J Infect Dis 1966;116:581–92.
12. Ball L, Mortimer RG, Cheney JM. Trichomoniasis: diagnosis, pathogenesis, treatment and control. In: Williams EI, editor. Proceeding of the 18th Annual Conference of the American Association of Bovine Practitioners. Des Moines (IA): 1984. p. 163–5.
13. BonDurant RH, Honiberg BM. Trichomonads of veterinary importance. In: Kreier JP, Baker JR, editors. Parasitic protozoa. 2nd edition. San Diego (CA): Academia Press; 1994. p. 111–88.
14. Strickland L, Edmondson M, Maxwell H, et al. Surface architectural anatomy of the penile and preputial epithelium of bulls. Clin Therio 2014;6:445–51.
15. Kimsey PB, Darien BJ, Kendrick JW, et al. Bovine trichomoniasis: diagnosis and control. J Am Vet Med Assoc 1980;177:616–9.

16. Skirrow SZ, BonDurant RH, Farley J, et al. Efficacy of ipronidazole against trichomoniasis in beef bulls. J Am Vet Med Assoc 1985;187:405–7.

17. Abbitt B, Meyerholz GW. *Trichomonas foetus* infection of range bulls in South Florida. Vet Med Small Anim Clin 1979;74:1339–42.

18. Hammond DM, Bartlett DE. Establishment of infection with *Trichomonas foetus* in bulls by experimental exposure. Am J Vet Res 1943;4:61–5.

19. Murname D. Field and laboratory observations on trichomoniasis of dairy cattle in Victoria. Aust Vet J 1959;35:80–3.

20. BonDurant RH. Diagnosis, treatment and control of bovine trichomoniasis. Compend Contin Educ Vet 1985;7:S179–86.

21. Parsonson IM, Clark BL, Dufty JH. Early pathogenesis and pathology of *Tritrichomonas foetus* infection in virgin heifers. J Comp Pathol 1976;86:59–66.

22. Rae DO, Crews JE. Tritrichomonas foetus. Vet Clin North Am Food Anim Pract 2006;22:595–611.

23. Mancebo OA, Russo AM, Carabajal LL, et al. Persistence of *Tritrichomonas foetus* in naturally infected cows and heifers in Argentina. Vet Parasitol 1995;59:7–11.

24. Alexander GI. An outbreak of bovine trichomoniasis in Queensland and its control. Aust Vet J 1953;29:61–6.

25. Skirrow SZ. Identification of trichomonad-carrier cows. J Am Vet Med Assoc 1987;191:553–4.

26. Goodger WJ, Skirrow SZ. Epidemiologic and economic analyses of an unusually long epizootic of trichomoniasis in a large California dairy herd. J Am Vet Med Assoc 1986;189:772–6.

27. Rae DO. Impact of trichomoniasis on the cow-calf producer's profitability. J Am Vet Med Assoc 1989;194:771–5.

28. Bartlett DE. *Trichomonas foetus* infection and bovine reproduction. J Am Vet Med Assoc 1947;8:343–52.

29. Clark BL, Dufty JH, Parsonson IM. The frequency of infertility and abortion in cows infected with *Tritrichomonas foetus* var. Brisbane. Aust Vet J 1986;63:31–2.

30. Skirrow SZ, BonDurant RH. Induced *Tritrichomonas foetus* infection in beef heifers. J Am Vet Med Assoc 1990;196:885–9.

31. Clark BL, Dufty JH, Parsonson IM. The effect of *Tritrichomonas foetus* infection on calving rates in beef cattle. Aust Vet J 1983;60:71–4.

32. Alstad AD, Krogh D, Fischer K, et al. Trichomoniasis in a beef herd. Vet Med 1984;79:708–9.

33. Barling KS, Field RW, Snowden KF, et al. Acute trichomoniasis and sub-optimal fertility in a cow/calf herd: an investigation and case management. Bov Pract 2005;39:1–5.

34. Mickelsen WD. Diagnosis of trichomoniasis: herd history and culture techniques. In: Williams EI, editor. Proceeding of the 17th Annual Conference of the American Association of Bovine Practitioners. Oklahoma City (OK): 1983. p. 134–5.

35. Mickelsen WD. The incidence of post-service pyometra in a herd of 597 beef cows infected with trichomoniasis. In: Proceedings for the Annual Conference of the Society for Theriogenology. Denver (CO): 1984. p. 245–8.

36. Villarroel A, Carpenter TE, BonDurant RH. Development of a simulation model to evaluate the effect of vaccination against *Tritrichomonas foetus* on reproductive efficiency in beef herds. J Am Vet Med Assoc 2004;65:770–5.

37. Ondrak JD, Keen JE, Rupp GP, et al. Repeated sampling and testing by culture and PCR to detect *Tritrichomonas foetus* carrier bulls in an infected Nebraska herd. J Am Vet Med Assoc 2010;237:1068–73.

38. Dennet DP, Reece RL, Barasa JO. Observations on the incidence and distribution of serotypes of *Tritrichomonas foetus* in beef cattle in North-Eastern Australia. Aust Vet J 1974;50:427–31.

39. Jin Y, Schumaker B, Logan J, et al. Risk factors associated with bovine trichomoniasis in beef cattle identified by a questionnaire. J Med Microbiol 2014;63: 896–902.

40. Mardones FO, Perez AM, Martinez A, et al. Risk factors associated with *Tritrichomonas foetus* infection in beef herds in the Province of Buenos Aires, Argentina. Vet Parasitol 2008;153:231–7.

41. Clark BL, Dufty JH, Parsonson IM. Studies on the transmission of *Tritrichomonas foetus*. Aust Vet J 1977;53:170–2.

42. Clark BL, White MB, Banfield JC. Diagnosis of *Trichomonas foetus* infection in bulls. Aust Vet J 1971;47:181–3.

43. Grotelueschen DM, Cheney J, Hudson DB, et al. Bovine trichomoniasis: results of a slaughter survey in Colorado and Nebraska. Theriogenology 1994;42:165–71.

44. Rodning SP, Wolfe DF, Carson RL, et al. Prevalence of *Tritrichomonas foetus* in several subpopulations of Alabama beef bulls. Theriogenology 2008;69:212–7.

45. Jones BM, Whitlock BK, Strickland LG, et al. Prevalence of *Tritrichomonas foetus* in Tennessee beef bulls [abstract]. Clin Therio 2015;7:333.

46. Yao C, Bardsley KD, Litzman EA, et al. *Tritrichomonas foetus* infection in beef bull populations in Wyoming. J Bacteriol Parasitol 2011;117. http://dx.doi.org/10. 4172/2155-9597.1000117.

47. Plebani M. The detection and prevention of errors in laboratory medicine. Ann Clin Biochem 2010;47:101–10.

48. Mukjufhi N, Irons PC, Michel A, et al. Evaluation of a PCR test for the diagnosis of *Tritrichomonas foetus* infection in bulls: effects of sample collection method, storage and transport medium on the test. Therio 2003;60:1269–78.

49. Peter D. Bovine venereal disease. In: Youngquist RS, editor. Current therapy in large animal theriogenology. 1st edition. Philadelphia: W.B. Saunders; 1997. p. 355–63.

50. Gregory MW, Ellis B, Redwood DW. Comparison of sampling methods for the detection of *Tritrichomonas foetus* infection in bulls. Vet Rec 1990;7:16.

51. Fitzgerald PR, Hammond DM, Miner ML, et al. Relative efficacy of various methods of obtaining preputial samples for diagnosis of trichomoniasis in bulls. Am J Vet Res 1952;13:452–7.

52. Sutka P, Katai PL. Rapid demonstration of bull trichomonadosis in unstained smear preparations from preputial scrapings. Acta Vet Hung 1969;19:385–9.

53. Tedesco LF, Errico F, Del Baglivi LP. Diagnosis of *Tritrichomonas foetus* infection in bulls using two sampling methods and a transport medium. Aust Vet J 1979;55: 322–4.

54. Parker S, Campbell J, Ribble C, et al. Comparison of two sampling tools for diagnosis of *Tritrichomonas foetus* in bulls and clinical interpretation of culture results. J Am Vet Med Assoc 1999;215:231–5.

55. Schonmann MJ, BonDurant RH, Gardner IA, et al. Comparison of sampling and culture methods for the diagnosis of *Tritrichomonas foetus* infection in bulls. Vet Rec 1994;134:620–2.

56. Hammond DM, Bishop VR, Jeffs G, et al. A quantitative study of *Trichomonas foetus* in preputial samples from infected bulls. Am J Vet Res 1950;11:308–14.

57. Hammond DM, Bartlett DE. The distribution of *Trichomonas foetus* in the preputial cavity of infected bulls. Am J Vet Res 1943;4:143–9.

58. BonDurant RH, Gajadhar A, Campero CM, et al. Preliminary characterization of a Tritrichomonas foetus-like protozoan isolated from preputial smegma of virgin bulls. Bov Pract 1999;33:124–7.

59. Clothier KA, Villanueva M, Torain A, et al. Effects of bacterial contamination of media on diagnosis of Tritrichomonas foetus by culture and real-time PCR. Vet Parasitol 2015;208:143–9.

60. Bryan LA, Campbell JR, Gajadhar AA. Effects of temperature on the survival of *Tritrichomonas foetus* in transport, Diamond's and InPouch TF media. Vet Rec 1999;144:227–32.

61. Cobo ER, Favetto PH, Lane VM, et al. Sensitivity and specificity of culture and PCR of smegma samples of bulls experimentally infected with *Tritrichomonas foetus*. Therio 2007;68:853–60.

62. Davidson JM, Ondrak JD, Anderson AA, et al. Evaluation of effects of high incubation temperatures on results of protozoal culture and real-time PCR testing for *Tritrichomonas foetus* inoculated in a commercially available self-contained culture media system. J Am Vet Med Assoc 2011;239:1589–93.

63. Clavijo A, Erol E, Sneed L, et al. The influence of temperature and simulated transport conditions of diagnostic samples on real-time polymerase chain reaction for detection of *Tritrichomonas foetus* DNA. J Vet Diagn Invest 2011;23: 982–5.

64. Kennedy JA, Pearl D, Tomky L, et al. Pooled polymerase chain reaction to detect *Tritrichomonas foetus* in beef bulls. J Vet Diagn Invest 2008;20:97–9.

65. Garcia Guerra A, Hill JE, Waldner CL, et al. Sensitivity of real-time polymerase chain reaction for Tritrichomonas fetus in direct individual and pooled preputial samples. Therio 2013;80:1097–103.

66. McKenna SLB, Dohoo IR. Using and interpreting diagnostic tests. Vet Clin North Am Food Anim Pract 2006;22:195–205.

67. Kvasnicka WG, Taylor REL, Huang JC, et al. Investigations of the incidence of bovine trichomoniasis in Nevada and of the efficacy of immunizing cattle with vaccines containing *Tritrichomonas foetus*. Therio 1989;31:963–71.

68. Hall MR, Kvasnicka WG, Hanks D, et al. Improved control of trichomoniasis with *Trichomonas foetus* vaccine. Agri Pract 1993;14:29–34.

Diagnosis and Control of Viral Diseases of Reproductive Importance

Infectious Bovine Rhinotracheitis and Bovine Viral Diarrhea

Benjamin W. Newcomer, DVM, PhD[a], Daniel Givens, DVM, PhD[b],*

KEYWORDS

- Biosecurity • Bovine herpesvirus • Bovine viral diarrhea virus • Surveillance
- Testing • Vaccination

KEY POINTS

- Both bovine viral diarrhea (BVDV) virus and bovine herpesvirus 1 can have significant negative reproductive impacts on cattle health.
- Vaccination is the primary control method for the viral pathogens in US cattle herds.
- Polyvalent, modified-live vaccines are recommended to provide optimal protection against various viral field strains.
- Of particular importance to BVDV control is the limitation of contacts of pregnant cattle with potential viral reservoirs during the critical first 125 days of gestation.

Viral infection and disease can have significant negative impacts on the reproductive efficiency of cattle herds in both the beef and the dairy industries. Consequences of infection range from abortion outbreaks that can affect a large proportion of the pregnant herd to more subtle syndromes (eg, impaired conception, early embryonic death) that may go unnoticed or undiagnosed. Diagnostic tests must be used in a way that conforms to the overall biosecurity program of the operation, and when applied correctly, should be viewed as an economic asset and not a liability. Control programs should be designed and implemented to prevent introduction and/or spread of the viral pathogens with particular attention to the periods in the

Drs B.W. Newcomer and M.D. Givens have received research funding from Boehringer Ingelheim Vetmedica, Inc and Zoetis.
[a] Department of Pathobiology, College of Veterinary Medicine, Auburn University, 127 Sugg Laboratory, Auburn, AL 36849-5516, USA; [b] Office of Academic Affairs, College of Veterinary Medicine, Auburn University, 217 Veterinary Education Center, Auburn, AL 36849-5536, USA
* Corresponding author.
E-mail address: givenmd@auburn.edu

production cycle when cattle are most susceptible to the consequences of disease. Such schemes must be implemented in harmony with the variance in management schemes and production goals of individual producers. This review focuses on (a) the potential reproductive consequences of bovine viral diarrhea (BVD) and infectious bovine rhinotracheitis (IBR); (b) surveillance schemes to assess the level of infection at the herd level and diagnostic assays for detection of infection in the individual; and (c) vaccination and biosecurity programs to prevent or mitigate the effects of infection in replacement heifers, the mature herd, and animals newly introduced to the farm.

REPRODUCTIVE CONSEQUENCES OF INFECTION WITH BOVINE VIRAL DIARRHEA VIRUS

Although capable of manifesting in any number of bodily systems, the reproductive consequences of BVD are the most costly on dairies and cow-calf operations.[1] Cattle that are infected shortly before the breeding period have reduced conception rates.[2,3] Decreased conception rates may result from impairment of fertilization or early embryonic death but may be, at least in part, mediated by alterations in ovarian function. Transient infection with bovine viral diarrhea virus (BVDV) can result in oophoritis and subsequent ovarian dysfunction,[4] resulting in impaired fertility and repeat breeder syndrome.

Viremia subsequent to infection of a naïve, pregnant animal allows the virus to readily cross the placenta of pregnant animals and infect the growing fetus; the effect on the growing fetus depends largely on the stage of gestation at which the infection occurs.[5] A naïve cow infected during the first month and a half of gestation may suffer early embryonic death, due to endometrial inflammation resulting from the viral infection or direct viral effects on the developing embryo. Infection between 3 and 5 months of gestation, while the fetus is undergoing the final stages of organogenesis, is associated with a variety of congenital defects, most commonly involving the central nervous system. Cerebellar hypoplasia is the most notable developmental defect, but other common defects include hydranencephaly, microphthalmia, hypotrichosis, and brachygnathism. If infection occurs after the completion of organogenesis and the development of fetal immunocompetence, the calf may mount a protective immune response as demonstrated by a precolostral antibody titer to BVDV. However, infection during this period can result in abortion of the pregnancy or, less commonly, the birth of weak calves.

The most important consequence of intrauterine infection is the creation of the persistently infected (PI) animal. In utero exposure to noncytopathic strains of BVDV before development of fetal immunocompetence (generally before 125 days of gestation) can result in a calf that is PI with the virus.[6] PI calves are often weak at birth, and most will die before 1 year of age. However, others may not show signs of disease but continuously shed virus and are epidemiologically important due to efficient transmission of BVDV. Superinfection of PI calves with homologous cytopathic strains of BVDV may result in mucosal disease, which is almost invariably fatal. Calves born to PI cows or heifers will consistently be PI themselves. Thus, preventing the creation of PI animals is essential to control of the virus.

Effects of infection in the bull are less noticeable than in female cows. Infectious virus is shed in the semen of transiently infected or PI bulls.[7] Although shed in lower levels, semen from transiently infected bulls, as well as from PI bulls, is capable of infecting naïve cattle, resulting in seroconversion and the potential birth of PI calves.[8,9] Less commonly, persistent testicular infection has been reported; such bulls consistently shed high amounts of live virus in the semen despite high serum antibody titers and a lack of viremia.[10,11] Although commonly overlooked, the bull should not be ignored when seeking to diagnose and control disease due to BVDV.

REPRODUCTIVE CONSEQUENCES OF INFECTION WITH BOVINE HERPESVIRUS 1

Like BVDV, bovine herpesvirus 1 (BHV-1) is capable of causing a variety of clinical reproductive syndromes. The virus is ubiquitous in cattle populations, and disease may be seen following acute infection or after viral recrudescence. Latency commonly occurs following natural infection or vaccination with attenuated strains; recrudescence is thought to occur following periods of stress. The genital forms of the disease, infectious pustular vulvovaginitis and infectious pustular balanoposthitis, were commonly seen in Europe but only rarely appreciated in the United States. Infected bulls shed live virus in the semen. Endometritis, infertility, and altered estrus cycles can be seen in cattle inseminated with infected semen.[12] Mucopurulent discharge may also be observed in cattle, and affected bulls may suffer from epididymitis.

More commonly, BHV-1 is associated with late-term abortions and infertility in North America.[13] Abortion generally occurs within a few weeks of exposure but may be delayed for up to 4 months if viral latency occurs in the placenta.[14] Recrudescence of the virus may subsequently infect the fetus, and thus, abortions may appear to be associated with vaccination if natural exposure occurred previously. Abortion is often accompanied by retained placenta, but subsequent infertility is not commonly seen. Occasionally, fetal infection results in the birth of stillborn or weak calves with increased mortality during the first week of life.

DIAGNOSIS
Herd Surveillance Testing

The presence of PI animals in the herd may often go unnoticed because such animals do not always show clinical signs and thus often serve as the viral reservoir to expose and infect susceptible herd mates. Consequently, herd surveillance testing at routine intervals is recommended to identify and cull PI animals from the herd. In the United States, herd surveillance for BHV-1 is less commonly used because the virus is often ubiquitous in cattle populations. The primary tests used for BVDV surveillance include the bulk tank milk (BTM) test on dairy operations and pooled ear-notch testing in nonlactating animals. In addition, feed trough sampling may be used to detect PI animals within a group of nonlactating animals, and sentinels can be used to detect circulation of either virus within the herd.

Bulk tank milk testing
The consistent shedding of high amounts of live virus in all bodily secretions, including milk, enables routine testing of BTM samples to readily identify herds containing lactating PI cows.[15] Testing BTM samples provides an economical, simple, and rapid way to determine the presence of PI animals in the lactating string.[16] Most commonly, somatic cells are collected from submitted BTM samples and subsequently tested by polymerase chain reaction (PCR) to detect viral RNA. Combining the testing of BTM samples by PCR and by virus isolation increases the sensitivity of detection[17] but adds expense and a delay in assay results. Although recommendations will vary between laboratories, PCR-based testing is sensitive enough to identify a single PI animal diluted 1:600 with milk from BVDV-negative animals.[17] When testing large herds, it is advised to contact the testing laboratory to determine their recommended number of cows per sample. String samples may be submitted in lieu of BTM samples when the number of total cows exceeds the recommended number of allowable cows per

sample. Specific laboratories should also be contacted for the desired specifics on sample handling and shipping. Alternatively, BTM samples may be assessed for the level of BVDV antibodies[18,19] or by using an antibody enzyme-linked immunosorbent assay (ELISA) test[20,21] for surveillance and determination of herd infection status. However, antibody-based surveillance is complicated by herd vaccination status, and results should be interpreted with caution in vaccinated herds.[22]

It is important to remember which animals are not included in the sample when testing a herd for BVDV. Obviously, only lactating animals will be tested; the status of replacement heifers, the most common class of animal brought onto dairy operations, will not be assessed until they enter the lactating herd. Bulls, dry cows, and cows in the hospital pen/string are groups commonly overlooked using BTM BVDV testing. Most cattle will be included in subsequent samples but transmission of the virus may occur before the PI animal is identified in future tests, especially in the case of introduced animals. Consequently, it is important to sample these animals by another method to assay their BVDV status, particularly in the face of an outbreak, or when the presence of a PI individual is suspected in the herd.

When a positive result on a BTM BVDV assay is encountered, additional testing is necessary to identify the source of the positive test result. The testing program that should be pursued will depend on the reason for the initial testing and the biosecurity/biocontainment goals of the dairy. At a minimum, the individual cow or cows responsible for the positive test and her offspring should be identified and removed from the herd (**Fig. 1**).

Pooled sample testing

The advent of molecular diagnostics has allowed the testing of pooled individual samples to detect the presence of PI animals within the tested group. Using PCR, pooling either blood[23,24] or ear-notch samples[25,26] provides a rapid and economical surveillance tool for BVDV. Using ear-notch samples has the benefit of being less invasive, and individual samples composing a positive pooled sample can be subsequently examined to positively identify the PI individual within the group. Pools of up to 100 samples have demonstrated high sensitivity in detecting PI animals, but the number of samples pooled may vary by laboratory depending on individual assay validation and the regional prevalence of disease. A smaller number of samples included in the pool become increasingly more cost-effective as the prevalence of disease increases because of the need for subsequent individual sample testing.[27] Pooled testing is currently the method of choice for BVDV surveillance testing in groups of nonlactating animals.

Antibody detection in sentinels

Screening sentinel animals for the presence of antibodies to BVDV has been proposed as a potential surveillance option for the detection of PI animals within the herd.[28,29] In one study involving 5 nonvaccinated calves of at least 6 months of age in 47 cattle groups, the presence of PI animals within the herd was accurately predicted if at least 2 sentinel animals had virus neutralization titers of 128 or greater.[30] However, in another study involving 27 cow-calf herds, finding a titer 1000 or greater in at least 3 of 10 sentinel calves accurately predicted the presence of a PI only 53% of the time.[31] In a surveillance program, sensitivity is valued over specificity; sensitivity of surveillance schemes involving antibody titers in sentinel animals is maximized by decreasing the threshold antibody titer or decreasing the number of calves required to have the threshold titer.[30] Precolostral antibody detection in dairy calves may be a more cost-effective surveillance tool than testing all calves for the presence of PI

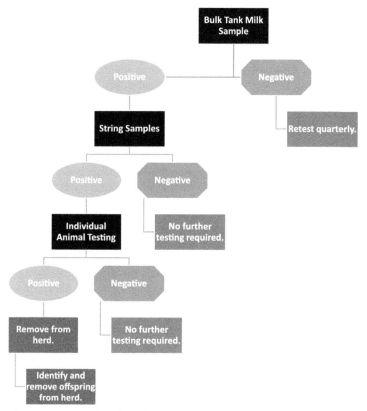

Fig. 1. Testing strategy to identify and remove animals PI with BVDV from the milking herd using BTM testing.

animals because more seropositive calves are likely to be born than PI calves in infected herds.[32] Precolostral surveillance has the added benefit of detecting circulating infections in nonlactating heifers that would be missed by BTM sampling.

Feed trough sampling

A diagnostic test using reverse transcription PCR (rtPCR) has been described for the detection of PI animals in a group of nonlactating animals that does not require individual animal handling.[33] By swabbing consumption surfaces within 6 hours after feeding and assaying the swabs by rtPCR, the investigators were able to detect the presence of PI animals in a larger group of cattle. The assay successfully differentiates between transient and persistent infection. The assay provides a potential alternative to the BTM BVDV test for use on beef cattle populations or in groups of replacement dairy heifers.

Individual Animal Testing

Mature animals

Individual animals are rarely tested for BHV-1 because the virus is nearly ubiquitous in North American cattle; exceptions are in the case of introduced animals or abortion outbreaks. Testing for BVDV in individual mature animals is most commonly performed to identify PI animals for removal from the herd, often after a clinical outbreak of BVD or following the detection of a PI animal on surveillance screening. Several tests are available, and selection of the appropriate test will be dictated by several factors, including the management system of the farm, financial constraints, and availability of tests at a given laboratory. Because not all available tests are appropriate for each clinical situation, care should be made when selecting a test in order to reach a successful solution quickly and efficiently.[34] Historically, isolation of live virus from tissues or secretions of infected animals is considered the "gold standard" diagnostic test for both BVDV and BHV-1 but is infrequently used in diagnostic laboratories due to the expense and time needed for the assay; isolation of virus from samples obtained from an animal at least 3 weeks apart is indicative of BVDV persistent infection.

Although molecular techniques have become the screening method of choice for BVDV and BHV-1, the demonstration of viral DNA does not confirm active infection. Most US cattle are latently infected with BHV-1, and disease most commonly results from viral recrudescence. The detection of BVDV antigen is preferred to confirm the PI status of individual animals. Commonly used antigen detection methods include antigen capture ELISAs (ACE) and immunohistochemistry (IHC) techniques. Additional testing may be warranted in certain circumstances due to the occurrence of false positives.[34] When pooled sampling detects a PI animal in the group, subsequent testing of the individual samples is used to positively identify the affected animal. Alternatively, several studies have demonstrated a high level of sensitivity for the commercial antigen capture ELISA kits when used as a screening test to detect PI animals.[35,36] Commercial ACE kits and IHC techniques rely on monoclonal antibodies targeting the E^{rns} glycoprotein of BVDV; consequently, the potential exists for a rare and uniquely divergent strain to escape detection by these tests.[37] Identification of mature PI cows necessitates the removal of any replacement offspring as they will also be PI.

Calves

Testing of individual calves for PI status is performed following a known or suspected exposure of the dam during pregnancy. Antigen detection assays are the most reliable methods for consistently detecting PI animals.[36] Identification of PI animals is ideally performed soon after birth to limit the potential exposure to naïve contacts. This identification is imperative in herds wherein PI calves will be in contact with other animals in early- to midgestation potentially resulting in the creation of additional PI animals such as in cow-calf herds with poorly defined calving seasons. Precolostral antibody titers to BVDV represent in utero exposure to the virus and may be useful in surveillance as described above but are less useful in identifying PI animals because such animals are immunotolerant to the virus.

Diagnosis of abortion

Diagnosis of bovine abortion can be challenging because a definitive diagnosis is obtained in only 20% to 30% of submitted cases. A recent review on ruminant abortion diagnostics is recommended for a complete discussion of the diagnostic workup.[38] When abortions due to BVDV or BHV-1 are suspected, submission of the aborted fetus and the entire placenta provide the best opportunity for establishing a diagnosis of viral infection. Both samples, but particularly the placenta, may be unavailable for submission for a variety of reasons, but it is important to communicate to the owner or herdsman the decreased opportunity for obtaining a diagnosis when either of these samples is unavailable. With the widespread use of viral vaccines in the United States, single serum samples from aborting dams are not often helpful in determining a diagnosis. An increase in titer as demonstrated in paired samples taken at least 4 weeks apart will be of greater benefit, but the results must be interpreted in light of the animal's vaccine history.

CONTROL
Vaccination

In North America, vaccination is the primary means of controlling reproductive losses due to the viral pathogens. Vaccination programs for BHV-1 and BVDV should have several goals: (1) prevention of acute disease in the vaccinate; (2) prevention of reproductive losses in the vaccinate; and in the case of BVDV, (3) prevention of the creation of PI animals. Fetal and abortive protection of vaccination against BHV-1 and BVDV is critical to the success of herd health programs, whereby eradication is not feasible or not practiced.[39] Although field protection is not complete,[40–42] challenge studies consistently demonstrate a significant decrease in fetal infection following virulent challenge for both BVDV (**Table 1**) and BHV-1 (**Table 2**) vaccines. A recent meta-analysis on the efficacy of BVDV vaccines to protect against reproductive loss found

Table 1
Primary studies to evaluate the efficacy of fetal protection of BVDV vaccination following viral challenge

Reference Number	Study Size	MLV/Inact	Interval (d)	Fetal Protection (%)
Brownlie et al,[73] 1995	18	Inact	25–90	100
Ficken et al,[74] 2006	58	MLV	370	100
Frey et al,[75] 2002	15	Inact/MLV	122	100
Givens et al,[76] 2012	29	MLV	102	100
Meyer et al,[77] 2012	22	MLV	120	100
Patel et al,[78] 2002	18	Inact	187	100
Rodning et al,[79] 2010	47	MLV	91	100
Schnackel et al,[80] 2007	65	MLV	110–150	98
Fairbanks et al,[81] 2004	55	MLV	120–132	97
Xue et al,[82] 2011	35	MLV	121	96
Ellsworth et al,[65] 2006	30	MLV	490	95
Kovacs et al,[83] 2003	35	MLV	88–146	95
Arenhart et al,[84] 2008	28	MLV	138	94
Brock & Grooms,[85] 1996	18	MLV	100–112	92
Dean et al,[86] 2003	36	MLV	121	92
Brock et al,[87] 2006	54	MLV	125–135	89
Mcclurkin et al,[88] 1975	27	Inact	30–60	89
Rodning et al,[79] 2010	28	Inact	91	89
Leyh et al,[89] 2011	50	MLV	124	85
Cortese et al,[90] 1998	18	MLV	107	83
Grooms et al,[91] 2007	29	Inact	69	79
Xue et al,[92] 2009	83	MLV	191–205	78
Ficken et al,[93] 2006	74	MLV	125–146	76
Harkness et al,[94] 1985	21	Inact	85–90	64
Brock & Cortese,[95] 2001	25	MLV	120–150	58

Study size describes the number of animals included in the study. MLV/Inact is the type of vaccine administered to experimental groups. Interval (d) is the interval in days between the administration of vaccine and the challenge of pregnant animals. Fetal protection is the percentage of vaccinates that produced calves free of infection.
Abbreviation: Inact, inactive.

Table 2
Primary studies to evaluate the efficacy of fetal protection of bovine herpesvirus 1 vaccination following viral challenge

Reference Number	Study Size	MLV/Inact	Interval	Fetal Protection (%)
Smith et al,[96] 1978	31	MLV	282–316	100
Givens et al,[76] 2012	29	MLV	102	100
Pospisil et al,[97] 1996	40	Inact	21	97
Saunders et al,[98] 1972	33	MLV	159–219	94
Cravens et al,[99] 1996	20	MLV	219	90
Zimmerman et al,[66] 2013	51	MLV	240–390	88
Zimmerman et al,[100] 2007	35	Inact	230	86
Ficken et al,[101] 2006	29	MLV	365	84

Study size describes the number of animals included in the study. MLV/Inact is the type of vaccine administered to experimental groups. Interval (d) is the interval in days between the administration of vaccine and the challenge of pregnant animals. Fetal protection is the percentage of vaccinates that produced calves free of infection.
Abbreviation: Inact, inactive.

that vaccination was associated with an overall decrease in abortions of nearly 50% and a nearly 85% decrease in fetal infection rate in vaccinates.[43] Consequently, a sound vaccination program will reduce reproductive losses but may not completely prevent all reproductive consequences of viral infection.

Selecting an appropriate vaccine type depends on the strengths and weaknesses of modified-live (MLV) or inactivated vaccines in light of the herd history and current management goals of the farm.[44] In general, MLV vaccines stimulate higher production of neutralizing antibodies and longer duration of protection than inactivated vaccines.[45,46] In addition to inducing significant antibody production, MLV vaccination also stimulates cell-mediated immunity.[47,48] Although peak immunity following vaccination with inactivated vaccines is seen only after the initial dosing schedule is complete, partial and complete protection from experimental BVDV challenge has been demonstrated at 3 and 5 days, respectively, after an initial dose of MLV vaccine.[49] Inactivated vaccines are generally safe for use in pregnant cattle with no, or unknown, vaccine history; however, several MLV vaccines have been developed for administration to pregnant cattle when label conditions are met. Even when used according to label conditions, MLV vaccines may be associated with subsequent abortions involving BHV-1 in a small number of pregnant cows (eg, 1 in 235 heifers aborted with detected BHV-1 in 1 study).[50] Because of demonstrated efficacy, the use of MLV vaccines is strongly encouraged when vaccinating nonpregnant cattle at least 30 days before breeding. Significant protection can still be achieved using inactivated vaccines: a meta-analysis of BVDV vaccines demonstrated a 34% decrease in abortion rate and a 76% reduction in fetal infection rate in vaccinated cattle compared with unvaccinated controls.[43]

The existence of multiple genotypes for both BVDV and BHV can pose a challenge to providing optimal vaccinal coverage. Both genotypes of BVDV (BVDV1 and BVDV2) are common in US cattle populations[51] and are clinically indistinguishable. Although BHV-1 has historically been the primary herpesvirus of concern in cattle, there is evidence that BHV-4[52–54] and BHV-5[55] may also cause reproductive disease in cattle populations. Although vaccination with heterologous strains provides some degree of protection against other genotypes,[56–59] immunity is generally inferior to vaccination with homologous strains or unable to prevent infection.[60–63] Currently, vaccines for BHV genotypes other than BHV-1 are not commercially available in the United States; however, polyvalent BVDV vaccines are commonplace. Inclusion of the 2 BVDV genotypes in a vaccine generally provides superior protection against the varied BVDV isolates to which cattle may be exposed. Thus, the use of vaccines containing type 1 and type 2 BVDV is recommended to help prevent disease caused by the varied strains encountered in the field.

Replacement heifers

Replacement heifers should receive their full complement of vaccinations for BVDV and BHV-1 at least 30 days before the onset of the breeding period. In a group of BVDV-challenged cattle near the time of breeding, conception rates were 78.6%, 44.4%, and 22.2% for cattle that seroconverted before, during, or after breeding, respectively.[2] When the second dose of an MLV polyvalent vaccine was given to 60 heifers seronegative to both BVDV and BHV-1 at least 10 days before synchronized natural breeding, no negative effects on reproductive performance were observed.[64] The researchers evaluated the duration of interestrus intervals, proportion of heifers responding to synchronization, serum progesterone concentrations, pregnancy rates, and pregnancies during the first 5 days of the breeding season. Consequently, vaccination of replacement heifers before the onset of breeding is both safe and effective. It is the authors' preference that replacement heifers be vaccinated using a multivalent MLV vaccine for optimal efficacy of protection.

Mature herd

Vaccination of the mature herd should be timed to match the peak of vaccinal immunity to the highest risk of reproductive loss due to viral challenge. In the cow-calf herd, revaccination is often performed annually, at least 2 weeks before the breeding season. Thus, after-vaccinal antibody titers are expected to persist through the breeding season and the crucial first 125 days of gestation. In dairy operations, cattle are typically in various stages of gestation so whole-herd vaccination schemes can be more problematic, particularly when MLV vaccines are used. Alternatively, an event-driven vaccination protocol may be desirable; cattle are vaccinated after a specific event (eg, dry-off, prebreeding) rather than a specific time of year. Most vaccines are labeled for annual revaccination, which may pose a problem for event-driven programs because the average calving interval on US dairies increases. Duration of fetal protection often extends beyond 12 months,[65,66] but adherence to all label directions is encouraged.

Biosecurity

Preventing the untimely introduction of BVDV and/or BHV-1 to naïve herds is essential to maintain herd health and limit reproductive losses in breeding female cows. Both viruses are spread through bodily secretions, including nasal exudate, genital secretions, semen, and respiratory droplets. In particular, PI animals shed high levels of infectious virus in all bodily secretions, which can be transmitted by fomites for a short period. Airborne transmission in the absence of direct contact is not a major route of transmission and occurs only over very short distances. However, it is recommended that groups more likely to contain individuals undergoing active infection (eg, young stock, introduced animals) not be housed adjacent to pregnant cattle whenever possible.

Cattle represent the major reservoir for spread of both viruses, although infection may be seen in multiple species. Cross-species transmission of BVDV has occurred in specific experimental situations,[67,68] although the risk of interspecies transmission remains largely uncharacterized. Prevention of exposure of pregnant cattle is a key factor to limiting reproductive losses from BHV-1 and BVDV.[69] Younger stock represents the cattle population most likely to be experiencing active infection with either virus; thus, limiting commingling and fence-line contact between these groups and pregnant cattle is recommended. Breeding bulls should also be protected from potential exposure because both viruses are capable of being passed in the semen following natural infection.[8,70]

Introduced animals

Introduced animals represent the greatest biosecurity risk for the introduction of infectious pathogens to a clean herd. Introduced cattle should be quarantined for a minimum of 3 weeks unless the animal has been shown to be free of active viral infection. The quarantine area should not be located adjacent to, or in contact with, areas holding pregnant cattle. Quarantining newly acquired animals is often overlooked or ignored by producers, but the risks posed to the reproductive health of the herd due to lack of quarantine should be effectively communicated.[71] Minimally, purchased animals should be tested to ensure they are not PI, preferably using an antigen detection assay as described above. It is important to note that most tests will not detect transient infections; thus, a quarantine period is still recommended even if the animal is shown not to be PI. Vaccination of introduced animals will depend on the vaccination history and gestational stage, if pregnant, of the animal. If the animal is not pregnant and has an unknown history, the authors prefer 2 doses of a multivalent, MLV administered per label instructions before introduction to the herd. If the animal is pregnant, a multivalent inactivated vaccine may be substituted.

Bred replacement heifers pose a potential double threat because the fetus may also serve as a reservoir of BVDV, even if the dam is not infected. An animal purchased in midgestation carrying a PI calf represents a significant threat for the introduction of BVDV even if the recommended quarantine period is observed for the dam. Currently, there is no practical way to determine the BVDV status of a gestating fetus; percutaneous aspiration of fetal fluids can be used to identify PI fetuses, but the procedure may be associated with increased fetal loss.[72] Consequently, testing of any newborn calves of introduced animals at the time of birth is a critical component of the biosecurity plan, particularly in cow-calf operations where the calf will likely not be weaned until dams are in midgestation of the next pregnancy,[69] creating the potential for additional PI births.

SUMMARY

Both BVDV and BHV-1 can have significant negative reproductive impacts on cattle health. Although latent BHV-1 infections are nearly universal, the potential for PI animals to silently introduce and/or spread BVDV within the herd warrants herd surveillance; molecular technologies have made such surveillance rapid and economical with minimal labor involvement. Introduced animals should also be BVDV tested. Vaccination is the primary control method for the viral pathogens in US cattle herds. Polyvalent, MLV vaccines are recommended to provide optimal protection against various viral field strains. However, the importance of biosecurity in the control of BVDV and BHV-1 cannot be overstated. Of particular importance to BVDV control is the limitation of contacts of pregnant cattle with potential viral reservoirs during the critical first 125 days of gestation. In addition, introduced animals should be quarantined and tested for persistent infection before introduction to the herd.

REFERENCES

1. Grooms DL. Reproductive consequences of infection with bovine viral diarrhea virus. Vet Clin North Am Food Anim Pract 2004;20:5–19.
2. Virakul P, Fahning ML, Joo HS, et al. Fertility of cows challenged with a cytopathic strain of bovine viral diarrhea virus during an outbreak of spontaneous infection with a noncytopathic strain. Theriogenology 1988;29:441–9.
3. McGowan MR, Kirkland PD, Richards SG, et al. Increased reproductive losses in cattle infected with bovine pestivirus around the time of insemination. Vet Rec 1993;133:39–43.
4. Grooms DL, Brock KV, Pate JL, et al. Changes in ovarian follicles following acute infection with bovine viral diarrhea virus. Theriogenology 1998;49:595–605.
5. Moennig V, Liess B. Pathogenesis of intrauterine infections with bovine viral diarrhea virus. Vet Clin North Am Food Anim Pract 1995;11:477–87.
6. McClurkin AW, Littledike ET, Cutlip RC, et al. Production of cattle immunotolerant to bovine viral diarrhea virus. Can J Comp Med 1984;48:156–61.
7. Kirkland PD, Richards SG, Rothwell JT, et al. Replication of bovine viral diarrhoea virus in the bovine reproductive tract and excretion of virus in semen during acute and chronic infections. Vet Rec 1991;128:587–90.
8. Kirkland PD, McGowan MR, Mackintosh SG, et al. Insemination of cattle with semen from a bull transiently infected with pestivirus. Vet Rec 1997;140:124–7.
9. Meyling A, Jensen AM. Transmission of bovine virus diarrhoea virus (BVDV) by artificial insemination (AI) with semen from a persistently-infected bull. Vet Microbiol 1988;17:97–105.
10. Voges H, Horner GW, Rowe S, et al. Persistent bovine pestivirus infection localized in the testes of an immuno-competent, non-viraemic bull. Vet Microbiol 1998;61:165–75.
11. Newcomer BW, Toohey-Kurth K, Zhang Y, et al. Laboratory diagnosis and transmissibility of bovine viral diarrhea virus from a bull with a persistent testicular infection. Vet Microbiol 2014;170:246–57.
12. Miller JM, van der Maaten MJ. Reproductive tract lesions in heifers after intrauterine inoculation with infectious bovine rhinotracheitis virus. Am J Vet Res 1984;45:790–4.
13. Yamini B, Mullaney TP, Patterson JS, et al. Causes of abortion in the North-Central United States: survey of 1618 cases (1983-2001). Bov Pract 2004;38:59–64.
14. Radostits OM, Gay CC, Hinchcliff KW, et al. Diseases associated with viruses and chlamydia - II. 10th edition. Edinburgh: Elsevier; 2007. p. 1306–438.
15. Radwan GS, Brock KV, Hogan JS, et al. Development of a PCR amplification assay as a screening test using bulk milk samples for identifying dairy herds infected with bovine viral diarrhea virus. Vet Microbiol 1995;44:77–91.
16. Hill FI, Reichel MP, Tisdall DJ. Use of molecular and milk production information for the cost-effective diagnosis of bovine viral diarrhoea infection in New Zealand dairy cattle. Vet Microbiol 2010;142:87–9.
17. Renshaw RW, Ray R, Dubovi EJ. Comparison of virus isolation and reverse transcription polymerase chain reaction assay for detection of bovine viral diarrhea virus in bulk milk tank samples. J Vet Diagn Invest 2000;12:184–6.
18. Niskanen R. Relationship between the levels of antibodies to bovine viral diarrhoea virus in bulk tank milk and the prevalence of cows exposed to the virus. Vet Rec 1993;133:341–4.

19. Graham DA, German A, McLaren IE, et al. Testing of bulk tank milk from Northern Ireland dairy herds for viral RNA and antibody to bovine viral diarrhoea virus. Vet Rec 2001;149:261–5.

20. Thobokwe G, Heuer C, Hayes DP. Validation of a bulk tank milk antibody ELISA to detect dairy herds likely infected with bovine viral diarrhoea virus in New Zealand. N Z Vet J 2004;52:394–400.

21. Beaudeau F, Assie S, Seegers H, et al. Assessing the within-herd prevalence of cows antibody-positive to bovine viral diarrhoea virus with a blocking ELISA on bulk tank milk. Vet Rec 2001;149:236–40.

22. Gonzalez AM, Arnaiz I, Eiras C, et al. Monitoring the bulk milk antibody response to bovine viral diarrhea in dairy herds vaccinated with inactivated vaccines. J Dairy Sci 2014;97:3684–8.

23. Munoz-Zanzi CA, Johnson WO, Thurmond MC, et al. Pooled-sample testing as a herd-screening tool for detection of bovine viral diarrhea virus persistently infected cattle. J Vet Diagn Invest 2000;12:195–203.

24. Larson RL, Miller RB, Kleiboeker SB, et al. Economic costs associated with two testing strategies for screening feeder calves for persistent infection with bovine viral diarrhea virus. J Am Vet Med Assoc 2005;226:249–54.

25. Kennedy JA. Diagnostic efficacy of a reverse transcriptase-polymerase chain reaction assay to screen cattle for persistent bovine viral diarrhea virus infection. J Am Vet Med Assoc 2006;229:1472–4.

26. Kennedy JA, Mortimer RG, Powers B. Reverse transcription-polymerase chain reaction on pooled samples to detect bovine viral diarrhea virus by using fresh ear-notch-sample supernatants. J Vet Diagn Invest 2006;18:89–93.

27. Yan L, Zhang S, Pace L, et al. Combination of reverse transcription real-time polymerase chain reaction and antigen capture enzyme-linked immunosorbent assay for the detection of animals persistently infected with Bovine viral diarrhea virus. J Vet Diagn Invest 2011;23:16–25.

28. Houe H, Baker JC, Maes RK, et al. Application of antibody titers against bovine viral diarrhea virus (BVDV) as a measure to detect herds with cattle persistently infected with BVDV. J Vet Diagn Invest 1995;7:327–32.

29. Pillars RB, Grooms DL. Serologic evaluation of five unvaccinated heifers to detect herds that have cattle persistently infected with bovine viral diarrhea virus. Am J Vet Res 2002;63:499–505.

30. Corbett EM, Grooms DL, Bolin SR, et al. Use of sentinel serology in a Bovine viral diarrhea virus eradication program. J Vet Diagn Invest 2011;23:511–5.

31. Waldner CL, Campbell JR. Use of serologic evaluation for antibodies against bovine viral diarrhea virus for detection of persistently infected calves in beef herds. Am J Vet Res 2005;66:825–34.

32. Schefers J, Munoz-Zanzi C, Collins JE, et al. Serological evaluation of precolostral serum samples to detect Bovine viral diarrhea virus infections in large commercial dairy herds. J Vet Diagn Invest 2008;20:625–8.

33. Givens MD, Marley MSD, Riddell KP, et al. A novel approach to bovine viral diarrhea virus surveillance. Proceedings of the 46th Annual Conference of the AABP. Wisconsin, September 19-21, 2013. p. 150.

34. Saliki JT, Dubovi EJ. Laboratory diagnosis of bovine viral diarrhea virus infections. Vet Clin North Am Food Anim Pract 2004;20:69–83.

35. Kuhne S, Schroeder C, Holmquist G, et al. Detection of bovine viral diarrhoea virus infected cattle–testing tissue samples derived from ear tagging using an Erns capture ELISA. J Vet Med B Infect Dis Vet Public Health 2005;52:272–7.

36. Edmondson MA, Givens MD, Walz PH, et al. Comparison of tests for detection of bovine viral diarrhea virus in diagnostic samples. J Vet Diagn Invest 2007;19: 376–81.

37. Gripshover EM, Givens MD, Ridpath JF, et al. Variation in E(rns) viral glycoprotein associated with failure of immunohistochemistry and commercial antigen capture ELISA to detect a field strain of bovine viral diarrhea virus. Vet Microbiol 2007;125:11–21.

38. Holler LD. Ruminant abortion diagnostics. Vet Clin North Am Food Anim Pract 2012;28:407–18.

39. Ridpath J. Preventive strategy for BVDV infection in North America. Jpn J Vet Res 2012;60(Suppl):S41–9.

40. Bolin SR, Lim A, Grotelueschen DM, et al. Genetic characterization of bovine viral diarrhea viruses isolated from persistently infected calves born to dams vaccinated against bovine viral diarrhea virus before breeding. Am J Vet Res 2009;70:86–91.

41. Blanchard PC, Ridpath JF, Walker JB, et al. An outbreak of late-term abortions, premature births, and congenital deformities associated with a bovine viral diarrhea virus 1 subtype b that induces thrombocytopenia. J Vet Diagn Invest 2010; 22:128–31.

42. O'Toole D, Miller MM, Cavender JL, et al. Pathology in practice: abortion in the heifers of this report was a result of BoHV-1 infection. J Am Vet Med Assoc 2012; 241:189–91.

43. Newcomer BW, Walz PH, Givens MD, et al. Efficacy of bovine viral diarrhea virus vaccination to prevent reproductive disease: a meta-analysis. Theriogenology 2015;83:360–5.

44. Kelling CL. Evolution of bovine viral diarrhea virus vaccines. Vet Clin North Am Food Anim Pract 2004;20:115–29.

45. Cortese VS, Whittaker R, Ellis J, et al. Specificity and duration of neutralizing antibodies induced in healthy cattle after administration of a modified-live virus vaccine against bovine viral diarrhea. Am J Vet Res 1998;59:848–50.

46. Ridpath JE, Neill JD, Endsley J, et al. Effect of passive immunity on the development of a protective immune response against bovine viral diarrhea virus in calves. Am J Vet Res 2003;64:65–9.

47. Platt R, Widel PW, Kesl LD, et al. Comparison of humoral and cellular immune responses to a pentavalent modified live virus vaccine in three age groups of calves with maternal antibodies, before and after BVDV type 2 challenge. Vaccine 2009;27:4508–19.

48. Woolums AR, Berghaus RD, Berghaus LJ, et al. Effect of calf age and administration route of initial multivalent modified-live virus vaccine on humoral and cell-mediated immune responses following subsequent administration of a booster vaccination at weaning in beef calves. Am J Vet Res 2013;74:343–54.

49. Brock KV, Widel P, Walz P, et al. Onset of protection from experimental infection with type 2 bovine viral diarrhea virus following vaccination with a modified-live vaccine. Vet Ther 2007;8:88–96.

50. Ellsworth MA, Brown MJ, Fergen BJ, et al. Safety of a modified-live combination vaccine against respiratory and reproductive diseases in pregnant cows. Vet Ther 2003;4:120–7.

51. Fulton RW, Whitley EM, Johnson BJ, et al. Prevalence of bovine viral diarrhea virus (BVDV) in persistently infected cattle and BVDV subtypes in affected cattle in beef herds in south central United States. Can J Vet Res 2009;73:283–91.

52. Czaplicki G, Thiry E. An association exists between bovine herpesvirus-4 sero-positivity and abortion in cows. Prev Vet Med 1998;33:235–40.
53. Deim Z, Szeredi L, Egyed L. Detection of bovine herpesvirus 4 DNA in aborted bovine fetuses. Can J Vet Res 2007;71:226–9.
54. Chastant-Maillard S. Impact of bovine herpesvirus 4 (BoHV-4) on reproduction. Transbound Emerg Dis 2015;62:245–51.
55. Kirkland PD, Poynting AJ, Gu X, et al. Infertility and venereal disease in cattle inseminated with semen containing bovine herpesvirus type 5. Vet Rec 2009; 165:111–3.
56. Fulton RW, Step DL, Ridpath JF, et al. Response of calves persistently infected with noncytopathic bovine viral diarrhea virus (BVDV) subtype 1b after vaccina-tion with heterologous BVDV strains in modified live virus vaccines and Man-nheimia haemolytica bacterin-toxoid. Vaccine 2003;21:2980–5.
57. Xue W, Mattick D, Smith L, et al. Vaccination with a modified-live bovine viral diarrhea virus (BVDV) type 1a vaccine completely protected calves against challenge with BVDV type 1b strains. Vaccine 2010;29:70–6.
58. Palomares RA, Givens MD, Wright JC, et al. Evaluation of the onset of protection induced by a modified-live virus vaccine in calves challenge inoculated with type 1b bovine viral diarrhea virus. Am J Vet Res 2012;73:567–74.
59. Del Medico Zajac MP, Puntel M, Zamorano PI, et al. BHV-1 vaccine induces cross-protection against BHV-5 disease in cattle. Res Vet Sci 2006;81:327–34.
60. van Oirschot JT, Bruschke CJ, van Rijn PA. Vaccination of cattle against bovine viral diarrhoea. Vet Microbiol 1999;64:169–83.
61. Van Campen H, Vorpahl P, Huzurbazar S, et al. A case report: evidence for type 2 bovine viral diarrhea virus (BVDV)-associated disease in beef herds vacci-nated with a modified-live type 1 BVDV vaccine. J Vet Diagn Invest 2000;12: 263–5.
62. Fulton RW, Ridpath JF, Confer AW, et al. Bovine viral diarrhoea virus antigenic diversity: impact on disease and vaccination programmes. Biologicals 2003; 31:89–95.
63. Spilki FR, Silva AD, Hubner S, et al. Partial protection induced by a BHV-1 re-combinant vaccine against challenge with BHV-5. Ann N Y Acad Sci 2004; 1026:247–50.
64. Walz PH, Edmondson MA, Riddell KP, et al. Effect of vaccination with a multiva-lent modified-live viral vaccine on reproductive performance in synchronized beef heifers. Theriogenology 2015;83:822–31.
65. Ellsworth MA, Fairbanks KK, Behan S, et al. Fetal protection following exposure to calves persistently infected with bovine viral diarrhea virus type 2 sixteen months after primary vaccination of the dams. Vet Ther 2006;7:295–304.
66. Zimmerman AD, Klein AL, Buterbaugh RE, et al. Protection against bovine herpesvirus type 1 (BHV-1) abortion following challenge 8 months or approxi-mately 1 year after vaccination. Bov Pract 2013;47:124–32.
67. Passler T, Walz PH, Ditchkoff SS, et al. Cohabitation of pregnant white-tailed deer and cattle persistently infected with bovine viral diarrhea virus results in persistently infected fawns. Vet Microbiol 2009;134:362–7.
68. Negron ME, Pogranichniy RM, Van AW, et al. Evaluation of horizontal transmis-sion of bovine viral diarrhea virus type 1a from experimentally infected white-tailed deer fawns (Odocoileus virginianus) to colostrum-deprived calves. Am J Vet Res 2012;73:257–62.
69. Smith DR, Grotelueschen DM. Biosecurity and biocontainment of bovine viral diarrhea virus. Vet Clin North Am Food Anim Pract 2004;20:131–49.

70. Rocha MA, Barbosa EF, Guimaraes SE, et al. A high sensitivity-nested PCR assay for BHV-1 detection in semen of naturally infected bulls. Vet Microbiol 1998;63:1–11.

71. Sanderson MW, Dargatz DA, Garry FB. Biosecurity practices of beef cow-calf producers. J Am Vet Med Assoc 2000;217:185–9.

72. Callan RJ, Schnackel JA, Van CH, et al. Percutaneous collection of fetal fluids for detection of bovine viral diarrhea virus infection in cattle. J Am Vet Med Assoc 2002;220:1348–52.

73. Brownlie J, Clarke MC, Hooper LB, et al. Protection of the bovine fetus from bovine viral diarrhoea virus by means of a new inactivated vaccine. Vet Rec 1995;137:58–62.

74. Ficken MD, Ellsworth MA, Tucker CM. Evaluation of the efficacy of a modified-live combination vaccine against bovine viral diarrhea virus types 1 and 2 challenge exposures in a one-year duration-of-immunity fetal protection study. Vet Ther 2006;7:283–94.

75. Frey HR, Eicken K, Grummer B, et al. Foetal protection against bovine virus diarrhoea virus after two-step vaccination. J Vet Med B Infect Dis Vet Public Health 2002;49:489–93.

76. Givens MD, Marley MS, Jones CA, et al. Protective effects against abortion and fetal infection following exposure to bovine viral diarrhea virus and bovine herpesvirus 1 during pregnancy in beef heifers that received two doses of a multivalent modified-live virus vaccine prior to breeding. J Am Vet Med Assoc 2012;241:484–95.

77. Meyer G, Deplanche M, Roux D, et al. Fetal protection against bovine viral diarrhoea type 1 virus infection after one administration of a live-attenuated vaccine. Vet J 2012;192:242–5.

78. Patel JR, Shilleto RW, Williams J, et al. Prevention of transplacental infection of bovine foetus by bovine viral diarrhoea virus through vaccination. Arch Virol 2002;147:2453–63.

79. Rodning SP, Marley MS, Zhang Y, et al. Comparison of three commercial vaccines for preventing persistent infection with bovine viral diarrhea virus. Theriogenology 2010;73:1154–63.

80. Schnackel JA, van Campen H, van Olphen A. Modified-live bovine viral diarrhea virus (BVDV) type 1a vaccine provides protection against fetal infection after challenge with either type 1b or type 2 BVDV. Bov Pract 2007;41:1–8.

81. Fairbanks KK, Rinehart CL, Ohnesorge WC, et al. Evaluation of fetal protection against experimental infection with type 1 and type 2 bovine viral diarrhea virus after vaccination of the dam with a bivalent modified-live virus vaccine. J Am Vet Med Assoc 2004;225:1898–904.

82. Xue W, Mattick D, Smith L. Protection from persistent infection with a bovine viral diarrhea virus (BVDV) type 1b strain by a modified-live vaccine containing BVDV types 1a and 2, infectious bovine rhinotracheitis virus, parainfluenza 3 virus and bovine respiratory syncytial virus. Vaccine 2011;29:4657–62.

83. Kovacs F, Magyar T, Rinehart C, et al. The live attenuated bovine viral diarrhea virus components of a multi-valent vaccine confer protection against fetal infection. Vet Microbiol 2003;96:117–31.

84. Arenhart S, da Silva LF, Henzel A, et al. Fetal protection against bovine viral diarrhea virus (BVDV) in pregnant cows previously immunized with an experimental attenuated vaccine. Pesquisa Veterinaria Brasileira 2008;28:461–70.

85. Brock KV, Grooms DL. Evaluation of a modiied-live bovine viral diarrhoea virus vaccine by fetal challenge. Proceedings of the Third ESVV Symposium on Pestivirus Infections. Lelystad, September 19-20, 1996. p. 177–9.

86. Dean HJ, Hunsaker BD, Bailey OD, et al. Prevention of persistent infection in calves by vaccination of dams with noncytopathic type-1 modified-live bovine viral diarrhea virus prior to breeding. Am J Vet Res 2003;64:530–7.

87. Brock KV, McCarty K, Chase CC, et al. Protection against fetal infection with either bovine viral diarrhea virus type 1 or type 2 using a noncytopathic type 1 modified-live virus vaccine. Vet Ther 2006;7:27–34.

88. Mcclurkin AW, Coria MF, Smith RL. Evaluation of acetylethyleneimine-killed bovine viral diarrhea-mucosal disease virus (BVD) vaccine for prevention of BVD infection of the fetus. Proc Annu Meet U S Anim Health Assoc 1975;(79): 114–23.

89. Leyh RD, Fulton RW, Stegner JE, et al. Fetal protection in heifers vaccinated with a modified-live virus vaccine containing bovine viral diarrhea virus subtypes 1a and 2a and exposed during gestation to cattle persistently infected with bovine viral diarrhea virus subtype 1b. Am J Vet Res 2011;72:367–75.

90. Cortese VS, Grooms DL, Ellis J, et al. Protection of pregnant cattle and their fetuses against infection with bovine viral diarrhea virus type 1 by use of a modified-live virus vaccine. Am J Vet Res 1998;59:1409–13.

91. Grooms DL, Bolin SR, Coe PH, et al. Fetal protection against continual exposure to bovine viral diarrhea virus following administration of a vaccine containing an inactivated bovine viral diarrhea virus fraction to cattle. Am J Vet Res 2007;68: 1417–22.

92. Xue W, Mattick D, Smith L, et al. Fetal protection against bovine viral diarrhea virus types 1 and 2 after the use of a modified-live virus vaccine. Can J Vet Res 2009;73:292–7.

93. Ficken MD, Ellsworth MA, Tucker CM, et al. Effects of modified-live bovine viral diarrhea virus vaccines containing either type 1 or types 1 and 2 BVDV on heifers and their offspring after challenge with noncytopathic type 2 BVDV during gestation. J Am Vet Med Assoc 2006;228:1559–64.

94. Harkness JW, Roeder PL, Drew T, et al. The efficacy of an experimental inactivated BVD-MD vaccine. Proceedings of the CEC seminar on research on animal husbandry. Ireland, October 30-31, 1985. p. 233–50.

95. Brock KV, Cortese VS. Experimental fetal challenge using type II bovine viral diarrhea virus in cattle vaccinated with modified-live virus vaccine. Vet Ther 2001;2:354–60.

96. Smith MW, Miller RB, Svoboda I, et al. Efficacy of an intranasal infectious bovine rhinotracheitis vaccine for the prevention of abortion in cattle. Can Vet J 1978; 19:63–71.

97. Pospisil Z, Krejci J, Machatkova M, et al. The efficacy of an inactivated IBR vaccine in the prevention of intra-uterine infection and its use in a disease-control programme. Zentralbl Veterinarmed B 1996;43:15–21.

98. Saunders JR, Olson SM, Radostits OM. Efficacy of an intramuscular infectious bovine rhinotraceitis vaccine against abortion due to the virus. Can Vet J 1972;13:273–8.

99. Cravens RL, Ellsworth MA, Sorensen CD, et al. Efficacy of a temperature-sensitive modified-live bovine herpesvirus type-1 vaccine against abortion and stillbirth in pregnant heifers. J Am Vet Med Assoc 1996;208:2031–4.

100. Zimmerman AD, Buterbaugh RE, Herbert JM, et al. Efficacy of bovine herpesvirus-1 inactivated vaccine against abortion and stillbirth in pregnant heifers. J Am Vet Med Assoc 2007;231:1386–9.
101. Ficken MD, Ellsworth MA, Tucker CM. Evaluation of the efficacy of a modified-live combination vaccine against abortion caused by virulent bovine herpesvirus type 1 in a one-year duration-of-immunity study. Vet Ther 2006;7:275–82.

Diagnosis and Control of Bovine Neosporosis

Milton M. McAllister, DVM, PhD

KEYWORDS

- Neospora caninum • Abortion • Transmission • Prevention • Parasite • Review

KEY POINTS

- Neosporosis is one of the most widespread and frequent causes of bovine abortion.
- The two major methods of parasite transmission to cattle are ingestion of oocysts shed by infected canids and transplacental transmission from infected dams.
- Effective vaccines have not yet been developed.
- Good management practices can help control neosporosis in herds, but complete eradication is usually impractical.
- The long-term key to avoid or reduce high infection prevalence, is to protect Total Mixed Rations and drinking water from contamination by canine feces.

PUTTING NEOSPOROSIS IN PERSPECTIVE

A recent analysis estimated that neosporosis costs the US dairy industry $546 million and the beef industry $111 million per year.[1]

Worldwide, neosporosis ranks among the most widespread and difficult-to-control causes of bovine abortion. For comparison, consider 4 other common infectious causes of abortion. Bovine *Brucellosis* has been eradicated from most wealthy nations; elsewhere, it may be possible to eliminate it from closed herds, and in other cases, abortion may be prevented or at least partially controlled by vaccination. Bovine *Pestivirus* (BVD virus) infection can be eliminated from closed herds and has even been eradicated from a few European countries, and vaccines are available in most countries. Bovine *Herpesvirus*-1 (IBR virus) has been eradicated from some European countries, and elsewhere, abortion can be prevented by vaccination. *Leptospirosis* control is challenging because there are many different serovars that may be transmitted by various wild or domestic animals; nevertheless, vaccines are available to provide short-term protection against the most important serovars, and antibiotic treatment can clear carrier cattle or entire herds from infection with bovine-adapted serovars.[2]

The author has nothing to disclose.
School of Animal & Veterinary Sciences, University of Adelaide, Roseworthy, South Australia 5371, Australia
E-mail address: milton.mcallister@adelaide.edu.au

In contrast, neosporosis occurs in all countries; no vaccine is currently available, and latent infections cannot be cleared by antimicrobials. Maintaining a closed herd cannot guarantee freedom from infection because the causative parasite may be transmitted in feedstuffs or water, and the parasite naturally cycles within wildlife.[3]

Critically, brucellosis and leptospirosis are zoonotic, whereas neosporosis is not. Furthermore, neosporosis is seldom if ever a cause of regional or international trade restrictions, unlike brucellosis, bovine pestivirus, and bovine herpesvirus. The economic importance of neosporosis lies simply within its effect on the reproductive performance of breeding cows.

CLINICAL MANIFESTATIONS OF BOVINE NEOSPOROSIS

Most infections in cattle are subclinical, but there are frequent exceptions. Abortion is the only major problem, which is generally not associated with other signs of illness in dams. Abortions may occur between 4 months of gestation and birth, but most occur in months 5 through 7. Neosporosis is not a significant cause of infertility or early embryonic resorption. Retained fetal membranes and metritis may be secondary complications that follow abortion.[4,5]

In addition to abortion, bovine neosporosis is associated with stillbirths or with the occasional birth of premature or neurologically impaired calves.[6–8] Clinically affected calves may have normal size or be notably small, and signs range from being neurologically moribund to having partial spinal deficits (**Fig. 1**) with poor conscious proprioception of the rear limbs and inadequate balance.

In dairy cattle, one of the costs associated with abortion (from any cause, not just from neosporosis) is reduced milk production. Reduced milk production is expected to occur because of interference with the timing and length of the lactation and dry periods, body conditioning, and udder health.

UNCLEAR ASSOCIATIONS WITH MILK PRODUCTION AND GROWTH RATES

When abortion has not occurred, there are contradictory studies regarding a possible effect of *Neospora* serologic status (ie, the presence of a detectable antibody titer) on milk production. However, the largest studies, involving thousands of dairy cattle and hundreds of herds, indicate that *Neospora* serologic status does not directly reduce milk production. A study in Ontario[9] concluded that loss of milk production was associated with abortion rather than with simply being seropositive, and a study in the

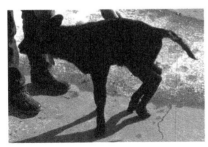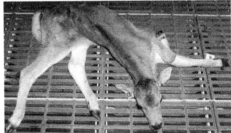

Fig. 1. Neurologic impairment in calves infected with *Neospora caninum*. The beef calf at left was born following a neosporosis abortion outbreak. It was undersized, had weak hindlimbs, and a conscious proprioceptive deficit that is here demonstrated by the dorsal placement of the left rear hoof. The dairy calf at right was unable to stand, maintain sternal recumbency, or elevate its head.

Netherlands[10] concluded that subclinical or endemic neosporosis is not associated with reduced milk production.

About 15 years ago, a research group in the United States reported that in comparison with uninfected herd mates, *Neospora*-seropositive steers had mildly decreased growth rates and feed efficiency, and increased average time spent in sick pens.[11,12] However, later studies in Canada and Argentina did not find these problems,[13–15] and there has been no further published evidence to support an effect on meat production.

THE CAUSATIVE PARASITE

Comparison with the familiar life cycle of a butterfly, which passes through egg, caterpillar, and chrysalis stages before emerging as a sexually competent adult, can help make the life stages of protozoa a bit easier to comprehend. Several microscopic forms of *Neospora caninum* reside inside of cells of infected animal hosts (**Fig. 2**). The parasite reproduces sexually within the intestinal tract of canid definitive hosts and is then shed in feces as environmentally hardy oocysts (pronounced Ō ō sists).

Intermediate hosts of *N caninum* are prey animals that become infected either by ingestion of oocysts that contaminate dust and water following decomposition of

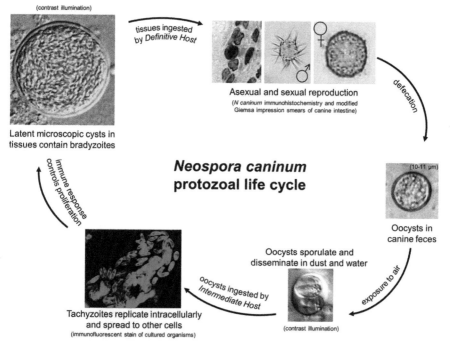

Fig. 2. *Neospora caninum* life stages. (*upper left*) Photomicrograph of a squash preparation showing a spherical, thick-walled cyst containing numerous bradyzoites; this latent stage survives in tissues for prolonged periods. (*upper right*) Asexual and sexual reproductive forms of the parasite that occur in canine intestine after ingestion of infected tissues. (*right*) Egg-like oocyst, shed in canine feces. (*bottom right*) Sporocysts containing sporozoites have developed within an oocyst, which is now infectious. (*bottom left*) Upon ingestion of infectious oocysts by an intermediate host animal, sporozoites are liberated by digestive juices, invade host cells, and become rapidly dividing tachyzoites; if unchecked by the immune response, tachyzoites may cause clinical disease. Otherwise, they convert to latent bradyzoites and the cycle is completed.

infected canine feces or by transplacental transmission from the mother. Regardless of the method of infection, there is an initial period of rapid asexual replication of *tachyzoites* within host cells, and then the host cells die as the tachyzoites rupture out and spread to infect new cells.

If clinical disease occurs, it is caused by tachyzoites. However, in most cases, tachyzoites fall under the control of the animal's immune response and then convert into relatively dormant *bradyzoites*, which reside within microscopic intracellular cysts. These cysts often endure for the life of the intermediate host. When an infected animal is preyed upon by a definitive host canid, then ingested bradyzoites become activated by gastric digestion, infect the canine intestinal tract, and the cycle is renewed.

RELATED ORGANISMS

Although there are several closely related parasites including *Toxoplasma gondii*, only *Neospora hughesi* shares *N caninum*'s genus name. *N hughesi* has been found in horses, in which it may cause spinal infections and ataxia, but much less is known about it. In this article, all further references to "*Neospora*" or "neosporosis" will be used to indicate the parasite *N caninum* and associated disease conditions, without further consideration of *Neospora hughesi* or other related parasites.

TRANSMISSION CYCLES IN CATTLE

There are at least 3 methods of transmission of *Neospora* infection to cattle (**Fig. 3**):

1. Cattle may become infected at any time by ingestion of oocysts. This occurrence may be referred to as horizontal transmission. Upon infection, there will be a period of tachyzoite proliferation, an antibody titer will develop, and then the organisms will convert into bradyzoites within latent intracellular cysts.
2. If a naive heifer or cow first ingests oocysts when she is pregnant, then the infection may breach the placenta and be transmitted to the developing fetus; this is termed

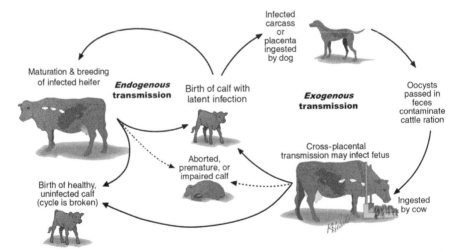

Fig. 3. Transmission of *Neospora caninum*. Cattle may become infected "horizontally" by ingestion of oocysts at any time of life (not only when pregnant). Congenital infection may result if infection is first acquired by a dam during pregnancy (exogenous transplacental transmission), or by reactivation of organisms from a latently infected dam (endogenous transplacental transmission). Artist: Kerry Helms.

exogenous transplacental transmission[16] (hereafter shortened to exogenous transmission). Exogenous transmission is a subtype of horizontal transmission in which both the dam and the offspring become infected from the same event.

3. If a female heifer or cow has a latent infection and later becomes pregnant, organisms may reactivate and cross the placenta; this is termed *endogenous transplacental transmission*[16] (hereafter shortened to endogenous transmission). Endogenous transmission may occur in multiple pregnancies of the same dam or may occur across several generations to transmit infection within maternal lines of cattle.

Confusingly, the *Neospora* literature often refers to "vertical" transmission. Technically, vertical transmission indicates transmission from mother to offspring, but this occurs in both endogenous and exogenous transmission; thus statements about vertical transmission are often ambiguous.

NEOSPOROSIS IN OTHER DOMESTIC ANIMALS AND IN WILDLIFE

As with cattle, *Neospora* infection in other animals is usually subclinical, but there are many exceptions. Dogs with clinical neosporosis may show a wide range of problems, such as hindlimb paresis or ataxia with muscle atrophy, myocarditis, dermatitis, or diarrhea. Clinical neosporosis in puppies may affect individuals or litters.[17]

Neosporosis abortion or neonatal illness is known to occur in a variety of large herbivores, including goat, sheep, llama, alpaca, several species of deer, lesser kudu, horse, and white rhinoceros.[3] Naturally occurring *Neospora* parasitism, but mostly without reports of disease, have been detected in adults of many other species of wild, feral, captive, and domestic animals, including rodents, lagomorphs, kangaroos, sparrows, parrots, and chickens. The possibility that these animals may serve as efficient intermediate hosts of the parasite, inducing patent infections when they are eaten by canids, is plausible but speculative.

Dogs, gray wolves, and Australian dingos (all subspecies of *Canis lupus*) and coyotes (*Canis latrans*) are known to be definitive hosts of *N caninum*.[18–21] Red foxes (*Vulpes vulpes*) have also been found to have small numbers of *N caninum* oocysts in feces and therefore may also be a definitive host[22]; however, experimental confirmation has not been achieved and thus the role of fox is uncertain.[23,24]

There is good evidence that *Neospora* actively cycles between gray wolves and their cervid prey.[19,25] However, deer also have high seroprevalence rates in regions without wolves, thus suggesting that coyotes and dogs may be sufficient to maintain this wild cycle. Dogs have been induced to shed *Neospora* oocysts after consuming hunter-killed white-tailed deer.[25]

EPIDEMIOLOGIC PATTERNS IN CATTLE

Three major patterns of neosporosis have been observed in herds of breeding cattle: abortion outbreaks (epidemic pattern), increased annual abortion losses (endemic pattern), and subclinical infections.

Epidemic Pattern

Outbreaks of neosporosis may occur in which a high proportion of pregnant cows abort within a short time period. Outbreaks are generally suspected to have resulted from an event in which the pregnant herd's feed or water has been contaminated with *Neospora* oocysts. This contamination is difficult to prove in retrospect; nevertheless, several lines of supporting evidence have been obtained from studies of outbreaks. Epidemic curves observed in outbreaks are consistent with point-source exposure events, such as contamination of a batch of mixed feeds, dietary supplements, or drinking water.[5,26,27] Specialized avidity serologic techniques have provided strong evidence that infections in cows were acquired recently in relation to the time of the abortion outbreak,[28–31] which is consistent with exogenous rather than endogenous transmission (see **Fig. 3**). Finally, epidemiologic studies have linked the odds of epidemic neosporosis with the presence and number of dogs on cattle farms, consistent with transmission to cattle by ingestion of oocysts.[32,33]

Experiments using oocysts are difficult, time-consuming, and expensive. First, infected tissues must be produced by inoculating animals (usually calves) with cultured organisms; then these tissues are fed to dogs to induce production of oocysts, and finally, the oocysts are administered to pregnant cows, which are followed to term. As a result, there have only been 3 small-scale experiments using oocysts in pregnant cattle,[34–36] so the following observations could use strengthening and refinement by additional investigation. Nevertheless, a pattern begins to emerge from examination of the combined results of the 3 available studies (**Table 1**). Administration of *Neospora* oocysts to 7 cows in the first trimester of pregnancy, even with the highest dose of 70,000 oocysts, did not result in transplacental infection of any calf. This transmission barrier began to break down a bit later in gestation; of 9 cows administered oocysts between 120 and 130 days of gestation, 6 gave birth to uninfected calves, but the other 3 had transplacental infection with 2 abortions (39–44 days after exposure) and 1 stillbirth. Another 7 cows were exposed in the late-second to early-third trimester, and 6 of their 7 calves were born with congenital infections, even with the lowest dose of approximately 127 oocysts, but were all clinically healthy. This experimental pattern roughly corresponds with the timing of neosporosis abortions in the field. This pattern also resembles transplacental toxoplasmosis in humans, in which the likelihood of transplacental transmission is lowest in the first trimester (but with the most severe consequences) and increases into the third trimester (and is often subclinical).[37] Thus, ingestion of *Neospora* oocysts by naive pregnant cows does appear to be capable of inducing an abortion outbreak, provided that exposure occurs

Table 1
Results of administration of *Neospora caninum* oocysts to pregnant cows, compiled from the only 3 published experiments of this type

	Day of gestation that oocysts were administered to cows		
	70	120–130	162–210
Number of cows that became infected and were followed to parturition	7	9	7
Number of offspring that became infected	0	3	6
Proportion of infected cows having infected offspring	0.00	0.33	0.86
Number of cows having abortions or stillbirths	0	3	0
Number of aborted fetuses or stillborn calves that were infected	—	3	—
Proportion of infected offspring that were aborted or stillborn	—	1.00	0.00

Data were included from all cows that became infected and that were followed until abortion or birth. All negative control cows gave birth to healthy uninfected calves.
Data from Refs.[34–36]

within an as-yet imprecisely defined gestational window of susceptibility, at a time when infection may cross the placenta but before the fetus has matured sufficiently to be able to defend itself (**Fig. 4**).

Endemic Pattern

In herds with endemic neosporosis, seropositive animals are often related along maternal lines that may span several generations.[38,39] Infected dams may give birth to one or more congenitally infected offspring, which in turn may enter the breeding herd and continue the cycle of endogenous transmission (see **Fig. 3**). There is a greater relative risk of abortion in *Neospora*-seropositive dams than in seronegative dams. For dairy cattle, a median relative risk of abortion of 3.5 was obtained from a compilation of numerous studies from 10 representative countries.[1] This relative risk indicates that seropositive dams are approximately 3.5 times more likely to suffer an abortion than are seronegative dams; for example, if the background rate of abortion in seronegative cattle is 2% or 3%, then about 7.0% to 10.5% of *Neospora*-seropositive cattle may abort. The data become more complicated when considering the effect of parity and of any previous abortions. For congenitally infected dams, the highest relative risk of having an abortion (7.4-fold in one study) occurs in the first pregnancy.[40] If the first parity is successful, then the relative risk of abortion drops considerably for future pregnancies, but if the heifer aborts her first pregnancy, then her risk of aborting future pregnancies remains high.[40]

In high seroprevalence dairy herds with year-round breeding programs, endemic abortions will occur more or less randomly throughout the year, although there may be minor seasonal fluctuations.[41] This problem may be so stable that the owner accepts it as normal for the herd, when in fact it represents a persistent drain upon profit.

It is possible for beef or dairy herds with endemic neosporosis, but which practice seasonal instead of year round breeding, to experience a pattern of abortion losses similar to an epidemic. Because most abortions occur between 5 and 7 months of gestation, annually increased losses in mid-gestation may cluster together within a short range of dates.

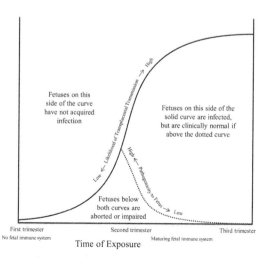

Fig. 4. Relation between the time of maternal exposure to *Neospora caninum* oocysts and the outcome of pregnancy in naive cattle.

Although endemic abortions are often assumed to be from endogenous transmission, horizontal transmission usually contributes to the maintenance of high seroprevalence in endemically infected herds.[42] Consistent with this, epidemiologic studies reveal statistical associations between the presence and number of dogs and the occurrence of *endemic* bovine neosporosis.[43,44] Because *Neospora* infection increases the likelihood of abortion and associated culling, a prolonged lack of horizontal transmission in a herd should result in the gradual depletion of seropositive animals, even if endogenous transmission were to occur in 100% of pregnancies (which is seldom the case). Horizontal transmission within endemic herds can occur as an irregular trickle that infects individual cattle at different times (perhaps from grazing), or as very infrequent exposure events that may infect a cohort of cattle (perhaps from contamination of a mixed ration or water).[42]

The efficiency of endogenous transmission, defined as the percentage of pregnancies of previously infected dams that give rise to congenitally infected offspring, has been the subject of many investigations. **Table 2** lists the 8 largest studies found in a literature search, each reporting the *Neospora* serologic status of at least 100 offspring of seropositive dams. Simple ratios (number of seropositive offspring/number of seropositive dams) vary between 41% and 86%, and the cumulative total provides an average of 63% efficiency of endogenous transmission. However, each of these studies included evidence of horizontal transmission (either postnatal or exogenous transplacental), which in 2 studies exceeded 20% per year.[45,46] Horizontal transmission causes upward skewing of the simple ratios that are used to calculate endogenous transmission, because some seronegative offspring will become seropositive from postnatal exposure, which gives the appearance of endogenous transmission.[42] One of the studies in **Table 2** provided a statistically corrected estimate of 45% for the rate of endogenous transmission, down from the listed simple calculation of 62%.[42] The true efficiency of endogenous transplacental transmission is likely to be somewhat lower than is reflected in the table, but a high degree of variability makes it impossible to be precise.

Table 2
Endogenous transplacental transmission rates of *Neospora caninum* in dairy cattle

Citation	Location	Seropositive Offspring/ Seropositive Dams	Simple Calculation of Endogenous Transmission Rate, %
Pan et al,[66] 2004	Ontario	252/619	41
Bartels et al,[42] 2007	Netherlands	325/526	62
Dijkstra et al,[67] 2003	Netherlands	363/500	73
Frössling et al,[68] 2005	Sweden	316/369	86
Romero & Frankena,[46] 2003	Costa Rica	168/285	59
Dijkstra et al,[45] 2001	Netherlands	163/204	80
Bergeron et al,[69] 2000	Quebec	64/144	44
Paré et al,[70] 1996	California	93/115	81
	Combined	1744/2762	63

Studies were included if they tested the offspring of at least 100 seropositive dams. These calculations have not been adjusted to account for horizontal transmission, which could cause upward skewing.

Endogenous transmission does not require that the dam herself was infected congenitally. This point was illustrated by an intensely investigated herd of beef cows that had suffered a neosporosis abortion outbreak. Avidity serology provided compelling evidence that most cows in the herd had acquired infection recently, consistent with a point source exposure event.[30] However, in the following 2 years, the calculated rate of endogenous transmission in that same herd was 85%. This finding is evidence that the initial episode of horizontal infection of pregnant dams, and the occurrence of exogenous transmission, later resulted in a high rate of endogenous transmission in those same cows.[47]

It is likely that long-term endogenous consequences of horizontally acquired *Neospora* infection in female cattle may depend on several variables, perhaps including the age and physiologic state of the animal at the time infection is acquired (eg, not pregnant, pregnant in early term without transmission to the fetus, or pregnant in later term with infection of the fetus), characteristics of the parasite strain, and infectious dose.

Although seropositive dams have a higher relative risk of abortion than do seronegative dams, this only holds true if the cows are not exposed to a horizontal challenge. Conversely, when herds of pregnant cattle have neosporosis abortion outbreaks, avidity serology shows that the previously uninfected cattle are at risk of aborting, whereas previously infected cattle appear to resist the horizontal challenge.[30,31,48] Experimental infectious challenge of latently infected, pregnant cattle also shows that they resist abortion.[49]

Subclinical Pattern

Overall, *Neospora*-seropositive dams have an increased relative risk of abortion compared with seronegative dams, but this does not hold true for every herd. A large-scale postnatal exposure event has been documented in which abortions were not noted.[50] A small number of studies have not shown a link between serologic status of dams and the relative risk for abortion. These circumstances are unlikely to be noticed unless performing serologic surveys.

EFFECT OF PRODUCTION TYPE

Overall, the prevalence of neosporosis is higher in dairy than in beef cattle.[1] This prevalence is probably related to production and management factors that affect the odds of exposure to the parasite, rather than a difference in susceptibility. Dairy cattle are more likely than beef cattle to be fed total mixed rations (TMR), which provide opportunities for point source exposure of herds to various ingested pathogens such as *Neospora* oocysts. Also, dairy cows require more feed and water than beef cows, increasing the opportunity to consume a larger dose of an infectious agent. Nevertheless, when they are seropositive, beef cows have a relative risk of abortion that is at least as high as for seropositive dairy cows.[1]

There are many more reports of abortion in European breeds of cattle (*Bos taurus taurus*) than in tropical Asian breeds (*Bos taurus indicus*). In one study, purebred Holsteins had a greater abortion risk than did Holstein-Zebu crosses.[4] Similarly, water buffalo (*Bubalus bubalis*) have infrequently been documented to suffer neosporosis abortion even though they may have a high prevalence of infection.[51] Because of this history of published reports, it is suspected that European cattle are more susceptible to neosporosis abortion in comparison with Asian cattle and water buffalo. However, it is also possible that abortions have simply been underinvestigated and underreported in tropical countries where zebu and buffalo are more common.

DIAGNOSIS

Neosporosis should be included in the differential diagnosis for either endemic or epidemic problems with bovine abortion, together with several other infectious and toxic causes of abortion, depending on the geographic location. Neosporosis abortions will not be associated with current or recent history of systemic illness in the dams, unlike some conditions such as nitrate poisoning, salmonellosis, or leptospirosis. Usually, the best diagnostic approach for an abortion problem is to perform a general workup, rather than to single out any one cause for diagnostic attention. For herds that clearly have an elevated proportion of abortions, diagnostic attempts have a good success rate. Conversely, results are often nondiagnostic for examinations of random abortions from herds that do not clearly have a significant abortion problem, and these may not be worth the trouble and expense of investigation.

So where should the line be drawn between normal background and elevated abortion losses? For dairy cattle, the US National Animal Health Monitoring Service (2007) has suggested a goal of 2% abortions per year, although stating that up to 5% was normal, with national averages of 5.0% for dairy cows and 3.3% for dairy heifers.[52] For beef cattle, the same service reports abortion prevalence of 0.5% for cows and 0.7% for replacement heifers.[53] Some investigators have suggested targets of 5% for dairy and 2% for beef, with annual abortion losses above this triggering investigation and corrective action.[54] Veterinarians should advise farmers on the establishment of targets that are appropriate for their situation.

Abortion diagnostics can be approached using serologic screening of dams to detect evidence of specific pathogens, or necropsy of aborted fetuses, or a combination of these. Serologic surveys have the advantage of being relatively easy to perform, but a disadvantage is that they can only detect evidence of a few specific agents. Examination of aborted fetuses provides the best opportunity to detect a wide variety of problems, not only common problems but also uncommon but important abortifacients such as *Salmonella dublin* and *Coxiella burnetti*. Disadvantages of this approach include the need to find aborted fetuses, the greater expense of examinations, and greater logistical issues in handling and shipping specimens.

Serologic Screening

At the time of abortion, affected dams usually can be expected to have a high level of specific antibodies against the causative pathogen. For example, it is possible for a single serologic examination of an aborting cow to provide a presumptive diagnosis of neosporosis or leptospirosis, but only if the result is quite high. Just what constitutes "quite high" for neosporosis will vary among diagnostic laboratories, because several different types of *Neospora* antibody detection methods are used, variously reported as titers, optical densities, or sample/positive ratios. As an example, the author considers an indirect fluorescent antibody test titer of 1:400 to be consistent with but not diagnostic of neosporosis abortion, 1:1600 as a likely association, and 1:6400 as a highly probable association. Keep in mind that the cutoff titer between a seronegative and a seropositive result can be set as low as 1:25, but that it is possible for a latently seropositive animal to abort from other causes.

The same serologic specimens can be used to examine titers for *Leptospira* serovars, viral antibody, or antigen tests, and for tests of other pathogens depending on regional considerations.

A more powerful serologic approach is to examine several dams that have *recently* aborted and compare them with a similar number of dams that have not aborted. The greater the number of animals tested, the greater the power of the comparison. For large herds, a rule of thumb is to test 10 or more animals per group. Results consistent with neosporosis, or of another condition such as leptospirosis, will show that most or all of the aborting dams are seropositive, whereas a lower proportion of the normal animals may be seropositive. There usually are seropositive animals in the normal group, because not every animal that is infected will abort. Statistical comparison can also be performed of the mean antibody levels in aborting and normal groups, with higher levels expected in clinically affected animals; this comparison may be essential in herds that have a very high seroprevalence (or, in the case of leptospirosis, to distinguish between infection and vaccination). Simple statistical procedures, such as the Fisher exact test (seropositive vs seronegative) or Mann-Whitney U test (level of titers), are sufficient for these comparisons, and many free online statistical calculators are available.

Examination of Aborted Fetuses

Necropsy of aborted fetuses provides the greatest chance for arriving at a diagnosis, regardless of the cause of the abortion problem. Diagnostic rates will be low when examining randomly lost fetuses within normal background levels of abortion, and many are presumed to have suffered genetic, placental, or hormonal defects. However, in the face of an abortion outbreak, the odds of achieving a meaningful diagnosis are much higher. Despite this, examination of more than one fetus is often needed. The diagnostic value of any one fetus cannot be guaranteed, in part because there is great variability between the time that the fetus dies and when it is expelled from the uterus, so that autolysis and putrefaction can be advanced. Nevertheless, accurate diagnosis has often been achieved from autolyzed or even mummified fetuses, so almost all fetuses have potential diagnostic value.

If there is convenient access to a veterinary diagnostic laboratory (VDL), then timely delivery of the entire chilled fetus may be the best option. When possible, include placenta (especially including cotyledons) and a serum sample from the aborting dam.

Alternatively, the veterinarian should examine the fetus, collect specimens, and ship these to a VDL. **Table 3** provides a general list of specimens to collect. Histology often

Table 3 Generally suggested specimens to send for bovine abortion diagnostics			
	Fresh Tissues	**Fluids**	**Formalin-fixed Tissues**
From head	Eyeball	—	Half of brain (even if soft) Cross-section of tongue
From thorax	Lung	Fetal fluid from any site (thorax, abdomen, or pericardium)	Lung Thymus Myocardium Diaphragmatic muscle
From abdomen	Liver Spleen Kidney	Abomasal fluid collected with sterile technique Fetal fluid if needed as listed above	Spleen Liver Adrenal Kidney
Placenta	+/−	—	Especially cotyledon
From dam	—	Serum	—
Information	Proportion affected; time course in herd; the presence of clinical signs in cows; a finding of icterus, mummification, or other lesions in fetus or placenta; recent movements, feed changes, or procedures; conditions suspected		

Specific consultation is recommended with the servicing VDL to correspond with the types of tests that they use.

provides the best value for money as a general surveillance technique that includes options to add additional tests using immunohistology and some types of polymerase chain reaction (PCR). For bacterial culture, abomasal fluid is an excellent specimen, easily collected using a syringe and needle without contamination, and transferred into a sterile vacuum tube or similar device for shipping. Abomasal fluid in part consists of swallowed fluid from the amnion and may contain pathogens that have caused placentitis or fetal pneumonia, yet abomasal fluid will remain free of the environmental contamination that affects the placenta upon abortion.

Safe secure packaging, chilling, and rapid shipment of biological specimens are essential, as is the inclusion of adequate information (something that is too often neglected!) (**Fig. 5**).

Aborted fetuses are often soft from autolysis, because fetal death typically occurs well in advance of expulsion. If the fetus is retained in the uterus for an unusually protracted period after death, then it may become dehydrated and shrunken; this "mummification" cannot occur with most bacterial infections, so neosporosis is one of the most common causes of this uncommon occurrence.[55] Other gross lesions of the fetus may be observed in a variety of abortifacient conditions that are beyond the scope of this discussion.

Examination of Farm Dogs

Diagnostic efforts in farm dogs are usually of questionable value, because there is not a clear strategy about what to do with the information. Serology can be performed. Seropositive dogs were infected at some time in the past, and they may have shed oocysts. However, the period to shed oocysts is usually (not always) less than 2 weeks, so seropositive dogs are not more likely to shed *Neospora* oocysts than are seronegative dogs. Seronegative dogs may be naive to the parasite and thus susceptible to acquiring infection and shedding oocysts. Parasitologic examination of canine feces may be attempted to observe oocysts, but because the period of shedding oocysts is likely to be brief, there is always a low likelihood of observing oocysts in any one specimen, whether the cattle herd has a high seroprevalence or not. The oocysts are about 10×11 μm in diameter (see **Fig. 2**), which presents approximately 2% of the surface area of *Toxocara canis* ova, so they are easily missed. Furthermore, oocysts of a closely related but nonpathogenic organism, *Hammondia heydorni*, are nearly identical in appearance (although 12×14 μm), so positive identification of *Neospora*-like oocysts must be confirmed by PCR or other specialized laboratory techniques. For comparison, oocysts of *Cryptosporidium parvum* in the feces of diarrheic calves are even smaller, 5×7 μm, and *Giardia* cysts in feces are about 9×13 μm.

WHY NEOSPOROSIS IS SO PREVALENT TODAY

Historically, all breeding cattle were managed extensively. Even dairy cattle were kept in small enough groups that could be milked by hand. *Neospora* oocysts in canine feces would be deposited in the great outdoors, where gradual weathering would have slowly disseminated the oocysts into the immediately surrounding dirt or surface water. Weeks or months later, individual cattle could become infected if they happened to graze the contaminated spots. Small groups of cattle might acquire infection by drinking together from a small water hole, but in larger bodies of water the dilutional effects would be too great to enable efficient transmission. As a result, *Neospora* would tend to infect individual animals. The prevalence of bovine neosporosis was probably much lower under those circumstances.

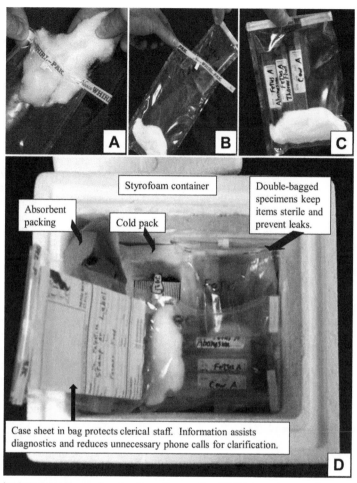

Fig. 5. Submitting specimens for abortion diagnostics. (*A*) Wet specimens of any type should be packaged within 2 containers, an inner primary and an outer secondary container, with absorbent material in between. Here, absorbent material is placed in the bottom of a biological specimen bag (not a zip-closing sandwich bag) to provide reliable secondary containment. (*B*) Tightly closed primary specimen containers are suitable for formalin specimens or fresh tissues. (*C*) Vacuum serum tubes are suitable sterile containers to hold liquid specimens including abomasal fluid, fetal fluids from thorax or abdomen, and serum from the aborting dam. (*D*) A package ready to be sealed and shipped.

In recent decades, and accelerating since the time that bovine neosporosis abortion was first described in 1988,[56,57] cattle enterprises are increasingly mechanized. Tractors and milking machines have enabled farmers to keep more and more cows in smaller and smaller spaces. As a consequence, it is no longer practical for large dairies to send cows to pasture during the day, but instead all feedstuffs are harvested and brought to the farm. Nutritional advances have led to the widespread adoption of TMR that contain a variety of feedstuffs and additives. One of the most commonly produced feedstuffs is silage, which decades ago tended to be stored within secure silo structures that could not be accessed by dogs or other animals. However, solid erect silos are expensive and can be slow to unload; as herd sizes began to increase, other

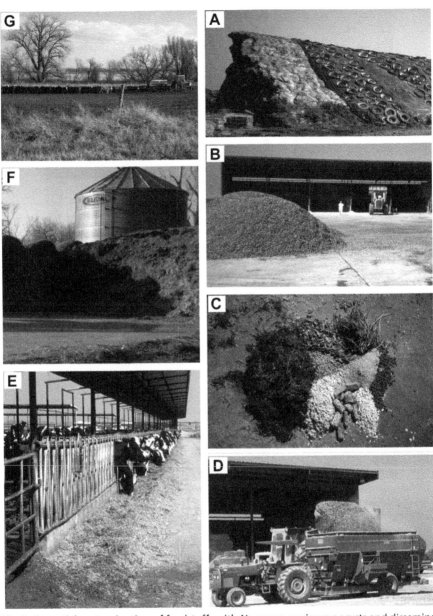

Fig. 6. Potential contamination of feedstuffs with *Neospora caninum* oocysts and dissemination in mixed rations. Representative dairy (*A–E*) and beef (*F, G*) farms are depicted that each had a recent neosporosis outbreak. Clockwise from upper right: (*A*) Above ground ensiling practices increase the opportunity for rodents to frequent or inhabit the silage, especially at the leading edge and around the sides, where discoloration reveals that anaerobic conditions have not been adequately maintained. When examined, rats and mice were flushed out of the silage pile. Dogs and other canids are attracted both to open silage and to rodents. (*B*) Examples of ration components piled in open bays or outside at a large dairy farm. (*C*) Various components of the mixed ration. (*D*) Use of a front-end loader and mixer wagon to prepare a TMR. If any component is contaminated with *Neospora* oocysts (or

forms of ensiling large amounts became more common, such as above ground or in pits. The variety of feedstuffs used in a typical TMR increased with computerization and development of least-cost ration analyses, and this in turn required that a greater variety of feedstuffs be purchased and stored until used. As a result of these technological advances and increases of scale, opportunities for widespread transmission of ingested pathogens have magnified (including *Neospora*, *Leptospira*, and *Salmonella*). Simply by contaminating a pile of exposed feedstuffs, a herd or pen of cattle may become exposed when the ingredient is mixed into a TMR and delivered for feeding (**Fig. 6**). If the cattle are not mature, or are not pregnant, or are not in a susceptible stage of pregnancy, then abortions do not occur. If some or most of the cattle happen to be in a susceptible stage of pregnancy, then abortions may occur (see **Fig. 4**). Either way, the prevalence of infection is augmented. Because infections last for life, and because many infected dams will endogenously transmit infections to future generations, the augmentation of seroprevalence has a prolonged effect.

In turn, maintaining a herd that has a high *Neospora* seroprevalence increases the opportunities for dogs or other canids to consume infected tissues, from either consuming placentas,[58] dead stock, or discarded offal, and then shed oocysts, thus increasing the frequency of environmental contamination and the associated likelihood of horizontal transmission.

CONTROL OPTIONS

The long-term key to avoid a high prevalence of infection, or to reduce a prevalence rate that is already high, lies in the protection of feedstuffs from contamination with canine feces. The historical, low-level, random acquisition of *Neospora* by grazing an infected spot of pasture cannot presently be prevented. It should be possible to reduce the prevalence of infection in intensively managed cattle, but not below the levels of infection that commonly occur in extensively managed cattle. Complete elimination of *Neospora* from a herd is not a recommended goal unless there are exceptional circumstances.

Feedstuffs used in mixed rations need to be better protected, so as to inhibit visits by dogs or wild canids. In small enterprises, this could be accomplished by maintaining feedstuffs in bins, silos, or behind closed doors. For large mechanized dairies, investment is needed to protect feedstuffs. The simplest solution may be use of dog-proof fencing. However, fences are no better than their gates, and it could become quite tiresome to have to manually open and close large gates for the heavy machinery involved in delivering feedstuffs, mixing rations, and feeding cattle. Gates could be left open during the day when predators are less likely to visit and operators are more likely to be aware. However, the best solution could be installation of automatic gates.

For operators that do not have a dedicated feed storage area, erection of electrified predator fencing around stored feeds could be used to inhibit canine access without the need to install permanent fencing.

---

other orally transmitted pathogens such as *Leptospira* or *Salmonella*), then it will become distributed throughout the TMR. (*E*) Feeding the TMR to a pen of dairy cows. Potential exists to deliver pathogens to many animals at a time. (*F*) This outdoor silage pile on a beef farm was not covered, and animal tracks and scats of many types were present, potentially increasing attractiveness to dogs and coyotes. (*G*) Provision of mixed silage and chopped hay to the beef cow herd, which were periodically brought in from winter pasture for supplemental feeding.

Similar consideration should be given to the protection of drinking water. The most likely sources of contamination would be small surface ponds or bogs, which could become contaminated with runoff from surrounding ground. Watering from elevated troughs should reduce risk and is a practical solution for most intensively managed herds.

Unfortunately, epidemiologic studies are clear that the presence of dogs on breeding cattle premises is a risk factor for bovine neosporosis, and therefore, removal of all dogs may be considered as a potentially effective method to reduce this risk. However, the author does *not* recommend a blanket ban on farm dogs and thinks that it is possible to reduce the risk of horizontal transmission of *Neospora* to cattle without the removal of all dogs. First, the farm should only keep the dogs that they really want on the property. Larger numbers of dogs on a property increase the risk of bovine neosporosis, and probably the greatest risk occurs when there are litters of puppies about. Compared with adult dogs, puppy litters are more likely to be naive to the parasite, and thus, they have greater potential to produce oocysts on first exposure to an infected meal. Therefore, breeding dogs and raising puppies on a cow-calf or dairy farm may be stretching luck a bit far. Second, be a good neighbor and keep an eye on where your dogs go and request the same in return. If unwanted stray dogs frequent your farm, then ask for help from local authorities. Third, even if a dog becomes infected and sheds *Neospora* oocysts for a period of time, this could be relatively unimportant as long as the dog's feces do not end up in the mixed ration; this gets back to the issue of fencing and the use of secure containers.

Another consideration is that some dogs will actively guard their territory and thereby reduce visits by wild and stray canids, thus providing some measure of protection from exposure to *Neospora*. Evidence consistent with this possibility was found for beef cattle,[59] in which exposure probably occurs in individual animals during grazing, rather than from mass exposure of a contaminated TMR. An infected working dog will only shed oocysts for a brief period, which is unlikely to infect a large number of grazing cattle. Afterward, the dog will probably be refractory to oocyst production,[60] while throughout its lifetime that same dog may reduce visits from many wild or feral canids.

What can an enterprise do if it already has a high prevalence of neosporosis abortions? In the author's opinion, any management strategy must include protection of feedstuffs. Without such protection, any reduction in the seroprevalence of cattle may not endure. However, if appropriate measures have been implemented to protect feedstuffs, and the farmer does not wish to wait for the seroprevalence to slowly reduce over the years, then consideration may be given to performing *Neospora* serology on all cows and heifer calves. Seropositive dams can be presumed to have a high (possibly 63%; **Table 2**) rate of endogenous transmission, so one possible method to speed a reduction in herd prevalence is to not retain heifer calves that are born to seropositive dams. A suggested variant of this strategy is to inseminate all seropositive dams using beef semen, and it has even been suggested that hybrid pregnancies are less susceptible to abortion.[61] A second but similar approach is to perform serology on all potential replacement heifers, regardless of the serologic status of their dams, and then retain only seronegative animals to enter the breeding herd; this serology could be performed from precolostral blood specimens obtained at birth, but more commonly, it would be performed after maternal immunity has waned, perhaps at 6 months of age.

Finally, if a seropositive cow or heifer has particularly valuable genetics, then the farmer may wish to consider using embryo transfer to ensure that endogenous transmission does not occur.[62] Surrogate cows should be selected after careful screening for *Neospora* and other unwanted pathogens such as bovine viral diarrhea virus, bovine-adapted *Leptospira* serovars (hardjo-bovis and hardjo prajitno), *S dublin*, and bovine leukemia virus.

No matter how well-designed and conscientiously practiced, neosporosis management programs may not achieve or sustain complete elimination of neosporosis from a herd. Certain factors are beyond control, such as whether a particular feedstuff or additive could have been contaminated before delivery, a stray or wild canid defecates in a pasture that is used for grazing or to make haylage, or if there is a chance contamination event of water. There may even be additional methods of parasite transmission that have not been described; for example, it is plausible that tissues of infected rodents could be chopped and mixed into a TMR, and such mechanically assisted carnivorism could be sufficient to infect cattle.

FUTURE PROSPECTS FOR VACCINES

Effective vaccines for bovine neosporosis are sorely needed. Although a killed vaccine was previously available in the United States, it was not reliable and is no longer in production.

A highly effective live-attenuated vaccine for a very similar condition of sheep, caused by *T gondii* rather than *N caninum*, has been used in New Zealand and parts of Europe since 1988.[63] There is good experimental evidence that bovine neosporosis could also be controlled by a similar vaccine containing attenuated organisms[64]; however, to date, none has been developed and commercialized. Government-sponsored research of animal diseases has been markedly curtailed in the United States[65] and currently tends to favor conditions that are bioterrorist threats, have zoonotic potential, or that restrict international trade. Neosporosis does not meet those funding criteria, despite its economic importance to the cattle industry in general and to intensive dairy enterprises in particular, and this has inhibited research efforts in the United States over the last 15 years.

Development of an effective neosporosis vaccine for dogs would also be a most welcome aid for the control of bovine neosporosis and could alleviate concerns about the traditional place of pet and working dogs around breeding cattle.

REFERENCES

1. Reichel MP, Alejandra Ayanegui-Alcérreca M, Gondim LF, et al. What is the global economic impact of Neospora caninum in cattle—the billion dollar question. Int J Parasitol 2013;43:133–42.

2. Mughini-Gras L, Bonfanti L, Natale A, et al. Application of an integrated outbreak management plan for the control of leptospirosis in dairy cattle herds. Epidemiol Infect 2014;142:1172–81.

3. Donahoe SL, Lindsay SA, Krockenberger M, et al. A review of neosporosis and pathologic findings of Neospora caninum infection in wildlife. Int J Parasitol Parasites Wildl 2015;4:216–38.

4. Asmare K, Regassa F, Robertson LJ, et al. Seroprevalence of Neospora caninum and associated risk factors in intensive or semi-intensively managed dairy and breeding cattle of Ethiopia. Vet Parasitol 2013;193:85–94.

5. Arnold LM. Investigation of an abortion epidemic due to Neospora caninum in a beef herd on pasture. Bov Pract 2013;47:1–6.

6. Parish SM, Maag-Miller L, Besser TE, et al. Myelitis associated with protozoal infection in newborn calves. J Am Vet Med Assoc 1987;191:1599–600.

7. O'Toole D, Jeffrey M. Congenital sporozoan encephalomyelitis in a calf. Vet Rec 1987;121:563–6.
8. Micheloud JF, Moore DP, Canal AM, et al. First report of congenital Neospora caninum encephalomyelitis in two newborn calves in the Argentinean Pampas. J Vet Sci Tech 2015;6:1000251.
9. Hobson JC, Duffield TF, Kelton D, et al. Neospora caninum serostatus and milk production of Holstein cattle. J Am Vet Med Assoc 2002;221:1160–4.
10. Bartels CJ, van Schaik G, Veldhuisen JP, et al. Effect of Neospora caninum-serostatus on culling, reproductive performance and milk production in Dutch dairy herds with and without a history of Neospora caninum-associated abortion epidemics. Prev Vet Med 2006;77:186–98.
11. Barling KS, McNeill JW, Thompson JA, et al. Association of serologic status for Neospora caninum with postweaning weight gain and carcass measurements in beef calves. J Am Vet Med Assoc 2000;217:1356–60.
12. Barling KS, Lunt DK, Snowden KF, et al. Association of serologic status for Neospora caninum and postweaning feed efficiency in beef steers. J Am Vet Med Assoc 2001;219:1259–62.
13. Waldner C, Wildman BK, Hill BW, et al. Determination of the seroprevalence of Neospora caninum in feedlot steers in Alberta. Can Vet J 2004;45:218–24.
14. Waldner C. Pre-colostral antibodies to Neospora caninum in beef calves following an abortion outbreak and associated fall weaning weights. Bov Pract 2002;36:81–5.
15. Moré G, Bacigalupe D, Basso W, et al. Serologic profiles for Sarcocystis sp. and Neospora caninum and productive performance in naturally infected beef calves. Parasitol Res 2010;106:689–93.
16. Trees AJ, Williams DJ. Endogenous and exogenous transplacental infection in Neospora caninum and Toxoplasma gondii. Trends Parasitol 2005;21:558–61.
17. Dubey JP. Neosporosis in dogs. CAB Reviews 2013;8(055):1–26.
18. McAllister MM, Dubey JP, Lindsay DS, et al. Dogs are definitive hosts of Neospora caninum. Int J Parasitol 1998;28:1473–8.
19. Dubey JP, Jenkins MC, Rajendran C, et al. Gray wolf (Canis lupus) is a natural definitive host for Neospora caninum. Vet Parasitol 2011;181:382–7.
20. King JS, Šlapeta J, Jenkins DJ, et al. Australian dingoes are definitive hosts of Neospora caninum. Int J Parasitol 2010;40:945–50.
21. Gondim LFP, McAllister MM, Pitt WC, et al. Coyotes (Canis latrans) are definitive hosts of Neospora caninum. Int J Parasitol 2004;34:159–61.
22. Wapenaar W, Jenkins MC, O'Handley RM, et al. Neospora caninum-like oocysts observed in feces of free-ranging red foxes (Vulpes vulpes) and coyotes (Canis latrans). J Parasitol 2006;92:1270–4.
23. Constantin EM, Schares G, Grossmann E, et al. Studies on the role of the red fox (Vulpes vulpes) as a potential definitive host of Neospora caninum. Berl Munch Tierarztl Wochenschr 2011;124:148–53 [in German].
24. Schares G, Heydorn AO, Cuppers A, et al. In contrast to dogs, red foxes (Vulpes vulpes) did not shed Neospora caninum upon feeding of intermediate host tissues. Parasitol Res 2002;88:44–52.
25. Gondim LFP, McAllister MM, Mateus-Pinilla NE, et al. Transmission of Neospora caninum between wild and domestic animals. J Parasitol 2004;90:1361–5.
26. McAllister MM, Huffman EM, Hietala SK, et al. Evidence suggesting a point source exposure in an outbreak of bovine abortion due to neosporosis. J Vet Diagn Invest 1996;8:355–7.

27. Yaeger MJ, Shawd-Wessels S, Leslie-Steen P. Neospora abortion storm in a mid-western dairy. J Vet Diagn Invest 1994;6:506–8.

28. Björkman C, Gondim LF, Naslund K, et al. IgG avidity pattern in cattle after ingestion of Neospora caninum oocysts. Vet Parasitol 2005;128:195–200.

29. Schares G, Barwald A, Staubach C, et al. p38-avidity-ELISA: examination of herds experiencing epidemic or endemic Neospora caninum-associated bovine abortion. Vet Parasitol 2002;106:293–305.

30. McAllister MM, Björkman C, Anderson-Sprecher R, et al. Evidence of point-source exposure to Neospora caninum and protective immunity in a herd of beef cows. J Am Vet Med Assoc 2000;217:881–7.

31. Jenkins MC, Caver JA, Björkman C, et al. Serological investigation of an outbreak of Neospora caninum-associated abortion in a dairy herd in southeastern United States. Vet Parasitol 2000;94:17–26.

32. Bartels CJ, Wouda W, Schukken YH. Risk factors for Neospora caninum-associated abortion storms in dairy herds in The Netherlands (1995 to 1997). Theriogenology 1999;52:247–57.

33. Dijkstra T, Barkema HW, Eysker M, et al. Natural transmission routes of Neospora caninum between farm dogs and cattle. Vet Parasitol 2002;105:99–104.

34. Trees AJ, McAllister MM, Guy CS, et al. Neospora caninum: oocyst challenge of pregnant cows. Vet Parasitol 2002;109:147–54.

35. Gondim LFP, McAllister MM, Anderson-Sprecher RC, et al. Transplacental transmission and abortion in cows administered Neospora caninum oocysts. J Parasitol 2004;90:1394–400.

36. McCann CM, McAllister MM, Gondim LF, et al. Neospora caninum in cattle: experimental infection with oocysts can result in exogenous transplacental infection, but not endogenous transplacental infection in the subsequent pregnancy. Int J Parasitol 2007;37:1631–9.

37. Desmonts G, Couvreur J. Congenital toxoplasmosis. A prospective study of 378 pregnancies. N Engl J Med 1974;290:1110–6.

38. Björkman C, Johansson O, Stenlund S, et al. Neospora species infection in a herd of dairy cattle. J Am Vet Med Assoc 1996;208:1441–4.

39. Paré J, Thurmond MC, Hietala SK. Neospora caninum antibodies in cows during pregnancy as a predictor of congenital infection and abortion. J Parasitol 1997; 83:82–7.

40. Thurmond MC, Hietala SK. Effect of congenitally acquired Neospora caninum infection on risk of abortion and subsequent abortions in dairy cattle. Am J Vet Res 1997;58:1381–5.

41. Thurmond MC, Anderson ML, Blanchard PC. Secular and seasonal trends of Neospora abortion in California dairy cows. J Parasitol 1995;81:364–7.

42. Bartels CJ, Huinink I, Beiboer ML, et al. Quantification of vertical and horizontal transmission of Neospora caninum infection in Dutch dairy herds. Vet Parasitol 2007;148:83–92.

43. Paré J, Fecteau G, Fortin M, et al. Seroepidemiologic study of Neospora caninum in dairy herds. J Am Vet Med Assoc 1998;213:1595–8.

44. Schares G, Barwald A, Staubach C, et al. Potential risk factors for bovine Neospora caninum infection in Germany are not under the control of the farmers. Parasitology 2004;129:301–9.

45. Dijkstra T, Barkema HW, Eysker M, et al. Evidence of post-natal transmission of Neospora caninum in Dutch dairy herds. Int J Parasitol 2001;31:209–15.

46. Romero JJ, Frankena K. The effect of the dam-calf relationship on serostatus to Neospora caninum on 20 Costa Rican dairy farms. Vet Parasitol 2003;114: 159–71.

47. Björkman C, McAllister MM, Frössling J, et al. Application of the Neospora caninum IgG avidity ELISA in assessment of chronic reproductive losses after an outbreak of neosporosis in a herd of beef cattle. J Vet Diagn Invest 2003;15:3–7.

48. McAllister MM, Wallace RL, Björkman C, et al. A probable source of Neospora caninum infection in an abortion outbreak in dairy cows. Bov Pract 2005;39: 69–74.

49. Williams DJ, Guy CS, Smith RF, et al. First demonstration of protective immunity against foetopathy in cattle with latent Neospora caninum infection. Int J Parasitol 2003;33:1059–65.

50. Dijkstra T, Barkema HW, Björkman C, et al. A high rate of seroconversion for Neospora caninum in a dairy herd without an obvious increased incidence of abortions. Vet Parasitol 2002;109:203–11.

51. Reichel MP, McAllister MM, Nasir A, et al. A review of Neospora caninum in water buffalo (Bubalus bubalis). Vet Parasitol 2015;212:75–9.

52. Anon. Dairy 2007. Part I: reference of dairy cattle health and management practices in the United States, 2007. Fort Collins (CO): USDA-APHIS-VS-NAHMS; 2007.

53. Anon. Part III: beef cow/calf health management. Fort Collins (CO): USDA-APHIS-VS; 2007.

54. Radostits OM, Leslie KE, Fetrow J. Herd health: food, animal, production medicine. 2nd edition. Philadelphia: W. B. Saunders Company; 1994.

55. Ghanem ME, Suzuki T, Akita M, et al. Neospora caninum and complex vertebral malformation as possible causes of bovine fetal mummification. Can Vet J 2009; 50:389–92.

56. Thilsted JP, Dubey JP. Neosporosis-like abortions in a herd of dairy cattle. J Vet Diagn Invest 1989;1:205–9.

57. Shivaprasad HL, Ely R, Dubey JP. A Neospora-like protozoon found in an aborted bovine placenta. Vet Parasitol 1989;34:145–8.

58. Dijkstra T, Eysker M, Schares G, et al. Dogs shed Neospora caninum oocysts after ingestion of naturally infected bovine placenta but not after ingestion of colostrum spiked with Neospora caninum tachyzoites. Int J Parasitol 2001;31:747–52.

59. Barling KS, Sherman M, Peterson MJ, et al. Spatial associations among density of cattle, abundance of wild canids, and seroprevalence to Neospora caninum in a population of beef calves. J Am Vet Med Assoc 2000;217:1361–5.

60. Gondim LF, McAllister MM, Gao L. Effects of host maturity and prior exposure history on the production of Neospora caninum oocysts by dogs. Vet Parasitol 2005; 134:33–9.

61. López-Gatius F, Santolaria P, Yániz JL, et al. The use of beef bull semen reduced the risk of abortion in Neospora-seropositive dairy cows. J Vet Med B Infect Dis Vet Public Health 2005;52:88–92.

62. Baillargeon P, Fecteau G, Paré J, et al. Evaluation of the embryo transfer procedure proposed by the International Embryo Transfer Society as a method of controlling vertical transmission of Neospora caninum in cattle. J Am Vet Med Assoc 2001;218:1803–6.

63. Buxton D, Innes EA. A commercial vaccine for ovine toxoplasmosis. Parasitology 1995;110(Suppl):S11–6.

64. Williams DJ, Guy CS, Smith RF, et al. Immunization of cattle with live tachyzoites of Neospora caninum confers protection against fetal death. Infect Immun 2007; 75:1343–8.

65. McAllister MM. Successful vaccines for naturally occurring protozoal diseases of animals should guide human vaccine research. A review of protozoal vaccines and their designs. Parasitology 2014;141:624–40.

66. Pan Y, Jansen GB, Duffield TF, et al. Genetic susceptibility to Neospora caninum infection in Holstein cattle in Ontario. J Dairy Sci 2004;87:3967–75.

67. Dijkstra T, Barkema HW, Eysker M, et al. Evaluation of a single serological screening of dairy herds for Neospora caninum antibodies. Vet Parasitol 2003; 110:161–9.

68. Frössling J, Uggla A, Björkman C. Prevalence and transmission of Neospora caninum within infected Swedish dairy herds. Vet Parasitol 2005;128:209–18.

69. Bergeron N, Fecteau G, Paré J, et al. Vertical and horizontal transmission of Neospora caninum in dairy herds in Québec. Can Vet J 2000;41:464–7.

70. Paré J, Thurmond MC, Hietala SK. Congenital Neospora caninum infection in dairy cattle and associated calfhood mortality. Can J Vet Res 1996;60:133–9.

Yearling Bull Breeding Soundness Examination
Special Considerations

Nora Schrag, DVM*, Robert L. Larson, DVM, PhD, ACT, ACVPM-Epi

KEYWORDS

- BSE • Breeding soundness examination • Yearling bull • Bull development
- Semen morphology • Semen quality

KEY POINTS

- Veterinarians should have the utmost confidence in their decisions when performing a breeding soundness examination (BSE) on yearling bulls.
- Veterinarians should confirm that young bulls submitted for a BSE have completed puberty before being classified as a satisfactory potential breeder.
- Care should be taken to detect congenital or inherited defects.
- Reporting results in a complete, easy-to-read format increases the clients' ability to market or use the bull in a manner that will be positive for their reputation and financial bottom line.

INTRODUCTION

Veterinarians should have the utmost confidence in their decisions when performing a breeding soundness examination (BSE) on yearling bulls. Accurate assessment is important for the bottom line of all interested parties: the buyer, the seller, and the veterinarian performing the BSE. The reputation of the client selling yearling bulls, as well as the reputation of the veterinarian testing them, is also important to recognize. This article is primarily aimed at those practitioners performing BSEs on large groups of yearling bulls before bull sales.

Yearling bull producers should be reminded that the value of BSE testing is to increase the percentage of cows in a breeding pasture that become pregnant in a defined breeding season. A field study demonstrated at least a 5% greater pregnancy percentage in cow herds exposed to bulls passing fertility test versus cow herds exposed to unselected bulls[1] (**Fig. 1**). This study also demonstrated that simply adding more bulls to the unselected population does not make up for this difference.[1]

The author has nothing to disclose.
Department of Clinical Sciences, Kansas State College of Veterinary Medicine, 1800 Denison Avenue, Manhattan, KS 66502, USA
* Corresponding author.
E-mail address: nschrag@vet.k-state.edu

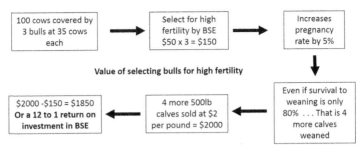

Fig. 1. Estimated economics of investment in BSEs.[1]

This article highlights special considerations when testing yearling bulls and thus improves practitioner confidence that their examination and classification are based on current research.

REPORTING

Efficient reporting allows for more successful communication of results with the client as well as aiding the veterinarian in being complete and efficient in their examination. Though the Society for Theriogenology (SFT) offers a standard form (**Fig. 2**), many practitioners prefer to use their own BSE reporting format.

Provided that a customized BSE reporting format displays equal or more information than is included in the SFT standard form, and improves recording efficiency and client communication, this seems like a reasonable approach. For large groups of bulls, it is often advantageous to input data electronically so that individual or group reports may be printed. This can be accomplished using the electronic BSE (eBSE) software offered by the SFT or by using other data processing software. For efficient

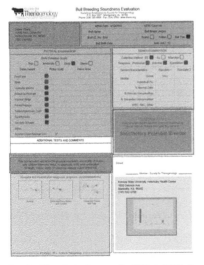

1. ID for Bull and Farm
2. Service capacity (libido and serving ability)
3. Physical Soundness
4. Semen quality
5. Classification

Assuming freedom from disease, bulls require these 3 attributes to be fertile
(Albert Barth)

Fig. 2. The SFT electronic BSE (eBSE) form created using the eBSE software. Data can be entered from an iPad. ID, identification. (*Courtesy of* Society for Theriogenology, with permission.)

communication, it is often best to have the information in list format for the bull producer and in individual format for buyers who purchase individual bulls.

The multiple bull report format abbreviates certain portions of an individual BSE form (**Fig. 3**). When using similar forms, important information not specifically mentioned in this form will be recorded for each bull in the comments section. It is assumed that for yearling bulls there would be no breeding history and that abnormal physical traits will be written in the comments. *The BSE itself is not abbreviated, it is simply the method of recording results that is streamlined.*

This article is structured around the BSE report to assure that information presented is relevant to the practitioner at the time of the examination.

Section 1: Identification

Yearlings often get a sale lot number that is different from their original identification (ID). For sale bulls, it is recommended that metal clip tags be inserted to facilitate having a permanent ID with which to write health papers after the sale.

Section 2: Sex Drive and Mating Ability

Sex drive and mating ability are not routinely examined by the veterinarian in the United States. Furthermore, libido or serving capacity tests are often inaccurate in yearlings due to their sexual inexperience.[2] It is the responsibility of the veterinarian to remind the client that this very important aspect is not being evaluated during the BSE.[3,4] This is particularly important for yearling bulls for whom a previous year's breeding performance is not available to provide any evidence about sex drive and

MULTIPLE BULL BREEDING SOUNDNESS EXAMINATION

Veterinary Health Center
AT KANSAS STATE UNIVERSITY
TO DISCOVER. TO TEACH. TO HEAL.

Owner: ____________
Ranch: ____________
Address: ____________
City: ________ State: ______ Zip: ______
Phone: ____________

18.6

Bull ID	Age	Scrotal	Motility	Normal	Proximal Droplets	Detached Heads	Head Defects	Midpiece Defects	Tail Defects	Comments	Satisfactory	Questionable	Deferred	Unsatisfactory

DVM Signature: ____________ Date: ____________

*The results of this bull evaluation should in no way be used as a legal document certifying or condemning fertility. Rather, it is an evaluation guide to utilize the knowledge we currently have to discourage use of potentially inefficient sires.

MULTIPLE BULL BREEDING SOUNDNESS EXAMINATION

4/15

Fig. 3. The BSE form formatted to improve efficiency when performing BSEs on a large number of bulls. (*Courtesy of* Kansas State University Veterinary Health Center, with permission.)

mating ability. When measured, approximately 10% of bulls have low service capacity, which is a measure of both physical soundness and libido.[4]

It cannot be assumed that bulls passing all other aspects of the BSE with above average scores will have good libido.[5] Because yearling bulls do require some experience to be efficient breeders, the owner's observation of breeding activity is extremely important. Time with cows is essential for the complete development of breeding instincts of young bulls. The simple presence of a dominant bull may be enough to suppress libido in a yearling.[4]

Section 3: Physical Soundness

One study demonstrated that the risk of injury to yearling bulls can be as high as 75%.[6] Although no cause for the extremely high risk of injury in the study could be identified and may not represent many situations, practitioners should be aware that injury to young bulls is common. Although long-term structural soundness is challenging to assess with high accuracy when bulls are evaluated as early as 12 months of age, at the very least, young bulls must be structurally sound at the beginning of their breeding careers.

Scrotal circumference

The importance and heritability of scrotal circumference has been documented in great detail elsewhere.[4,7–13] In addition, a study indicated that a high plane of nutrition shows some benefit for testicular development but only when applied before 6 months of age.[14] Other studies show that enhanced nutrition early in life only had a transient effect on scrotal circumference, with bulls fed higher caloric diets having a larger scrotal size at 1 year of age compared with bulls on a control diet but by the time of maturity having no difference.[15] Nutrition after weaning (6–12 months of age) seems to have minimal influence on mature scrotal size.[14]

There are breed differences in average scrotal circumference (**Table 1**) and these averages have changed with time.[16] However, at present, no breed-specific standards have been recommended for use in the United States when performing a BSE. Due to the importance and high heritability of testicular size, veterinarians should encourage bull producers to apply selection pressure to improve average scrotal circumference, especially in herds in which average circumference is low.

Table 1			
Scrotal circumference by breed			
Breed	**Number of Bulls**	**Mean Scrotal Circumference (cm) Corrected to 365 Days of Age**	**Standard Deviation (cm)**
Angus	3004	34.62	2.21
Charolais	1469	34.55	2.82
Gelbvieh	190	34.41	2.63
Hereford	272	33.93	2.41
Limousin	290	31.52	2.22
Salers	31	31.84	2.84
Shorthorn	66	33.03	1.60
Simmental	1050	36.06	2.50
Speckle Park	55	32.04	1.77

Adapted from Guerra AG, Hendrick S, Barth AD. Increase in average testis size of Canadian beef bulls. Can Vet J 2013;54(5):485–90.

Body condition, rate of gain

Because of perceived preference by buyers, many bulls are developed at a relatively high rate of daily weight gain so that they can be sold as heavily conditioned yearlings. It is not uncommon to perform a BSE on yearling bulls with body conditions of 7 and greater. It has been shown that average daily gains of approximately 1 to 1.6 kg/d (2.2–3.5 lb/d) did not result in excessive fat accumulation in the scrotum, increased scrotal temperature, or reduction in sperm production and semen quality, and could be considered safe targets for growing beef bulls.[4,14] In light of other research showing a high incidence of osteoarthritis in bull management systems that use these types of daily weight gain, perhaps further evaluation of the safety of this rate of gain is indicated.[17] Excessive energy intake in young bulls may result in laminitis, abnormal bone and cartilage growth, and increased risk of rumenitis, which may lead to the development of vesicular gland infections.[18]

Eyes

Vision is an essential part of the bulls' ability to detect heat.[4] This is a judgment call for each practitioner because it is difficult to predict how much of a scar due to infectious bovine keratoconjunctivitis (pinkeye) will interfere with heat detection and how much this corneal scar will change with time. Remember that the individual signing a BSE form that classifies a bull as satisfactory needs to be comfortable that the bull does not have evidence of visual deficiencies that will prevent it from detecting cows in heat. Any eye lesion should be noted on the report, regardless of how this bull is classified.

Feet and legs

In a study that examined bones in the hind limb of 46 bulls slaughtered at the end of a growth-testing period, 97.8% had lesions in their joints or growth plates.[17] Bulls in the study were raised from 6 to 12 months of age on diets that resulted in average daily growth of 1 to 1.6 kg/d (2.2–3.5 lb/d). One notable characteristic of the management of bulls in this particular study was that the bulls were raised on concrete with straw bedding rather than on dirt. In another study that compared bone lesions to history of poor performance in adult bulls demonstrated that poor performance was highly associated with hind limb osteoarthritis lesions.[19] These studies raise the question of what frequency and severity of joint lesions should be tolerated in the development of yearling bulls considering the importance of long-term structural and breeding soundness.

Despite evidence that structural soundness of feet and legs should be emphasized in yearling bulls, it can be very challenging to make this evaluation in a bull at 12 months of age. Many osteoarthritis lesions are not detectable at the time of BSE and corkscrew claw often becomes noticeable at 18 months of age or older but is not apparent at 12 months.[4] However, if detectable, deficiencies should be noted at time of the BSE.

Testicles, inguinal rings, scrotum, spermatic cord, epididymis, vesicular glands, penis, prepuce

There are a variety of abnormalities that can be associated with reproductive tract structures in yearling bulls (**Table 2**).[4,20–23] Heritability is high for some of these defects and they have various effects on fertility. The importance of recognizing these types of defects during a BSE cannot be overemphasized.

Current research has made use of thermography to further study the effects of thermoregulation in testicular development. One study showed that as the testicles develop the ability of the vascular cone to regulate heat changes

Table 2
Anatomic defects in yearling bulls

Location	Defect	Description
Testicles	Testicular hyperplasia	Often associated with hypoplasia of the contralateral testicle
		Often satisfactory semen quality
	Young bulls with unusually large scrotal circumference 40–45 cm	Several possibilities: (1) normal in all respects, (2) normal testicles but poor semen quality for unrelated reason, (3) orchitis or duct aplasia results in testicular degeneration, (4) scrotal development lags behind testicular development and semen quality is poor for several months until scrotum lengthens and the scrotum has a neck
	Testicular hypoplasia	Difficult to distinguish from degeneration
		Can be heritable and can be caused by zeranol (Ralgro, Intervet Inc d/b/a Merck Animal Health, Summit, NJ) exposure
	Cryptorchidism	Heritable, sterile if bilateral
		Discourage use if unilateral due to heritability
Inguinal rings	Scrotal hernia	Interferes with thermoregulation, heritable
Scrotum	Short scrotum Prominent caudal frenulum of scrotum Rotated scrotum	Usually not problematic unless interferes with thermoregulation
		If thermoregulation is affected, poor semen quality results
Cord	Vascular malformations of spermatic cord	Variable semen quality
Ductules	Blind ending efferent ductules	Relatively common, degree it affects fertility is variable
		Bulls can initially be fertile, then decline in fertility because granuloma formation completely obstructs the ducts
Epididymis	Epididymal aplasia	0.35% reported in study of Red Danish bulls
		Hereditable, but older bulls can acquire this defect due to injury and subsequent granuloma formation
	Cystic appendix epididymis	Develops slowly and does not block movement of sperm
		Semen quality is unaffected
Vesicular glands	Hypoplasia, aplasia, cysts, and duplication of vesicular glands	Congenital
		One documented bull had normal morphology but poor motility that remained unchanged for 3 mo
Penis	Spiral deviation	May be heritable
		Commonly assumed that spiral deviation during electroejaculation is not significant
		Scientific evidence is lacking
	Dorsal deviation	Simply overshooting the cow with a normal penis is more common than a dorsal deviation
		Very inefficient breeders
	Rainbow deviation	Rare
		More commonly caused by failure of complete erection due to a vascular shunt
	Congenitally short penis	Minimal >20 cm is needed for breeding
	Persistent frenulum	Common, fertility not affected if frenulum is transected
		Heritable, use in purebred herd is concerning
	Hypospadia	Congenital or due to trauma such as wart removal
Prepuce	Preputial eversion	Commonly thought to be more prone to injury
		Evidence is lacking

Data from Refs.[4,20–23]

dramatically. Bulls with decreased thermoregulatory development had decreased semen quality.[24] However, at this time, thermography cannot be used to predict semen quality.

Section 4: Semen Quality

Collection

Semen collection techniques for young bulls do not differ appreciably from techniques used in mature bulls. In some situations, a smaller-sized probe can be effective and may be necessary for atraumatic insertion. As with older bulls, manual stimulation of accessory glands per rectum before ejaculation greatly facilitates collection success and decreases collection time. Care should be taken to begin stimulation slowly and to maintain a steady rate and rhythm while gradually increasing stimulation intensity tailored to the bull's reaction. In the author's experience, yearling bulls that have indeed completed puberty and are properly stimulated collect as easily as adult bulls. However, young bulls in an early to intermediate stage of pubertal development may present a semen collection challenge to the practitioner. Welfare should be considered when attempting to collect a semen sample from young bulls. If 3 attempts using an electroejaculator fail to produce a sample, further collection attempts should be postponed to a later date. Although aspermia is possible, especially in a young unproven bull, it is very rare.[4] Failure to collect a sample on a single collection day is unlikely to indicate aspermia and more likely to indicate unsuccessful collection.

Because of some concerns expressed about animal welfare issues related to electroejaculation, alternatives have been studied. Transrectal massage was found suitable when compared with artificial vagina collection of semen with the disadvantage of massage being that lower volume of semen was collected.[25] The other disadvantages of transrectal massage included that the penis was less likely to protrude; more time was required to obtain a sample; and semen samples had lower percent motile sperm, lower sperm concentration, and lower percent live sperm when compared with electroejaculator collection.[26] Morphology did not differ between the methods.[26] At this time, appropriately performed electroejaculation seems to be a reasonable way to collect yearling bulls in an efficient manner in the field.

Response

Extension is absolutely essential to properly assess young bulls due to the frequency that warts, persistent frenulums, and other abnormalities of the penis may be encountered. Studies involving a large number of bulls over several years have reported frequency of persistent frenulum from 4.4% to 16.5%, with frequency in 11-month-old bulls higher than in older bulls.[27,28] A persistent penile frenulum can generally be treated by simple transection. Use of bulls with this defect in purebred herds should only be done after consideration of the heritability of this defect; however, use of bulls with this corrected defect in commercial herds that do not retain bulls for breeding should not cause concerns.

One study diagnosed penile warts 1.8% to 2.8% of all bulls tested.[27,28] The effectiveness of vaccine strategies to reduce penile warts in humans has been documented.[29] The potential for DNA-based vaccines against bovine papillomavirus shows promise but is not currently available.[30] Current therapy for warts involves debulking plus or minus the use of cryotherapy or laser. Both commercial and autogenous wart vaccination are commonly used, though scientific evidence of efficacy in cattle is lacking.

Semen motility

When examining motility there are no differences between yearlings and adults, other than the sample concentration may be less. If sperm cell concentration in the semen sample is very dilute, motility may need to be assessed on an individual sperm level.

Sperm cell morphology

In discussions among practitioners, it is not uncommon to hear the opinion that proximal droplets do not mean anything in a young bull. This opinion stems from experiences checking bulls that have large numbers of proximal droplets and then have normal semen morphology within a relatively short time period. According to current literature, there is reason to believe that proximal droplets in young bulls are equally detrimental to fertility as they are in older bulls. However, there is evidence that often, but not always, these bulls will have high-quality semen after a short time period. The following short review of spermatogenesis should help clarify some of the normal physiology affecting the incidence of proximal droplets, as well as other defects associated with young bull semen quality.

Fig. 4 illustrates that morphologically defective spermatids can acquire their defects during spermatogenesis in the testicle, or during maturation and storage in the epididymis.[4] The 3 defects that can be associated with disturbances of epididymal maturation or storage can also be caused by a disturbance during spermatogenesis.[4] For example, a defective spermatid that has a proximal droplet may have acquired this defect due to a disturbance of spermatogenesis when the proximal droplet was formed in testicular tissue, or it may have acquired it during a disrupted maturation phase (eg, low testosterone) in the epididymis. Because the same defect has 2 separate causes, it seems reasonable that the prognosis for recovery may differ based on cause. If the problem is immature spermatogenesis, this will likely improve as the bull matures. If the problem is low testosterone, this may also improve fairly rapidly in a young bull as he completes puberty. Attaining and maintaining adequate testosterone level is important in the production of morphologically normal sperm.[4,31]

Similarly, when an excessive percentage of free heads is identified, the problem could be due to a defective formation of the head–tail junction in the seminiferous tubules of the testicle, or it could be due to long storage time in the epididymis causing this inherently weak structure to break down.[4]

Simple distal midpiece reflexes are most likely created during sperm storage in the epididymis, unlike other midpiece defects that are created in the testicle during the formation of the spermatid.[4,31]

Classification of morphologic defects has been described in many different ways. Current literature suggests that all classification systems have limits and morphology should be performed in a way that specifically differentiates defects.[4]

Two problems with assessment of sperm morphology are evident: the human variability factor, including staining technique; and the lack of scientifically tested cut-points for the various morphological defects. Staining, training and counting differences, notwithstanding, because of the lack of a true gold-standard sperm morphology evaluation system it is difficult to support or refute the superiority of one system of sperm morphology evaluation over the other.
—Barth and Oko (1989)[32]

Although counting each of the 20-plus defects separately is not practical in field settings, defects can be differentiated in a way that groups them by location and pathogenesis, allowing more accurate assessment of the bull's relative maturity. The

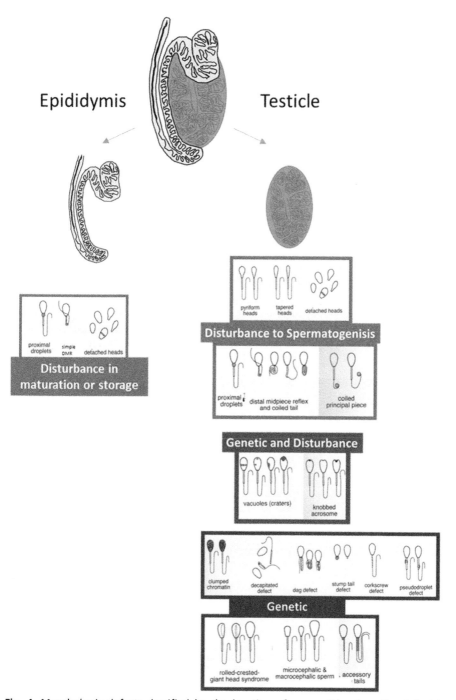

Fig. 4. Morphologic defects classified by the location of spermatids when the defect is created. (*Adapted from* Barth AD. Bull breeding soundness. 3rd edition. Saskatoon, SK: Western Canadian Association of Bovine Practitioners; 2013.)

details of morphologic classification of defects do not differ from adult bulls and are beyond the scope of this article.

Potential for automated standardized systems for describing morphology exist. One such system is the Trumorph, another is BullMate. Currently neither are validated or available for use in the field.[33,34] Regardless of technique used, it is important to remember a few key points about yearling bull morphology:

1. BSEs are performed on young bulls to put genetic pressure on the herd and breed to mature early.
2. Puberty resembles disturbed spermatogenesis.[4]
3. The cause of reduced normal semen morphology is likely immaturity.
4. Many, but not all, young bulls will improve with time because age is likely the problem causing the abnormal sperm cells.

Young bulls can have significant variation in performance and some individuals take longer to learn how to mate; however, semen quality and quantity are likely the most important limiting factors for breeding success.[4]

Round cells

Round cells can be of spermatogenic or nonspermatogenic origin. On eosin-nigrosin stained slides, round cells appear as bright white objects larger than the spermatid heads. Because all round cells with an intact membrane will look the same on eosin-nigrosin stained slides, it is important to use a differential stain such as modified Giemsa (Diff Quick) to differentiate immature spermatids from inflammatory leukocytes (**Fig. 5**).[35]

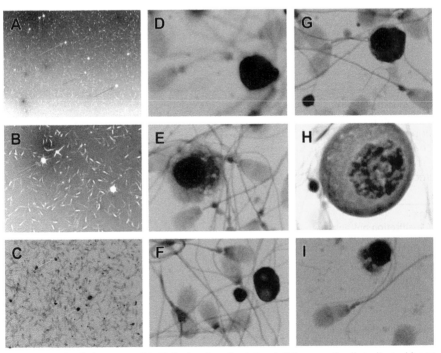

Fig. 5. Round cells in semen. (*A, B*) Eosin-nigrosin stained slide, round cells indicated by arrows. (*C*) Diff Quik stained slide, round cells indicated by arrows. (*D–I*) Immature spermatids, Diff Quik stained.

Box 1
Interpretation parameters for leukocytes found in bovine semen

Steps to quantify leukocytes in bull semen samples after standard dilution using hemocytometer

1. Count the number of leukocytes per field in 20 fields ($400\times$ magnification)

2. Average the count per field (ie, total number of leukocytes/20)

3. Determine maximum average count compatible with a satisfactory breeder
   Less than 1 equals normal
   1 to 5 equals monitor for other indications of reproductive tract inflammation
   Greater than 5 equals not-satisfactory

If leukocytes are identified, the practitioner must determine if the number observed will affect semen quality. Up to 1 leukocyte per $400\times$ field after averaging 20 fields is considered normal, whereas greater than an average of 5 leukocytes per $400\times$ field is associated with poor semen quality[36] (**Box 1**).

This method of assessment of leukocyte effect on semen has been validated in dogs, horses, and now bulls.[36] It also seems that morphologically abnormal sperm attract leukocytes, so it seems reasonable that bulls with a high percentage of morphologic changes also are more likely to have elevated numbers of leukocytes present in their semen.[36]

Section 6: Classification

The percentage of yearling bulls that pass their BSE varies greatly between and within population subsets and by month of age.[12,27,37] The goal of every practitioner should simply be to be as accurate and consistent as possible. The final classification of a bull is important both for identifying individuals likely to breed cows very efficiently and also for putting genetic selection pressure on the group to mature earlier (**Box 2**).

It may be tempting to get distracted by the pressure some owners may put on a practitioner to pass a young bull. At times, owners need to be reminded that individual assessments are not only about a particular bull. Each assessment is part of an ongoing and broad strategy to exert pressure on the herd to select for young age at puberty and high fertility. Properly performed yearling bull BSEs put pressure on the genetic pool for highly fertile early maturing bulls.

The goal to produce highly fertile bulls that reach puberty at a young age is facilitated by identifying animals that are producing semen with greater than 70% normal

---

Box 2
Classification options for bulls based on their breeding soundness examination

Classification

- Satisfactory: shows evidence of high fertility potential; this is not a guarantee of future fertility, observe breeding, watch for returns to heat

- Deferred: shows evidence of immaturity and is likely (but not guaranteed) to improve with time

- Questionable: may be capable of settling some cows but does not show evidence of being highly fertile

- Unsatisfactory: shows evidence of significant decrease in fertility; using this bull for efficient breeding is not recommended

---

morphology and pass all other criteria to be classified as satisfactory by a herd-specific target-age. The selection pressure put on group (ie, herd and/or breed) genetics to have highly fertile early maturing animals is perhaps the most important reason to check bulls at a young age. If it were not for this, the decision to fertility check might as well be delayed until just before turnout.

SUMMARY

Do a complete examination, specifically watching for congenital or inherited defects. Select for early maturing bulls by selecting bulls with large scrotal circumference and normal semen morphology by 12 months of age, and report BSE results in a clear and efficient manner. A properly performed yearling bull BSE should benefit the financial bottom line as well as the reputation of both the veterinarian and the client.

REFERENCES

1. Wiltbank JN, Parish NR. Pregnancy rate in cows and heifers bred to bulls selected for semen quality. Theriogenology 1986;25(6):779–83.
2. Parkinson TJ. Evaluation of fertility and infertility in natural service bulls. Vet J 2004;168(3):215–29.
3. Menegassi SRO, Barcellos JOJ, Peripolli V, et al. Behavioral assessment during breeding soundness evaluation of beef bulls in Rio Grande do Sul. Anim Reprod 2011;8(3–4):77–80.
4. Barth AD. Bull breeding soundness. 3rd edition. Saskatchewan: Western Canadian Association of Bovine Practitioners; 2013.
5. Scheepers SM, Annandale CH, Webb EC. Relationship between production characteristics and breeding potential of 25-month old extensively managed Bonsmara bulls. S Afr J Anim Sci 2010;40(3):163–72.
6. Ellis RW, Rupp GP, Chenoweth PJ, et al. Fertility of yearling beef bulls during mating. Theriogenology 2005;64(3):657–78.
7. Kastelic JP, Thundathil JC. Breeding soundness evaluation and semen analysis for predicting bull fertility. Reprod Domest Anim 2008;43:368–73.
8. Gipson TA, Vogt DW, Ellersieck MR, et al. Genetic and phenotypic parameter estimates for scrotal circumference and semen traits in young beef bulls. Theriogenology 1987;28(5):547–55.
9. Hafla AN, Lancaster PA, Carstens GE, et al. Relationships between feed efficiency, scrotal circumference, and semen quality traits in yearling bulls. J Anim Sci 2012;90(11):3937–44.
10. Kastelic JP, Cook RB, Pierson RA, et al. Relationships among scrotal and testicular characteristics, sperm production, and seminal quality in 129 beef bulls. Can J Vet Res 2001;65(2):111–5.
11. Smith BA, Brinks JS, Richardson GV. Relationships of sire scrotal circumference to offspring reproduction and growth. J Anim Sci 1989;67(11):2881–5.
12. Arteaga A, Baracaldo M, Barth AD. The proportion of beef bulls in western Canada with mature spermiograms at 11 to 15 months of age. Can Vet J 2001;42(10):783–7.
13. Smith MF, Parish N, Wiltbank JN. Selecting bulls for fertility. Beef Cattle Research in Texas; 1981. p. 86–8.
14. Brito LF, Barth AD, Wilde RE, et al. Effect of growth rate from 6 to 16 months of age on sexual development and reproductive function in beef bulls. Theriogenology 2012;77(7):1398–405.

15. Harstine BR, Maquivar M, Helser LA, et al. Effects of dietary energy on sexual maturation and sperm production in Holstein bulls. J Anim Sci 2015;93(6): 2759–66.
16. Guerra AG, Hendrick S, Barth AD. Increase in average testis size of Canadian beef bulls. Can Vet J 2013;54(5):485–90.
17. Dutra F, Carlsten J, Ekman S. Hind limb skeletal lesions in 12-month-old bulls of beef breeds. Zentralbl Veterinarmed A 1999;46(8):489–508.
18. Barth AD. Pubertal development of Bos taurus beef bulls. Le Médecin vétérinaire du Québec 2004;34(1–2):54–5.
19. Persson Y, Soderquist L, Ekman S. Joint disorder; a contributory cause to reproductive failure in beef bulls? Acta Vet Scand 2007;49:31.
20. Blockey MA, Taylor EG. Observations on spiral deviation of the penis in beef bulls. Aust Vet J 1984;61(5):141–5.
21. Elmore RG, Breuer J, Youngquist RS, et al. Breeding soundness examinations in 18 closely related inbred Angus bulls. Theriogenology 1978;10(5):355–63.
22. Blom E. Segmental aplasia of the Wolffian duct in the bull. A congenital and most probably hereditary defect overlooked in the past. Riproduzione animale e fecondazione artificiale; 1972. p. 57–63.
23. Barth AD. Congenital and acquired abnormalities of the scrotum, testes and epididymides of bulls. Large Anim Vet Rounds 2006;6(4).
24. Brito LF, Barth AD, Wilde RE, et al. Testicular vascular cone development and its association with scrotal temperature, semen quality, and sperm production in beef bulls. Anim Reprod Sci 2012;134(3–4):135–40.
25. Sylla L, Palombi C, Stradaioli G, et al. Effect of semen collection by transrectal massage of accessory sexual glands or artificial vagina on the outcome of breeding soundness examinations of Italian yearling beef bulls. Theriogenology 2015;83(5):779–85.
26. Palmer CW, Brito LF, Arteaga AA, et al. Comparison of electroejaculation and transrectal massage for semen collection in range and yearling feedlot beef bulls. Anim Reprod Sci 2005;87(1–2):25–31.
27. Bruner KA, McCraw RL, Whitacre MD, et al. Breeding soundness examination of 1,952 yearling beef bulls in North Carolina. Theriogenology 1995;44(1):129–45.
28. Spitzer JC, Hopkins FM, Webster HW, et al. Breeding soundness examination of yearling beef bulls. J Am Vet Med Assoc 1988;193(9):1075–9.
29. Brotherton JML. Human papillomavirus vaccination: where are we now? J Paediatr Child Health 2014;50(12):959–65.
30. Lima EG, Lira RC, Jesus ALS, et al. Development of a DNA-based vaccine strategy against bovine papillomavirus infection, involving the E5 or L2 gene. Genet Mol Res 2014;13(1):1121–6.
31. Tang WH, Jiang H, Ma LL, et al. Relationship of sperm morphology with reproductive hormone levels in infertile men. Zhonghua Nan Ke Xue 2012;18(3):243–7 [in Chinese].
32. Barth A, Oko R. Abnormal morphology of bovine spermatozoa (1st ed.). Ames: Iowa State University Press; 1989.
33. Soler C, Garcia-Molina A, Contell J, et al. The Trumorph® system: the new universal technique for the observation and analysis of the morphology of living sperm [corrected]. Anim Reprod Sci 2015;158:1–10.
34. Palmer CW, Barth AD. Comparison of the BullMate (TM) sperm quality analyzer with conventional means of assessing the semen quality and breeding soundness of beef bulls. Anim Reprod Sci 2003;77(3–4):173–85.

35. Johanisson E, Campana A, Luthi R, et al. Evaluation of 'round cells' in semen analysis: a comparative study. Hum Reprod Update 2000;6(4):404–12.
36. Zart AL, Jurgielewicz VC, Fernandes CE. Seminal leucocytary profile in beef bulls. Reprod Domest Anim 2014;49(5):719–24.
37. Kennedy SP, Spitzer JC, Hopkins FM, et al. Breeding soundness evaluations of 3648 yearling beef bulls using the 1993 Society for Theriogenology guidelines. Theriogenology 2002;58(5):947–61.

Management and Breeding Soundness of Mature Bulls

Colin W. Palmer, DVM, MVSc

KEYWORDS

- Breeding soundness • Bulls • Spermatogenesis • Sperm morphology

KEY POINTS

- Mature bulls must be managed appropriately year-round to ensure that they are ready for the short and intense breeding season.
- Bulls housed or pastured in groups should be of similar age and moved from pasture to paddock with a view to social hierarchy.
- Mature bulls may be joined with females at up to 1:40 (bull:female), but must be observed for social dominance, libido, and injury-related issues.

INTRODUCTION

The management of young, growing bulls differs from that of mature bulls. Growth rate, growth performance, puberty, and conformational attributes are the focus of seed stock bull producers. Congenital and developmental faults are more likely to be detected at or before the first breeding soundness evaluation resulting in those affected being culled. Mature bulls, those 2 years of age and older, have or soon will be purchased by the end-user with most being used by the commercial beef cow-calf sector. By 2 years of age, *Bos taurus* bulls have generally achieved their mature frame size, have or will soon reach their maximal scrotal circumference, and will weigh at least 85% of their lifetime maximal weight. At one time, it was common practice for beef bulls to be held back to enter the breeding bull market as 2-year-olds for the simple reason that yearling and long yearling bulls were just not considered to be mature enough. Through increased selection pressure, more intensive feeding programs, and calving seasons for seedstock cattle that are a few to several months in advance of their commercial neighbors, bull suppliers have been able to offer bulls for sale as yearlings. In reality these "yearling" bulls typically range in age from 12 to 18 months, with the older bulls being more desirable, as they are physically larger and more likely to be classified as satisfactory potential breeders on a breeding

The author has nothing to disclose.
Department of Large Animal Clinical Sciences, Western College of Veterinary Medicine, University of Saskatchewan, 52 Campus Drive, Saskatoon, Saskatchewan S7N 5B4, Canada
E-mail address: colin.palmer@usask.ca

Vet Clin Food Anim 32 (2016) 479–495
http://dx.doi.org/10.1016/j.cvfa.2016.01.014
0749-0720/16/$ – see front matter © 2016 Elsevier Inc. All rights reserved.

soundness evaluation. Depending on a number of factors, which can largely be distilled down to the basic market forces of supply and demand, 2-year-old bulls can be hard to find by would-be purchasers but offer the advantage of being able to breed more cows, and with increased age most structural faults should be evident.

In actual dollar value, bulls represent one of the largest inputs on a cow-calf operation. **Table 1** shows a listing of those costs using 4 different purchase prices. Values of course vary depending on the herd and price fluctuations typical of the industry; however, the author has attempted to assign a number to each category with the assumption that the bull will sire 30 calves per year and will remain in the herd for 4 years. The total cost is divided by the number of calves sired by each bull to determine the bull cost per calf. The example calculations assume that each bull will sire equivalent calves with no consideration for any additional genetic value. For instance, bulls that sire calves with heavier weaning weights, produce superior daughters, or achieve higher pregnancy rates earlier in the breeding season and, therefore, have heavier calves at weaning would provide additional value compared with bulls that did not achieve these characteristics. However, using these or similar calculations is a good start. By considering the costs on a per-calf basis, producers can then consider if more expensive bulls are worth it for their herds and can also look for ways to maximize the economic return on their investments.

BULL MANAGEMENT

Given the value of breeding bulls within the cow-calf enterprise, there is a surprisingly limited amount of bull-specific management information in the scientific literature. For the most part, management practices that are used in the cow herd should be the same for bulls, but with an understanding that there are specific social dominance, housing, and feeding issues that are unique.

Bulls should be processed within 1 of 2 months of the breeding season, which should include a breeding soundness evaluation, annual revaccination, and hoof trimming if needed. Ensuring these procedures are completed well in advance of the breeding season will allow time for replacement bulls to be sourced and for any short-term lameness to be resolved before commencement of breeding.

Nutrition

Information regarding the current feeding regimen should accompany every animal being relocated to a new facility. Bulls that have been grazing on pasture and will be turned into the breeding field soon should ideally remain on pasture, or be fed a

Table 1
Costs per calf associated with purchasing and maintaining a beef bull using 4 different purchase prices and assuming the bull will remain in the herd for 4 years

Purchase Price	$3000	$4000	$5000	$6000
Salvage value	$1500	$1500	$1500	$1500
Yardage, feed, pasture/year	$1000	$1000	$1000	$1000
Veterinary costs/year	$100	$100	$100	$100
Death loss (10%/y × 4 y)	$1200	$1600	$2000	$2400
Total Cost (4 y)	$7100	$8500	$9900	$11300
Number of calves sired (30 calves per bull per year)	120	120	120	120
Bull cost/calf	$59.17	$70.83	$82.50	$94.17

good-quality grass hay. Legume feeds with a high bloat risk should be avoided or carefully introduced if the feeding period will be extended. Bulls that have been conditioned for a show and are still on a high-energy ration should be continued on a similar diet. If a grain concentrate was being fed, then the same or similar feed should be purchased even if the goal is to transition the bull onto another ration. Rapid changes in diet can cause rumen acidosis, precipitating systemic illness, lameness, and even death. Feed the concentrate at 50% to 70% of what he was being fed and try to maintain the same daily feeding schedule reducing the quantity gradually until the desired amount is reached. The remainder of the ration should be good-quality hay with a total ration protein content of at least 12%.

Hard-working bulls normally lose some condition throughout the breeding season, but excessive weight loss should be avoided. It is common for bulls, especially those with a body condition score in excess of 7.0 to 7.5 (9-point scale), to lose up to 2 cm of scrotal circumference between the beginning and end of breeding season. Breeding seasons of not more than 2 or 3 months are not only important for calving management, but also provide several months to restore condition for the next breeding season. Encouraging weighing and body condition scoring of bulls is sound advice. Breeding bulls should have a body condition score of 6 to 7 (9-point scale) at the onset of the breeding season.[1] In the author's opinion, Charolais, Angus, and Hereford bulls with an average frame size should weigh in the range of 1800 to 2100 pounds (820–950 kg) at the time of turnout and sport the look of a well-muscled athlete. Too heavy and they are more prone to feet and leg injury; too light and they will not have enough condition to sustain them for the breeding season. Bulls will usually consume 30% to 50% more feed than cows; therefore, the risk of bloat is compounded, especially if feed quality or quantity are inconsistent. Feeding an ionophore to improve feed efficiency and reduce the risk of bloat is recommended. Depending on a combination of breed, individual characteristics, and ranch management, overfeeding can be as much of a problem as underfeeding. Selection for "easy fleshing" animals has undoubtedly resulted in mature animals that will gain weight with surprisingly limited resources, especially if they are sedentary. Bulls older than 12 to 18 months may have a tendency to accumulate fat in the scrotal neck, which can negatively affect spermatogenesis.[2] Minerals and vitamins are essential to proper nutrition. Deficiencies of zinc, and vitamins A and E have been shown to have a direct, negative effect on testicular function. Other deficiencies may have an indirect effect via disturbances in gonadotropin release from the pituitary that are integral in the regulation of spermatogenesis.[3]

In cold climates, consideration must be given to increasing feed quantity and quality during winter months, as maintenance requirements dictate. Providing easy access to fresh water at all times will help to maintain bulls in adequate condition. Limiting water will also limit feed intake, and having to walk a considerable distance to water will use additional energy. Adequate bedding and shelter from the wind are crucial for preventing scrotal frost bite.

Vaccination

The general recommendation is to vaccinate breeding bulls with the same vaccines used in the cow herd. Special consideration should be given to vaccinating bulls with a footrot vaccine in regions where it is a common occurrence. Even short-term bouts of lameness can not only prevent a bull from breeding, but can have long-lasting negative effects on spermatogenesis. Although not usually considered necessary in mature cattle, annual or even biennial revaccination with a multivalent clostridial vaccine is a sound and inexpensive practice because of the potential for fighting-related injuries among mature bulls.

Campylobacteriosis and Trichomoniasis may be of concern in some herds and geographic regions. Mature bulls are capable of sustaining the causative organisms within the deep crenulations of their prepuce where they may remain infected for years. Neither the respective causative bacteria *Campylobacter fetus* subspecies *venerealis* nor the causative protozoan *Tritrichomonas foetus* subspecies *venerealis* cause disease in bulls, but are conclusively linked to pregnancy loss in infected females. Oil adjuvanted, as opposed to aluminum hydroxide adjuvanted, *Campylobacter* vaccines have been shown to be protective for cows[4] and a double vaccination scheme was reportedly successful in clearing the infection from a high percentage of mature bulls.[5] Control of Trichomoniasis has been historically most effective when suspect bulls are identified through diligent testing and isolated from clean herds; and nonpregnant females are identified and culled. Immunization with *T foetus* whole-cell antigens prevented infection in experimentally challenged bulls[6] and was effective in clearing *T foetus* from infected bulls.[7]

Bovine viral diarrhea virus (BVDV) can be transmitted via the semen of persistently infected (PI) and acutely infected bulls.[8,9] Persistently infected bulls acquire the virus in utero before their immune systems are competent. Once believed to be impossible, PI bulls are capable of normal growth performance and survival to adulthood to spread the virus via semen and other bodily fluids. Infection acquired after birth may present in 1 of 3 ways. Bulls may be transiently infected and shed the virus in semen for up to 28 days. This can occur following infection at any age in naïve animals.[10] Acute infection has been associated with reduced sperm concentration, poor sperm motility, and an increase in sperm morphologic abnormalities.[11] Prolonged and persistent testicular BVDV infections follow acute infection in prepubertal bulls. Prolonged testicular infections have been reported to persist for more than 2 years before clearance; however, transmission of the virus to susceptible females has not been reported. In contrast, persistent testicular infection is associated with consistent shedding of infective virus in the semen for several months, but to date has been reported only in 2 dairy bulls with shedding occurring when they were younger than 2 years of age. Both were non-viremic at the time of assessment, but maintained a high level of circulating antibody. The persistence of BVDV in prolonged and persistent infections is believed to be due to incompetent testicular immune defenses at the time of infection.[11] The current recommendation is that bulls should be vaccinated according to label instructions with a cytopathic modified live BVDV vaccine.[12]

Parasite Control

External and internal parasite control efforts should be consistent with the cow herd. Dosages should be consistent with the body weight of the bulls as with any other class of cattle.

Flies can be irritating to all classes of cattle. Horn flies seem to have an affinity for bulls, gathering in large numbers on the withers and topline. Control measures include insecticide-containing back rubbing devices and repellant sprays, pour-ons, and tags. Pyrethrin-containing sprays are now in popular use and have been shown to have no negative effects on bull fertility when used appropriately.[13]

Social Dominance

Social hierarchy is determined whenever bulls are mixed. Bull studs house bulls individually largely to reduce the risk of fighting-related injuries; however, this level of segregation is not always practical in ranch settings. When group-penning bulls, it is a good idea to introduce new individuals to a group by assembling both new and existing group members together in a new paddock. This practice seems to reduce the fighting pressure on the newest members of the group, as bulls tend to exhibit hierarchal fighting behavior whenever they are given a new space. Seniority and to a lesser extent age determine social ranking with the social dominance order established in the paddock remaining the same in the breeding field within groups of bulls of similar age.[14] Under most circumstances, it is not a good idea to mix age groups of bulls, for example, 2-years-olds with 4-year or older bulls, as the older bulls are more likely to inhibit the breeding activity of the younger bulls, especially when fewer females are displaying estrus. Breeding interference did not occur when 2-year-old bulls were pastured together and pregnancy rates were higher than the mixed-age breeding groups. Social dominance order was much more likely to remain stable among the bulls of similar age with few disruptions of breeding activity.[14]

BULL-TO-FEMALE RATIO

A common recommendation is 1 bull to 25 or 30 females for bulls 2 years old or older, and 1 bull to 15 or 20 females for bulls younger than 2.[1,15] Considering the data presented in **Table 1**, increasing the number of females per bull would decrease the bull cost per calf. Ratios as low as 1:60 (bull:female) probably will not have a negative effect on conception rates[15,16]; however, this may be applicable only in specific situations. Social dominance order in multisire breeding situations and libido are 2 potential limiting factors to the breeding potential of a bull. Add to that the potential for bull injury, which could easily result in the number of eligible females per bull increasing dramatically. For example, 2 bulls placed with 80 cows. If one bull becomes injured in the first week of the breeding season and is not replaced that could leave potentially 60 or more cows for the remaining bull to breed. Use of such low ratios warrants daily observation of breeding activity and only bulls with high libido and sperm-producing capability should be used.

A series of studies designed to provide scientific recommendations on bull selection and mating practices in Australia used DNA parentage testing and generated some interesting results from Brahman-type cattle. Of 235 bulls evaluated, 58% sired 10% or fewer calves whereas 6% sired no calves. Fourteen percent sired more than 30% of the calves in their respective mating groups. Moreover, breeding performance was moderately repeatable across years in most of the pastures. Multiple regression models showed that breeding performance was variably influenced by a number of factors, including sheath depth (an issue in Brahman bulls), scrotal circumference, sexual ability in serving capacity testing, sperm motility, and sperm morphology, but the models explained only 35% to 57% of the variation in calf output.[17] The behavior of *Bos indicus* cattle in various libido and serving capacity tests can be quite different from that of *B taurus* cattle, with *B indicus* generally considered to be less efficient breeders. In the final paper in the series, however, it was reported that in multiple-sire mating using reproductively sound mature Brahman bulls at 1:40 (bull:female) did not affect herd fertility in comparison with higher ratios. Furthermore, the 1:40 group was contained in what most would consider a large pasture covering 60 km^2.[18]

Certainly there is scientific evidence to support larger numbers of females per breeding bull, and with the advent of DNA parentage testing and genomics research new avenues are sure to be explored. Bulls must be relied on to perform very effectively for a 6- to 8-week period each year, so they must be in excellent physical condition. Given our current knowledge, mature bulls with ample semen production and libido can be used at a ratio as low as 1 bull to 40 females. Lower ratios are possible; however, despite our best efforts, injury rates remain high, and without replacement bulls conception rates are sure to suffer when the proportion of bulls in the herd is too low during a period of intense breeding activity.

THE BREEDING SOUNDNESS EVALUATION

The intent of a bull-breeding soundness evaluation (BSE) is to identify subfertile bulls and must address not only semen quality, but the bull's ability to successfully breed cows. Those performing a complete BSE are obligated to include a thorough physical, and reproductive tract and semen examination.[19] Anything less is not acceptable. To ensure quality and consistency, it is best that a standardized format is followed so that all of the appropriate information is gathered. Bull BSE standards, forms, and educational documents are produced by at least 3 separate organizations in existence today. Their standards are very similar and differ only on select criteria considered relevant in the jurisdiction in which they are used. Bull BSE standards are reviewed periodically by these organizations and will continue to evolve as science and technology dictate. The current Society for Theriogenology (SFT) standards were adopted in 1993[19,20] and are the accepted format in use by veterinarians in the United States and many other parts of the world. The standards set forth by the Western Canadian Association of Bovine Practitioners (WCABP) were adopted by veterinarians in Canada in 1993 and differ from the SFT standards on minimum percent motile sperm threshold (60% and 30%, respectively), the use of age and breed minimum acceptable scrotal circumferences, and the classification of bulls that do not meet the criteria for satisfactory. The BSE standards in use in Australia were put forth by the Australian Cattle Veterinarians; the most substantial difference between this system and the others is the inclusion of a service capacity test.[19] Both the SFT and WCABP systems of bull BSE do not specifically address libido and mating ability, with the WCABP leaving room on their form to record the owner's observations.

PHYSICAL EXAMINATION

The bull owner should convey the reason for the BSE, including a relevant history. Generally, only healthy bulls are presented for a BSE; therefore, an all systems style complete examination is not warranted. Breeding bulls must be able to move with ease, detect females in estrus, and be able to mount and complete service. The bull should be observed as he moves up the chute to the examination area. General condition, any lameness, and any abnormal body movement suggestive of pain should be noted. Once in the examination area, the bull should be restrained so as to limit side-to-side and back-forth movement for the remainder of the examination. The examiner should confirm the bull's identification, age, and breed. A systematic general inspection should be done to determine body condition score, to determine if vision appears normal, and to inspect the feet and legs. Congenital defects are more apt to be noticed in young bulls. Some defects, including corkscrew claw, poor foot conformation, and hoof changes associated with laminitis may not be evident until the bull is at least 3 years of age.

Inspection of the scrotum and its contents is an integral part of the physical examination and is most effectively performed from the rear of the animal. The testes should be symmetric, ovoid in shape, have a resilient texture, and be freely movable within the scrotum. Any scars, scabs, or thickening of the scrotum should be noted.[21,22] The epididymides should be easily palpable and symmetric. The cauda or tail, located at the base of the testis, should be firm, not hard, with no distinct swellings or lumps. Epididymitis, either primary or secondary to orchitis, may be a cause of pain, swelling, and discoloration of affected tissues. Common causes of primary epididymitis and orchitis are trauma and bacterial infection. Because the cauda is the principal storage area for mature sperm, a palpably smaller duct may be suggestive of an impairment of sperm production or nonpatency of the tubular genital system upstream.[23] Complete occlusion of the tubular pathway results in the accumulation of sperm, the formation of a spermatocele, and ultimately epithelial rupture with extravasation of sperm into the surrounding tissue. Sperm are recognized as foreign by the immune system with the eventual outcome being granuloma formation. Granulomas are usually found at the apex of the testis in the caput or head of the epididymis, occurring as a result of occlusion of one or more efferent ductules.[23]

Scrotal circumference is an easily measured, highly heritable, fertility-associated trait that is positively correlated with sperm production.[24] Scrotal circumference had positive linear regressions with the percentage of progressively motile sperm and epididymal sperm reserves and a negative linear regression with testicular-origin (primary) sperm defects.[25] Waldner and colleagues[26] reported that cows exposed to bulls with smaller scrotal circumferences (≤34 cm), regardless of breed, were less likely to be pregnant and those that were pregnant required more time to become pregnant. The lack of breeding success was attributed to a decrease in the proportion of morphologically normal sperm and potentially lower numbers of sperm in the ejaculate. Using the volume of a sphere calculation and knowing that each centimeter of scrotal circumference equates to 50 g of testicular tissue,[27] a bull with a 38-cm scrotal circumference has 3 times as much testicular weight as a bull with a 30-cm scrotal circumference, which equates to 3 times as much sperm-producing capacity. More sperm production means that more cows can be successfully mated within a given time period.

A scrotal circumference measurement may be obtained by grasping the scrotum around the scrotal neck with the thumb and forefingers positioned laterally (**Fig. 1**). Next, by sliding the hand down the scrotal neck and squeezing firmly, the testes should be forced, but not squashed, ventrally into the scrotum. The scrotal tape is placed at the widest point on the scrotum and pulled to a moderate tension to obtain the scrotal circumference.[21] The tape should be repositioned and measurement retaken to ensure its accuracy. The interpretation of moderate tension has been a source of error, which led to the development of scrotal tapes with spring-scale mechanisms. The Reliabull (Lane Manufacturing, Inc, Denver, CO) is one such tape marketed today that applies 5 pounds of tension when used according to instructions.[22]

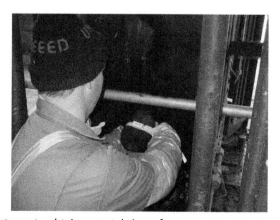

Fig. 1. The correct way to obtain a scrotal circumference measurement.

The internal genitalia are examined transrectally. Accessory sex glands that contribute to semen in the bulls include the ductus deferens, ampullae, seminal vesicles, prostate, and the bulbourethral glands.[28] Seminal vesiculitis is the most common abnormality involving the accessory glands and they should be palpated carefully to assess texture and size.[29] The seminal vesicles are easily identifiable as lobulated glands that diverge laterally from the anterior end of pelvic urethra. They vary in size from 8 to 15 cm long and approximately half as wide. Abnormalities include substantial asymmetry, abscesses, adhesions, fibrosis, and evidence of pain. Effort should be made to identify the paired ampullae that are located between the seminal vesicles. They surround the ductus deferens and are 10 to 15 cm and 5 to 8 mm in diameter.[30] They are rarely abnormal, but are very important when using transrectal massage to facilitate semen collection. Too often examiners overlook the internal inguinal rings. They may be palpated transrectally at a point 15 to 20 cm ventral from the pelvic brim and 5 to 15 cm lateral from the midline. Enlarged rings may allow the examiner to insert 3 or more fingers and are believed to predispose the animal to an inguinal hernia.[22,30]

SEMEN COLLECTION AND EVALUATION
Sperm Production

All veterinarians offering BSE of bulls should develop a firm understanding of spermatogenesis. All is well when the semen sample looks normal and the bull can be easily classified as a "satisfactory" breeder; however, when abnormalities are detected questions arise as to the cause and the prognosis for improvement. Understanding the cause of the abnormality, the nature of the abnormality, the prognosis, and, of course, the effect of the abnormality on fertility are integral components of a breeding soundness assessment.

The testes are encapsulated by the 2-layered testicular capsule consisting of the inner tunica albuginea and the outer visceral vaginal tunic. The inner tan-colored testicular mass, or parenchyma, is composed of numerous seminiferous tubules and supporting interstitial tissue consisting of blood vessels, lymphatics, nerves, connective tissue, and testosterone-producing Leydig cells. Sperm are produced within the highly convoluted seminiferous tubules connected at both ends to the rete tubules located in the central part of the testis. The seminiferous tubules are lined by a basement membrane closely attached to the tubular epithelium referred to as the germinal epithelium. The most prominent cells forming the germinal epithelium are the highly specialized Sertoli cells responsible for nourishing, supporting, and regulating sperm production. The Sertoli cells also produce the fluid that will carry the sperm through the testicular tubular system. Between adjacent Sertoli cells is a complex of tight junctions forming what is referred to as the basal compartment. The tight junctions together with the myoid cells located outside of the basement membrane form the blood-testis barrier necessary for protecting the germ cells from the body's immune systems.[28,31] Moving centrally toward the lumen of the tubule are the deep and peripheral adluminal compartments where more developed germ cells are found.

Spermatogenesis begins with the type A and B spermatogonia that undergo 3 mitotic divisions each to form the primary spermatocytes. Spermatogonia and primary spermatocytes are found in the basal compartment with eventual movement of the primary spermatocytes into the deep adluminal compartment where they give rise to the secondary spermatocytes and round spermatids. Through a complex series of changes involving nuclear condensation, formation of the acrosome and elongation of the tail, the round spermatids are transformed into spermatids. Elongated spermatids are positioned in the peripheral adluminal compartment within deep invaginations into the Sertoli cell cytoplasm for final maturation processes before being released into the tubular lumen as spermatozoa. Once released, spermatozoa, also referred to simply as sperm, flow through the seminiferous tubule to the rete tubules located within the central region of the testis then into the efferent ducts converging into the singular tube of the head (caput) of the epididymis located adjacent to apex or the testis. The sperm make their way from the caput through the body (corpus) and eventually reach the tail (cauda) of the epididymis. During epididymal transit, final maturational changes occur to enable the sperm to be fertile, including gaining the capacity for progressive motility, final condensation of the nucleus, and further modification of the acrosome. Resorption of seminiferous tubule fluid also occurs and sperm are transitioned to a metabolically limited environment to preserve energy reserves. The epididymides of the bull are approximately 40-m long with a transit time of 8 to 11 days, shorter if sperm are depleted from storage. Sperm are stored in the tail of the epididymis, but it is only the distal one-third of the epididymis that is capable of supplying sperm to the ductus deferens and urethra at the time of ejaculation. Stored sperm are not motile, but will become motile when an appropriate buffer or seminal fluid is added. Sperm production is a continuous process, with storage capacity extending in to the ductus deferens and ampulla of the tubular genital system. Ejaculation will reduce stored inventory; however, without ejaculation excess, senescent sperm are normally shed during urination. Sperm can be stored in the tubular storage system for several weeks.[28,31]

From the primordial type A spermatogonia until spermatozoa are released into the tubular lumen requires nearly 62 days. With the addition of 8 to 11 days of epididymal maturation, the total time requirement is more than 70 days.[31]

Semen Collection

Semen may be obtained via transrectal massage of the ampullae, pelvic urethra, and prostate; aspiration from the vagina of a recently bred cow; use of an artificial vagina; or electroejaculation. Collection with an artificial vagina requires tractable bulls, adequate facilities, additional personnel, mount animals, and perhaps the most time-consuming requirement is that nearly all bulls will require some training and patient handling. With the exception of bulls that are collected frequently at bull studs, electroejaculation is the most popular method for collecting semen from bulls in North America. The key advantage of electroejaculation is the ability to obtain a high-quality, representative semen sample very fast and efficiently. The only detractor is that there is a mild to modest amount of pain associated with the procedure; however, it is short-lived and can be ameliorated by using a gentle stimulation technique.[32]

Electrical stimulation is supplied by the electroejaculator unit and delivered to a probe placed in the rectum. Rectal probes have electrodes facing ventrad that lie adjacent to the accessory sex glands and pelvic urethra. Following the examination of the internal genitalia, the examiner may apply a gentle back and forth massage of the rectum, thereby relaxing the anal sphincter to enable placement of the rectal probe. Massage directed specifically at the ampullae, seminal vesicles, and pelvic urethra will sexually excite the bull and has been shown to shorten the duration of electrical stimulation required to obtain a semen sample.[32] Rectal probes vary in diameter to accommodate the various sizes of bulls. To ensure that good contact is maintained between the electrodes and adjacent tissues, the examiner should choose the largest probe that can be comfortably placed in the bull's rectum.

During the electroejaculation process, the examiner should make every effort to achieve penile protrusion. If this does not occur, an assistant can push on the sigmoid flexure just caudal to the scrotum while the operator attempts to grasp the glans penis as it protrudes. A surgical gauze sponge held in the palm of the hand is a safe and effective grasping tool facilitating full extension of the penis. Warts, abrasions, and penile deviations may be evident following penile protrusion. Corkscrew deviations occurring as a result of electroejaculation are a common occurrence and are not considered pathologic, but other deviations are abnormal. Preputial scarring, adhesions, and stenosis are common following preputial lacerations and may prevent full erection. Firm masses are often palpable in the penile sheath indicative of these lesions.

Semen collection is facilitated by the use of a commercially available semen collection handle, in which can be placed a disposable, plastic semen collection funnel attached to a plastic tube. Collection tubes should be kept warm until just before semen is collected. Clear preseminal fluid should not be collected, as it dilutes the sample and, because of chilling, will negatively affect sperm motility if the collection process is prolonged. When the ejaculated fluid becomes cloudy and white, the collection cone should be placed over the penis and a sample obtained. Most mature bulls can be collected very easily with a modest amount of electrical stimulation. A few cases are challenging and will require a variation in collection technique. A common cause of difficulty in mature bulls is the use of a rectal probe that is simply too small - the very large 90-mm probe (Lane Manufacturing, Inc, Denver CO) is indispensable in these cases. Not all bulls can be successfully collected using electroejaculation, and a bull that is difficult to collect will often be difficult to collect at subsequent attempts.

Semen Evaluation

Sperm concentration, motility, and morphology have all been considered important determinants of fertility.[33–38] Density or concentration of the ejaculate is often recorded, but its only real value is as an indicator that the bull is capable of producing a high-quality ejaculate and that the semen collection procedure was appropriate. Electroejaculation is not an appropriate way to assess sperm-producing capability because the volume and density of the semen sample vary with the collection technique. Instead, sperm-producing capability is assessed indirectly by measuring the scrotal circumference. Healthy, mature bulls should produce a milklike, creamy ejaculate; the most concentrated samples appear grainy in appearance and contain 1 billion or more sperm per millimeter.[39] Concentrated margarine-yellow or golden-colored semen samples are a common, normal occurrence associated with the presence of riboflavin. Urine contamination will also cause yellow discoloration; however, urine has a diluting effect. Tainted samples tend to smell of urine or may be confirmed by using a blood urea nitrogen test strip. Depending on the quantity, blood contamination will cause variable discoloration ranging from slight pink to nearly blood red. Both blood and urine negatively affect sperm viability.[40]

Sperm motility is assessed by 1 or 2 approaches. Gross motility or gross wave motion is the fastest and simplest, requiring only the placement of a large drop of semen on a warm microscope slide, which is then viewed using bright field microscopy at ×40 to ×125 magnification. Usually, observation of 1 or 2 fields is all that is necessary; however, gross motility must be interpreted with a view to what it represents. The visual effect of wave motion does not represent only motile sperm, but is generated by a combination of sperm concentration; progressive motility and the rate of speed of the motile sperm. As a result, dilute samples may have a high proportion of motile sperm, but dark swirls typical of a very good gross motility classification are absent. Another common occurrence is when samples become chilled; sperm concentration and motility may be adequate, but the rate of motility has slowed considerably. See gross motility classifications in **Table 2**. Therefore, it is accepted practice that if gross

Table 2 Descriptors for gross motility		
Motility	**Abbreviation**	**Description**
Very Good	VG	Rapid dark swirls
Good	G	Slower swirls and eddies
Fair	F	No swirls, prominent individual cell motion
Poor	P	Little or no individual cell motion

motility is classified as good or very good, the examiner is assured that there are no issues with sperm motility and no further assessment of motility is required. However, if the sample has fair or poor gross motility, then individual motility should be assessed to look for possible reasons for those outcomes. Individual motility or percent progressively motile sperm (**Table 3**) is determined by placing a 2-mm to 4-mm drop of semen on a clean, warm microscope slide and viewing at $\times 200$ to $\times 400$ magnification. Individual sperm are more easily observed when phase contrast is used versus bright field microscopy. Veterinary practices offering bull BSEs should make the modest investment to upgrade their microscopes with phase contrast for the individual motility objective.[39] Individual motility is usually estimated by observing the proportion of sperm moving versus those that are immotile or barely motile. Observing several fields and averaging the proportions of motile sperm recorded generates a much more reliable estimate.[37] Sperm motility can be easily affected by heating, chilling, and contamination with urine or other fluids or soaps, for example. Recording a poor motility classification should always be substantiated by sperm morphology and perhaps vitality (proportion of live sperm). For example, distal midpiece reflexes, or a high percentage of dead sperm are common causes of true poor motility. Bowed midpieces are not a morphologic abnormality, but rather represent sample chilling or contamination affecting sperm membrane integrity. If a finding of poor motility cannot be substantiated, then a second sample should be evaluated. The minimum acceptable individual motility percentage is 30% for the SFT system and 60% for the WCABP system.

Evaluation of sperm morphology begins with a well-prepared smear. Eosin-nigrosin is the most popular stain in use for evaluating bull sperm and is widely available. Eosin penetrates damaged sperm membranes to stain dead and nonviable cells pink; hence, it is referred to as a vitality stain. Nigrosin provides a dark purple background, enhancing the appearance of both live and nonviable cells. Live sperm do not take up the eosin stain and appear white; half-stained sperm are protected by the acrosomal membrane in the anterior end, but eosin has managed to penetrate distal to the equatorial region. Half-stained sperm are of course nonviable, but are common when

Table 3 Descriptors for individual motility		
Motility	**Abbreviation**	**Description[a]**
Very Good	VG	80%–100%
Good	G	60%–79%
Fair	F	40%–59%
Poor	P	<40%

[a] Percent progressively motile sperm.

semen smears are prepared under less than ideal conditions. When semen samples are handled correctly and there are no morphologic defects affecting sperm motility, the proportion of sperm staining live and the percent progressively motile are very positively correlated.[22]

To prepare a semen smear, place a 4- to 5-mm drop of stain at one end of the slide. The stain should always be placed first to limit exposure of the sperm to the damaging effects of chilling and desiccation before fixing with stain. Place a slightly smaller drop of semen adjacent to the stain and immediately mix the 2 together. Wooden stir sticks work well for obtaining droplets of semen and mixing. Using the stir stick, spread the mixture down the length of slide in a stopping and starting fashion to create thick and thin areas of stain. This will help provide the ideal area to count approximately 10 to 20 sperm per microscope field once the slide is dry. Smears should be dried as quickly as possible to prevent the occurrence of bowed tails, an artifactual occurrence due to the hypotonic nature of eosin-nigrosin. This may be accomplished by the use of a slide warmer and by blowing on the slides to speed drying. Differential counts of sperm morphology are done will oil immersion, bright field microscopy at $\times 1000$ magnification, and are made easier by using cell counters. Counting 100 sperm cells will be sufficiently representative if few abnormalities are recorded. When many abnormalities are encountered, it is advised to count at least 300 cells to improve the reliability of the morphology assessment.[22] When using cell counters, 2 keys may be pushed at once for sperm having more than 1 defect, but only 1 cell is counted in the total, hence the proportion of defects is recorded as defects per 100 cells versus number of defective sperm per 100 cells counted.

There are approximately 25 different morphologic sperm defects[22] with images and descriptions widely available in texts, manuals, and information sheets. Use of a good-quality microscope and careful preparation of smears combined with systematic study of each sperm cell form the foundation of a sound sperm morphology evaluation. Diadem vacuoles, tapered heads, and to some degree distal midpiece reflexes, to name a few, are missed or misclassified by inexperienced observers. Sending stained smears to a more experienced colleague for a second opinion is a great way to improve one's assessment skills. Developing an understanding of the pathogenesis of abnormal sperm morphology is necessary for both diagnosis and prognosis.

PATHOGENESIS OF ABNORMAL SPERM MORPHOLOGY

To be classified as a satisfactory breeder, a bull must have greater than 70% morphologically normal sperm. While most unsatisfactory spermiograms exhibit a variety of morphologic defects, occasionally there are smears in which only 1 defect is present. In these cases it is advisable to be more cautious, as a preponderance of a single defect may be indicative of a more serious problem that very well could worsen. As such, spermiograms with more than either 20% sperm head defects, 20% proximal droplets; 25% acrosome or 25% tail abnormalities should not be considered satisfactory.[39]

Morphologically, abnormal sperm are indeed common and at least a few are noted in nearly every semen evaluation with little to no effect on fertility. Large proportions of abnormal sperm are suggestive of a widespread problem affecting extensive areas within several seminiferous tubules. These events are often referred to as disturbances or insults to spermatogenesis. Genetics, toxins, nutritional deficiencies, infectious diseases and seasonal change alone or in combination have been implicated, but by far the 2 most common insults to spermatogenesis in bulls of all ages are heat and stress.[41]

The testes are maintained at 4°C cooler than the body temperature by their external location in the scrotum and the cooling of arterial blood through the countercurrent heat exchange mechanism created by the pampiniform plexus located at the apex of the testis.[42] Dermatitis (including frostbite), orchitis, trauma, and systemic illness have all been shown to interfere with thermoregulation of the testes; nonetheless, the most common cause of abnormal thermoregulation is fat deposition in the scrotal neck associated with obesity[43] (see **Fig. 2**). Not all obese bulls deposit fat in the neck of the scrotum and not all bulls within a given breed will deposit fat similarly; however, fat bulls regardless of breed are more likely to exhibit poor semen quality. Bulls that are 2 years of age and older are most at risk with the blame residing with the prevailing notion that fat bulls are more visually appealing at shows and sales.[42] Younger, more rapidly growing bulls are less likely to have fat deposition in the scrotal neck. The testes function on the brink of hypoxia such that increases in ambient temperature lead to increases in cell metabolism, hence the true effect of increased temperature is hypoxia.[44] The effect on spermatogenesis can range from what might be called an insult to spermatogenesis associated with 20% to 50% morphologically abnormal sperm on the smear to what is referred to as testicular degeneration. Testicular degeneration is a term used to describe a loss of scrotal circumference, softening of the testicles, and a substantial increase in the number of morphologically abnormal sperm; often greater than 80%. These changes are a result of widespread loss of germinal layers affecting most, if not all, of the seminiferous tubules. If the Sertoli cells and spermatogonia remain intact, then there is a good chance that spermatogenesis will return to normal, but several weeks to months will be required. More severe or longstanding degenerative changes may never resolve.[43]

Stress caused by illness, injury, pain, hunger, or inclement weather affects testicular function indirectly through the release of cortisol. Cortisol suppresses luteinizing hormone and follicle-stimulating hormone secretion, which in turn decreases testosterone production by the Leydig cells. Sertoli cell function is under endocrine control; therefore, any change in hormone production affects spermatogenesis. Bulls on the show circuit, are lame, or are experiencing a long period of inclement weather are sufficiently stressed to show an effect on sperm morphology. A good rule of thumb is that to have an effect, the stress usually needs to be at least of 3 or 4 days' duration.

The last 18 days of spermatogenesis (called spermiogenesis) is when round spermatids are transformed into elongated spermatids, then finally spermatozoa are ready for release into the tubule lumen. Spermatids are the most vulnerable of the germ cell types to insults; therefore, morphologic changes are most likely to occur during this time period. Cells in meiosis are also very sensitive to insults, but tend to degenerate,

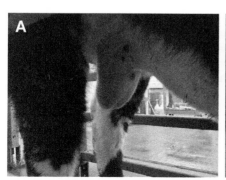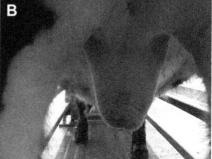

Fig. 2. Bull with excessive fat in the neck of the scrotum (*A*) Front/side view. (*B*) Rear view.

leaving spaces in the germinal epithelium with the end result being fewer sperm produced.[31] Remarkably, heat and stress showed little difference in the type of sperm defects and the sequence of their appearance. Following either scrotal insulation for 4 days or the administration of 20 mg dexamethasone intramuscularly daily for 7 days to mimic stress, the percentage of normal sperm reached the lowest at 3 weeks and returned to pretreatment levels by 6 weeks after the treatments began.[45]

Morphologic abnormalities have been classified according to where the defect was thought to originate, or whether or not the defect was known at the time of classification to have an effect on fertility. Such systems were perhaps suitable in their day, but are confusing and not practical for the practicing veterinarian.[22] Instead, effort should be made to understand the cause and significance of the most prevalent defects. A differential count of the sperm defects also should be done to determine the potential impact on fertility. Knowing whether a sperm defect may be compensated for by increasing the dose, thereby increasing the quantity of normal sperm versus a non-compensable defect that cannot be compensated for by increasing the sperm dosage is an important next step. For example, sperm lacking progressive motility are compensable. Detached heads, distal midpiece reflexes, and coiled principal pieces will not be transported through the cervix or will be removed before they reach the oviduct. Sperm with the knobbed acrosome defect can travel normally to the ovum, but are unable to penetrate the zona pellucida; therefore, normal sperm may compensate.[22,46] Provided the head shape has not been distorted, sperm with nuclear vacuoles are able to penetrate the zona pellucida, thereby preventing access to other sperm. Increasing the dose in such cases will not increase the odds that a normal sperm will be more likely to fertilize the ovum.[22,46,47] Continued research will help advance our knowledge on the true effect of selected sperm defects on fertility. An important finding has been that sperm possessing proximal droplets will not attach to the ovum in vitro and, surprisingly, otherwise normal-appearing sperm in the same ejaculate also exhibit a reduced ability to bind to ova.[22]

SUMMARY

To be classified as a satisfactory potential breeder using either the WCABP or SFT systems, a bull must be physically sound including achieving the minimum scrotal circumference and must have greater than 70% morphologically normal sperm with greater than 60% (WCABP) or greater than 30% (SFT) progressively motile sperm. In addition, the WCABP system has questionable, decision-deferred, and unsatisfactory categories, whereas the SFT system has unsatisfactory and classification-deferred categories. Each organization provides criteria for classification in these categories.

Mature bulls must be managed appropriately year-round to ensure that they are ready for the short and intense breeding season. Bulls house or pastured in groups should be of similar age and moved from pasture to paddock with a view to social hierarchy. Mature bulls may be joined with females at up to 1:40 (bull:female), but must be observed for social dominance, libido, and injury-related issues.

REFERENCES

1. King EH. Management of breeding bull batteries. In: Hopper RM, editor. Bovine reproduction. Ames (IA): Wiley Blackwell; 2015. p. 92–6.
2. Brito LFC. Bull development: sexual development and puberty in bulls. In: Hopper RM, editor. Bovine reproduction. Ames (IA): Wiley Blackwell; 2015. p. 41–57.

3. Setchell BP. Spermatogenesis and spermatozoa. In: Austin C, Short R, editors. Reproduction in mammals, 1: germ cells and fertilization. 2nd edition. Cambridge (United Kingdom): Cambridge University Press; 1994. p. 1363.

4. Cobo E, Cipolla A, Morsella C, et al. Effect of two commercial vaccines to campylobacter fetus subspecies on heifers naturally challenged. J Vet Med B Infect Dis Vet Public Health 2003;50:75–80.

5. Vasquez LA, Ball L, Bennet BW, et al. Bovine genital campylobacteriosis (vibriosis): vaccination of experimentally infected bulls. Am J Vet Res 1983;44:1553–7.

6. Cobo ER, Corbeil LB, Gershwin LJ, et al. Preputial cellular and antibody responses of bulls vaccinated and/or challenged with tritrichomonas foetus. Vaccine 2010;28:361–70.

7. Cobo ER, Corbeil LB, BonDurant RH. Immunity to infections in the lower genital tract of bulls. J Reprod Immunol 2011;89:55–61.

8. Kirkland PD, McGowan MR, Mackintosh SG. The outcome of widespread use of semen from a bull persistently infected with pestivirus. Vet Rec 1994;135:527–9.

9. Kirkland PD, McGowan MR, Mackintosh SG, et al. Insemination of cattle with semen from a bull transiently infected with pestivirus. Vet Rec 1997;140:124–7.

10. Newcomer BW, Toohey-Kurth K, Zhang Y, et al. Laboratory diagnosis and transmissibility of bovine viral diarrhea virus from a bull with a persistent testicular infection. Vet Microbiol 2014;170:246–7.

11. Paton DJ, Goodey R, Brockman S, et al. Evaluation of the quality and virological status of semen from bulls acutely infected with BVDV. Vet Rec 1989;124:63.

12. Givens M. Assessment of available vaccines for bulls to prevent transmission of reproductive pathogens. Clinical Theriogenology 2012;4:308–13.

13. Stewart JL, Shipley CF, Ireland FA, et al. Long-term effects of clinical applications of pyrethrin and cyfluthrin, a synthetic pyrethroid, on bull reproductive parameters. Clinical Theriogenology 2015;7:309.

14. Blockey MAdeB. Observations on group mating of bulls at pasture. Appl Anim Ethol 1979;5:15–34.

15. Rupp GP, Ball L, Shoop MC, et al. Reproductive efficiency of bulls in natural service: effects of male to female ratio and single- vs multiple-sire breeding groups. J Am Vet Med Assoc 1977;171:639–42.

16. Petherick JC. A review of some factors affecting the expression of libido in beef cattle, and individual bull and herd fertility. Appl Anim Behav Sci 2005;90: 185–205.

17. Holroyd RG, Doogan VJ, De Faveri J, et al. Bull selection and use in northern Australia 4. Calf output and predictors of fertility in multiple-sire herds. Anim Reprod Sci 2002;71:67–79.

18. Fordyce G, Fitzpatrick LA, Cooper NJ, et al. Bull selection and use in northern Australia 5. Social behaviour and management. Anim Reprod Sci 2002;71:81–9.

19. Hopper RM. Breeding soundness in the bull: concepts and historical perspective. In: Hopper RM, editor. Bovine reproduction. Ames (IA): Wiley Blackwell; 2015. p. 58–67.

20. Alexander JH. Bull breeding soundness evaluation: a practitioner's perspective. Theriogenology 2008;70:469–72.

21. Monke DR. Examination of the bovine scrotum, testicles, and epididymides–part I. Compend Contin Educ Pract Vet 1987;9:F252–5.

22. Barth AD. Bull breeding soundness. 3rd edition. Saskatoon (SK): Western Canadian Association of Bovine Practitioners; 2013. p. 14–49.

23. Monke DR. Examination of the bovine scrotum, testicles and epididymides–part II. Compend Contin Educ Pract Vet 1987;9:F277–83.

24. Steffen D. Genetic causes of bull infertility. Vet Clin North Am 1997;13:243–53.
25. Kastelic JP, Cook RB, Pierson RA, et al. Relationships among scrotal and testicular characteristics, sperm production and seminal quality in 129 beef bulls. Can J Vet Res 2001;65:111–5.
26. Waldner CL, Kennedy RI, Palmer CW. A description of the findings from bull breeding soundness evaluations and their association with pregnancy outcomes in a study of western Canadian beef herds. Theriogenology 2010;74:871–83.
27. Coulter GH, Keller DG. Scrotal circumference of young beef bulls: relationship to paired-testes weight, effect of breed and predictability. Can J Anim Sci 1982;62: 133–9.
28. Senger PL. The organization and function of the male reproductive system. In: Senger PL, editor. Pathways to pregnancy and parturition. 2nd edition. Pullman (WA): Current Conceptions, Inc; 2003. p. 44–79.
29. Alexander J. Evaluation of breeding soundness: the physical examination. In: Hopper RM, editor. Bovine reproduction. Ames (IA): Wiley Blackwell; 2015. p. 64–7.
30. Cates WF. Examination of the bull for breeding soundness. Vet Clin North Am 1983;5:157–67.
31. Barth AD, Oko RJ. Normal bovine spermatogenesis and sperm maturation. In: Barth AD, Oko RJ, editors. Abnormal morphology of bovine spermatozoa. Ames (IA): Iowa State University Press; 1989. p. 19–88.
32. Palmer CW. Welfare aspects of theriogenology: investigating alternatives to electroejaculation of bulls. Theriogenology 2005;64:469–79.
33. Larsen RE, Littell R, Rooks E, et al. Bull influences on conception percentage and calving date in angus, Hereford, Brahman and Senepol single-sire herds. Theriogenology 1990;34:549–68.
34. Peet RL, Kluck P, McCarth M. Infertility in 2 Murray grey bulls associated with abaxial and swollen midpiece sperm defects. Aust Vet J 1998;65:359–60.
35. Barth AD, Oko RJ. Introduction. In: Barth AD, Oko RJ, editors. Abnormal morphology of bovine spermatozoa. Ames (IA): Iowa State University Press; 1989. p. 3–7.
36. Soderquist L, Janson L, Larsson K, et al. Sperm morphology and fertility in AI bulls. Zentralbl Veterinarmed A 1991;38:534–43.
37. Foote RH. Fertility estimation: a review of past experience and future prospects. Anim Reprod Sci 2003;75:119–39.
38. Clarke RH, O'Neill GH, Hewetson RW, et al. The predictability of fertility from semen scores. Aust Vet J 1973;49:498.
39. Barth AD. Evaluation of potential breeding soundness of the bull. In: Youngquist RS, editor. Current therapy in large animal theriogenology. Philadelphia: W.B. Saunders; 1997. p. 222–36.
40. Hopper RM, King EH. Evaluation of breeding soundness: basic examination of the semen. In: Hopper RM, editor. Bovine reproduction. Ames (IA): Wiley Blackwell; 2015. p. 68–78.
41. Johnson WH. The significance to bull fertility of morphologically abnormal sperm. Vet Clin North Am 1997;13:255–82.
42. Barth AD, Cates WF, Harland RJ. The effect of amount of body fat and loss of fat on breeding soundness classification of beef bulls. Can Vet J 1995;36:758–64.
43. Barth A. Testicular degeneration. In: Hopper RM, editor. Bovine reproduction. Ames (IA): Wiley Blackwell; 2015. p. 103–8.
44. Waites GMH, Setchell BP. Effects of local heating on blood flow and metabolism in the testis of the conscious ram. J Reprod Fertil 1964;8:339.

45. Barth AD, Bowman PA. The sequential appearance of sperm abnormalities after scrotal insulation or dexamethasone treatment in bulls. Can Vet J 1994;34: 93–102.
46. Kastelic JP, Thundathil JC. Breeding soundness evaluation and semen analysis for predicting bull fertility. Reprod Domest Anim 2008;43(Suppl 2):368–73.
47. Saake R, Nadir S, Nebel R. Relationship of semen quality to sperm transport, fertilization, and embryo quality in ruminants. Theriogenology 1994;41:45.

Management of Male Reproductive Tract Injuries and Disease

Richard M. Hopper, DVM

KEYWORDS

- Bull • Urogenital • Surgery • Penis • Prepuce • Scrotum • Trauma

KEY POINTS

- The replacement cost of many breeding bulls justifies treatment of injuries if there is a reasonable prognosis for success.
- Some of the conditions described are amiable to medical treatment, and there are time-tested surgical techniques for others.
- Early recognition and immediate initiation of treatment decrease the potential for further damage from secondary infection and fibrosis, thus, improving prognosis and decreasing the time to recovery/return to function.
- Surgical procedures that cannot be performed in a chute can be performed with tilt table restraint coupled with heavy sedation and regional analgesia.
- The correct estimation of prognosis is of importance as an animal identified as having a condition with a poor prognosis can be culled in such a manner as to maximum salvage value.

INTRODUCTION

Injuries to the reproductive tract are a frequent occurrence and carry the potential of ending the functional use of a bull. Elite breeding bulls of high genetic potential have always been of a sufficient economic value to justify efforts at medical and surgical restoration. However, even bulls selected for use in commercial herds require a significant purchase price investment representing an economic threshold for which even extensive treatment is justified in many situations.

The knowledgeable cowman understands the value of a Veterinary Breeding Soundness Examination (VBSE) performed before each breeding season and the need to closely observe bulls during the breeding season. Indeed it is through these

The author has nothing to disclose.
Theriogenology, Food Animal Medicine & Ambulatory, Department of Pathobiology & Population Medicine, College of Veterinary Medicine, Mississippi State University, 4561 South Montgomery, Starkville, MS 39759, USA
E-mail address: hopper@cvm.msstate.edu

Vet Clin Food Anim 32 (2016) 497–510
http://dx.doi.org/10.1016/j.cvfa.2016.01.015
0749-0720/16/$ – see front matter © 2016 Elsevier Inc. All rights reserved.
vetfood.theclinics.com

two distinct activities that virtually all reproductive tract maladies can be identified. During a properly performed routine VBSE as directed by the standards of the Society for Theriogenology, fibropapillomas, hair rings, minor preputial injury, and vesicular adenitis should be identified. The observant cowman who checks his or her bulls daily and observes mating activity should notice problems that lead him or her to seek veterinary intervention, which in turn should lead to the identification of such maladies as penile hematoma, preputial prolapse, phimosis, paraphimosis, or an injury that has led to a denervation, vascular shunt, or deviation.

HEMATOMA OF THE PENIS

Hematoma of the penis is probably the most common injury of the penis. This injury occurs when the penis misses the intended target, hits the cow's perineum, and bends. Although it usually occurs in young inexperienced bulls,[1–4] it can also occur in the older bull, which, because of orthopedic injury or pain, has altered his approach during mounting. The hematoma is due to rupture of the tunica albuginea and the subsequent hemorrhage from the corpus cavernosum. The initial volume of blood escaping is less than 250 mL,[1] but the size of the resultant hematoma varies as each subsequent erection results in further hemorrhage. Thus, the hematoma may range in size from 15 to 30 cm. The resultant swelling occurs in the sheath over and cranial to the rudimentary teats.

A prolapsed prepuce often results secondary to a penile hematoma, and this in fact may be the owner's reason for seeking help. Diagnosis may be aided with ultrasound. Do not attempt to aspirate the swelling as inadvertent introduction of bacteria can convert a hematoma to an abscess. It has been reported that smaller (<20 cm) hematomas respond almost as well to conservative medical therapy as they do to surgery, but larger (>20 cm) hematomas have a much better response (75%–80% vs 33%) with surgery[5]; so medical therapy is a viable option for small hematomas and a reasonable alternative for any bull whose value prohibits an investment in surgery.

Regardless of which treatment plan is followed, systemic antibiotic treatment should be instituted immediately. Medical treatment consists of a continuation of antibiotics (procaine penicillin: 44,000 IU/kg, intramuscularly, twice a day), hydrotherapy, and sexual rest. If surgery is to be performed, 5 to 7 days after occurrence has been shown to be the optimal time frame.[6] Given that the owner or attendant typically may not notice this problem for 2 to 3 days and that patients should be starved for 36 to 48 hours before surgery, surgery must be scheduled immediately in an attempt to fit that best time frame and avoid the clot organization and fibrosis that begins to occur 10 days after injury.

Once the decision is made to attempt surgical correction, antibiotic therapy is instituted if not already begun and feed is removed. The bull is starved for 36 to 48 hours and water withheld overnight. General anesthesia can be used, or regional anesthesia coupled with heavy sedation may be selected.[7] Either way the bull is placed in right lateral recumbency on a tilt table with the left hind leg pulled back and up and fastened securely. The surgical area is prepped, and a 20- to 25-cm vertical incision is made just cranial to the rudimentary teat. Careful dissection, attention to hemostasis, and manual removal of the blood clot follows. Lavage with a warm saline plus povidone-iodine (Betadine Prep Solution) aids in the removal of additional clots and, coupled with blunt dissection, identification of the lesion (**Fig. 1**). Careful blunt or manual dissection is not just preferred over scalpel or scissor dissection but mandatory as injury to the area vasculature and nerves must be avoided. Specifically, the area near the dorsal nerve of the penis must be avoided. Because identification of this

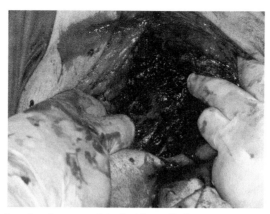

Fig. 1. Rent in tunica albuginea associated with penile hematoma.

area can be confusing as penile manipulation changes the anatomic context, it is useful to identify the urethra, which is on the ventral aspect of the penis and, thus, 180° from the dorsum.

After the tear or rent is identified, carefully lavage the area again and debride the often tattered edges of the rent. This debridement must be minimal as excessive removal of tissue complicates closure and following healing there is the potential that the bull will have trouble extending his penis. Closure of the defect with No. 1 PGA in a bootlace pattern is the long-standing recommendation and justifiably so, as there is enough wound tension to make simple interrupted suture patterns problematic. The elastic layers over the penis can be closed with 3-0 chromic gut in a simple continuous pattern. The penis is then returned to its normal position; the subcutaneous tissues are closed with 0 chromic gut, and the skin can be closed with a 6-mm Braunamid typically with a Ford interlocking pattern. Antibiotics are continued for 5 to 7 days. The bull should have 60 to 90 days of sexual rest following surgery. Seroma formation occurs often enough that it probably should not be considered a true complication.

Complications include abscess, suture dehiscence, permanent analgesia to the penis, and reoccurrence during the subsequent breeding seasons.[8] Permanent analgesia, that is, loss of sensation, likely results from the initial injury rather than from the surgery.

PREPUTIAL INJURY

Preputial prolapse is alternatively a predisposing factor for or result of trauma and bruising of the prepuce. It is more common in the Brahman-influenced breeds because of their pendulous sheath, redundant preputial tissue, and larger preputial orifice.[1,9–11] Polled breeds typically lack the preputial retractor muscle, thus, exacerbating the condition when combining genetics with the Brahman. Minor trauma with prolapse (grade 1) can be treated with various medications and wrapped. More extensive trauma with swelling and the presence of necrotic tissue (grades 2–4) requires surgical correction because these cases result in fibrosis of the preputial tissue if not correctly resolved. In any case, medical treatment should be instituted as soon as possible either as the primary method of management or as a necessary precursor for surgery.

Before bandaging the prepuce, the wounds should be cleaned and an attempt should be made to replace the prolapse. This can be facilitated with hydrotherapy (water hose spray, showerhead spray, or soaking) (**Fig. 2**). Soaking the prolapsed prepuce in a hypertonic solution (The author adds both salt and sugar so that the solution will be very hypertonic without being too irritating) with povidone iodine also serves to aid in the debridement of the tissue. Then after drying, an ointment is applied. The author prefers the petrolatum, tetracycline, and scarlet red oil mixture (Petercillin-Auburn)[1] for severely traumatized, necrotic wounds. The author uses less irritating ointments or mixtures for less affected tissue or after several days of treatment when the tissue is less swollen. Options for this are commercially available udder balms, intramammary infusion ointments, or sugardine (Betadine + sugar). A 6- to 10-in rigid plastic tube (milk line or equine nasogastric tubes can be used) is then placed within the prepuce to allow urination, and the prepuce is wrapped with elasticon (**Fig. 3**). In addition to facilitating urination, the placement of the tube helps decrease the circumferential scarring of the preputial orifice, which results in phimosis. Bandage change intervals are dictated by the extent of damage, the bull's tolerance for the bandage, and whether or not you can completely replace the prepuce within the sheath. Following resolution of swelling due to infection and/or inflammation, a decision can be made to return the bull to use or to initiate surgical correction.

Often a client will choose to cull rather than allow treatment. Because these bulls are the victims of severe price discrimination, the author will offer a salvage-type procedure. A large swine rectal (prolapse) ring or short length of polyvinyl chloride (PVC) pipe is placed within the preputial lumen dorsal to the lesion, and a band is placed around the prepuce over the pipe. This technique will amputate the damaged prepuce, but fibrosis and stenosis will likely occur. Alternatively holes can be drilled in the PVC pipe before placement; rather than a band, heavy (6 mm) Braunamid is used in an overlapping pattern that serves to both fix the tube and provide for hemostasis when the end of the prepuce is amputated. This technique is the ring amputation procedure and can be performed with the bull standing, using local analgesia and chute restraint. This procedure usually results in some degree of stricture and also may be considered for the client that desires a more economical option than treatment followed with surgical correction by circumcision. It should be noted that correction with the circumcision technique remains an option for bulls in which the ring amputation resulted in a stricture.

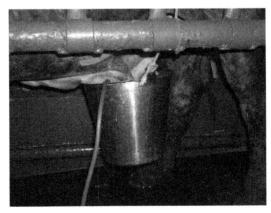

Fig. 2. Soaking prepuce.

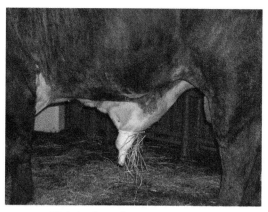

Fig. 3. Bandaged prepuce with tube for urine egress.

The surgical technique that is advocated by the author is the circumcision or reefing technique. This procedure can be performed with regional analgesia and sedation. Before surgery, the bull is starved for 36 to 48 hours and water withheld overnight. The bull is placed in right lateral recumbency, and the hair of the sheath is clipped. The penis is extended and maintained in extension with towel forceps that engage the apical ligament. The penis and prepuce are prepped (NO alcohol) and draped. Apply a tourniquet using 1-in Penrose tubing proximal to the area to be transected. The amount of prepuce to be resected is then determined (the remaining prepuce must be a minimum length of 1.5 times the free portion)[12]; marker sutures are placed to ensure that tissues are returned to the proper alignment, and 2 circumferential incisions are made. These incisions are joined with a longitudinal incision. These incisions are to be very superficial so that with careful, sharp dissection, underlying tissue, blood vessels, and lymphatics will be spared. The area of fibrosis should be included in the tissue removed. Following dissection and tourniquet removal (the tourniquet can be maintained safely for up to 1 hour), hemorrhage is controlled by vessel ligation and/or cautery. When hemostasis is achieved, lavage the area with a warm solution of sterile saline with 50 mL Betadine Prep Solution added per liter. The edges are sutured with a simple continuous subcuticular pattern using your choice of 2-0 absorbable suture material.

Do not use one continuous suture pattern, but instead end the pattern and restart in 3 stages to avoid a constrictive (purse-string) effect. Do not close dead space. Close the skin with a row of staples or your choice of suture patterns with 0 chromic gut. Then suture in place the Penrose tubing over the end of the penis. Apply an antibiotic ointment to the wound, and place the free end of the Penrose tubing into a 6- to 10-in rigid tube. The penis and prepuce are carefully returned into the sheath and bandaged. The bandage can stay on as long as a week; the staples can be removed in 2 weeks. A support wrap (bull diaper) can be used to protect the bandage and prevent pendulous swelling.

Preputial injuries that occur on bulls of English or Continental (*Bos taurus*) breeds typically result in stricture-induced phimosis (inability to extend the penis out of the prepuce) rather than prolapse and, therefore, represent a different sort of challenge. If the penis is forcefully extended but not immediately repaired and replaced within the sheath, paraphimosis (protrusion of the penis with an inability to retract the penis into the prepuce) may result. The preputial cavity can be lavaged with an antiseptic solution followed by application of an ointment of your choice. Second intention healing will result in functional recovery in many bulls. After 60 to 90 days, ascertain the extent of remaining fibrosis and whether or not the penis can be extended (some bulls that can extend will still require surgery). For bulls with residual phimosis, the scar tissue must be removed to allow easy, painless, and full extension of the penis. Unlike the Brahman-influenced bull, *Bos taurus* bulls rarely have enough preputial tissue to allow for a circumcision. A scar revision technique is used. Following regional analgesia and preparation as described previously, an elliptical incision that includes the scar is made. The incision is made on whatever plane necessary to facilitate dissection of the scar but closed on a longitudinal plane (**Fig. 4**). Closure technique is crucial. A bootlace pattern is initiated distally (on the extended penis) and then continued proximally.

After completion, the penis is released and allowed to return back within the prepuce BEFORE the suture ends are tied.[1] Tightening and tying off the suture before this will prevent retraction. A Penrose drain is sutured to the end of the penis to facilitate urine drainage as described in the previous technique, but bandaging is usually not required. The sutures can be removed in 2 weeks or an absorbable suture can be used. The penis should be extended and examined before return to service.

In the case of either a circumcision or scar revision, the bulls should receive 3 months of sexual rest before return to service.

Paraphimosis with resultant injury from penile exposure can be managed with a combination of medical and surgical therapy. Because of the inability to completely retract the penis, significant damage to the epithelial layers of the penis occurs (**Fig. 5**). Soaking the affected areas, as described previously for preputial prolapse, should occur immediately and continued daily until the normal appearance of the tissue returns. In between the daily therapeutic soaking, the penis is covered with stockinette that has been coated in a suitable ointment (the author's preference is one of the commercially available bag balms). Realize that 3 to 4 weeks of medical management is often required before the tissue is healed and surgery can be performed. Once the superficial layers are healed, a scar revision procedure to allow the penis to resume normal retraction/extension can be performed (**Fig. 6**).

FIBROPAPILLOMA (WARTS)

Fibropapilloma or warts are a common finding in young cattle younger than 24 months. Group housing of young bulls along with a predisposition for homosexual behavior both increase the incidence and add to the possibility that the penis will be among the affected locations. Penile warts are usually identified at the time of a VBSE[9] or by an owner that notices a young bull that is reluctant or unable to breed (**Fig. 7**). Bulls may present with either a phimosis or paraphimosis.

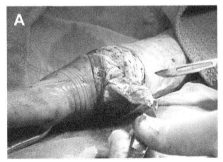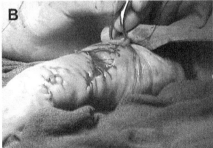

Fig. 4. (*A, B*) Scar revision incision and closure with bootlace suture pattern.

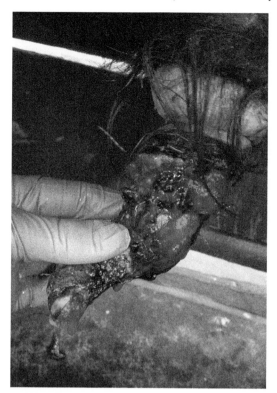

Fig. 5. Paraphimosis on admission.

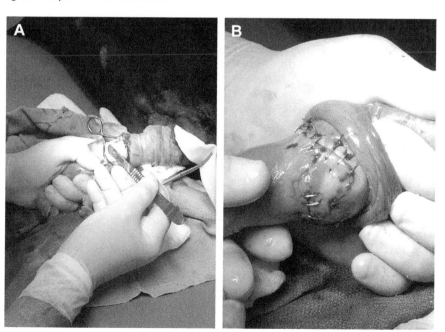

Fig. 6. (*A, B*) Images of a scar resection/revision that allows retraction of penis (note that the fibrosis that prohibited the penis from retraction into the prepuce is on the free portion of the penis and bootlace suture closure was not necessary).

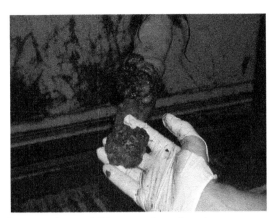

Fig. 7. Severe penile warts that prohibits retraction of penis.

Careful surgical removal whether by excision, cryotherapy, use of a laser, alone, or in conjunction with immunization is a management option. Immunization can be accomplished with the use of a commercial wart vaccine; in fact, the author personally recommends the use of a wart vaccine for bulls being prepared for shipment to bull test stations where they would be housed with multiple bulls from multiple sources. When this is a continuous herd problem, utilization of an autogenous vaccine is a useful management tool.[7]

HAIR RING

Although far less common than warts, the presence of a hair ring also occurs because of homosexual behavior and group housing of young bulls. Accumulation of hair during riding and the continuous action of riding, extension, and retraction of the penis serves to create a tight band of hair. These bands are typically identified during a VBSE, and treatment is simply removal and application of a suitable ointment. Careful examination to determine the depth of the lesion and possible damage to the urethra[9] is warranted. Small fistulae will typically heal, but those that are larger or more proximally located should be closed with a simple interrupted pattern using 3-0 chromic catgut. Denervation is also possible but certainly rare.

TESTICULAR INJURY

Trauma to the scrotum often results in rupture of the vaginal tunic, which leads to hemorrhage, swelling, and permanent damage to the testicle. Diagnosis is typically straightforward based on palpable differences between the affected and unaffected testes. The use of ultrasound and thermography can aid in establishing the prognosis. Cases that present shortly after injury may not have had significant changes to the spermiogram yet and cryopreservation of semen can be attempted for a short period of time. Studies in which scrotal insulation is applied reveal that spermatogenesis is altered within hours[13–15] of a thermal insult and abnormally high temperatures as measured by thermography will persist for at least 3 weeks after a testicle has been removed.[16]

The primary goal of management is based on salvaging the function of the contralateral testicle. To this end, the thermoregulatory process of the contralateral testicle must be preserved. Chronic thermal insult results in testicular degeneration, so surgical removal (hemi-castration) should be performed as soon as reasonably possible. However, the administration of antibiotics and a nonsteroidal antiinflammatory drug can be initiated as soon as the diagnosis is made, while awaiting surgery. Cold-water hydrotherapy may also be helpful in decreasing damage to the contralateral testicle while the bull awaits surgery and during the postsurgical recovery period.[17]

The technique for hemilateral or unilateral castration is straightforward and can be performed on the bull with a combination of sedation, good restraint, and local anesthesia. If the bull is to be placed in lateral recumbency on a tilt table, he should be starved for 48 hours and water withheld overnight. Antibiotics are begun the day before surgery and continued for at least 5 days after surgery. A local anesthetic can be injected into the neck of the scrotum, infiltrating the spermatic cord.[18] The surgical area is prepared for aseptic surgery, as the scrotum will be closed. An elliptical incision the length of the testicle, taking care to leave the parietal tunic intact, will provide excellent exposure and serve to minimize dead space following removal of the testicle and closure. After blunt dissection to free the testicle, the parietal tunic is excised to expose the testicle and the spermatic cord. The cremaster muscle is transected, and the spermatic artery and vein are double ligated with an absorbable suture (No. 0 or larger). Remove most of the parietal tunic, leaving only enough to suture over the cord stump. The cord can be closed with No. 0 absorbable suture followed by closer of the dead space with the same suture material. The incision can then be closed with a No. 2 Braunamid using a suture pattern of your choice. Placing a Penrose drain seems to be associated with an increase incidence of infection and is contraindicated; allowing exercise as opposed to stall confinement will limit postsurgical swelling.

VESICULAR ADENITIS

Vesicular adenitis, which is often and incorrectly referred to as seminal vesiculitis, is most commonly encountered in yearling bulls at the time of VBSE and is typically manifested by enlarged vesicular glands and pus (white blood cells [WBCs]) in the ejaculate.[19] The administration of systemic antibiotics, specifically a single tulathromycin injection or 2 tilmicosin injections 3 days apart (both at label dose), have been shown to be effective as have intraglandular injections of procaine penicillin (at 10% the recommended parental dose in an injection volume of 6 mL).[20] The same study also reported that a significant number of young bulls will recover without treatment.

Thus, the most reasonable management approach for young bulls diagnosed with this condition at VBSE is the administration of one of the aforementioned systemic antibiotics followed by a VBSE recheck in 30 to 45 days. Note WBCs in an ejaculate can be identified, as they are about 1.5 times the width of a bovine sperm head. However, if there is a question as to identification, you can stain a semen sample with Giemsatype (Diff-Quik) stain.

For cases that are nonresponsive to systemic treatment, an intraglandular antibiotic treatment can be used. Additionally, chemical ablation of the entire vesicle can be accomplished with the injection of 15 to 40 mL of 4% formaldehyde solution into the gland.[21]

Intraglandular injection can be most easily performed following epidural analgesia, by first placing a 12-gauge needle through the skin in the ischiorectal fossa. This placement will facilitate the passage of a long (40–44 cm) 18- or 16-gauge needle (**Fig. 8**). Those with a stylet will be easier to direct. Successful results of intraglandular antibiotic injection have been documented,[20,22] and an informal survey of

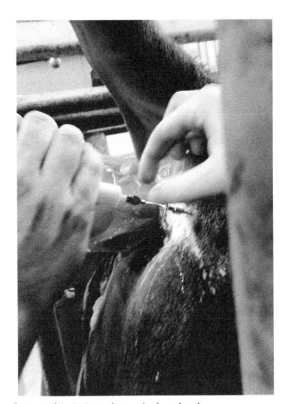

Fig. 8. Injection of an antibiotic into the vesicular gland.

veterinarians who have used the intraglandular injection of 4% formaldehyde reveals that it is a very good option for refractory cases (Dwight Wolfe, DVM, MS, Auburn, AL, Mike Thompson, DVM, Holly Springs, MS, Gary Warner, DVM, Elgin, TX, personal communication, 2015).

LESS FREQUENTLY OCCURRING INJURIES

Although most cavernosal shunts and penile deviations are developmental, some can result from breeding injuries. Shunts can occur following penile hematoma (regardless of treatment vs nontreatment), and penile deviation can follow an injury to the free portion of the penis that results in fibrosis. Likewise, denervation of the penis can follow any injury in which the dorsum of the penis is involved.

Observation of the breeding act is useful in the diagnosis of these 3 conditions. A bull with a cavernosal shunt will lose his erection, whereas those with a penile deviation or denervation will typically miss the vulva and do not achieve intromission.

Spiral and ventral deviations of the penis typically result because of abnormalities of the apical ligament.[23] A ventral deviation can occur following an injury to the free portion of the penis (**Fig. 9**). This deviation, as with those of a developmental cause, can be repaired with a fascia lata implant technique described by Walker and Young.[24] A rectangular strip of fascia is harvested from the bull, cleaned (areolar tissue removed), and placed between the apical ligament and the tunica albuginea. Alternatively, synthetic surgical mesh material can be used to substitute for the fascia implant.

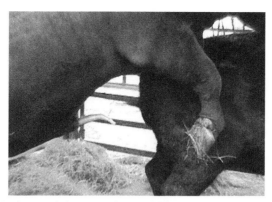

Fig. 9. A ventral deviation of the penis, first identified at annual VBSE at 5 years of age.

Utilization of the mesh has the obvious advantage of removing the time-consuming fascia-harvesting step. However, problems with postoperative infection with the mesh materials of the day along with dissatisfaction with the apical ligament strip technique were the impetus stated by Walker and Young[24] for the development of this technique. Thus, the fascia lata technique is described; those who prefer to can easily modify the technique to use surgical mesh.

The bull is starved for 48 hours and water withheld overnight. Depending on its degree of fractiousness, the bull is sedated with 10 to 20 mg xylazine and 10 mg acepromazine intravenously. With the bull restrained and standing, the surgical site, an area on the upper left hind limb, is prepped because the bull will later be placed in lateral recumbency on his right side. A local block using an inverted L injection pattern is administered. A 15- to 20-cm incision is then made using the patella and greater trochanter as anatomic guides, with the incision being midway between. When the fascia lata is exposed, remove a rectangle-shaped section. Removing a section that is 3 cm wide by 15 cm long will provide more than enough tissue for your graft (**Fig. 10**).

Place the tissue in saline maintaining sterility, and suture the edges of the fascia with a continuous pattern using any No. 1 or 2 dissolvable suture. Failure to do so will result in painful muscle herniation. The skin can be closed with a No. 3 Braunamid using a Ford interlocking pattern. The harvested tissue is then prepared by rinsing in the saline and removing any attached tissue.

The bull can then be prepared for the placing of this graft material. As with the other surgeries described, general anesthesia can be used or, alternatively, regional anesthesia with heavy sedation is an option. The bull is placed on a tilt table in right lateral recumbency, and the preputial area is clipped and prepped. The penis is then extended and the apical ligament identified and grasped with towel forceps. The penis is prepared with Betadine Surgical Scrub, rinsed with sterile water or saline, and dried. Unlike when performing a circumcision, a tourniquet is not used, as you will want to be able to easily visualize the area vasculature. An incision is made on the central dorsal aspect of the penis from a point 3 cm from the tip and extending 20 cm proximally. With careful dissection, identify the apical ligament and incise through it for its entire length. This incision will expose the tunica albuginea; this is where the fascia or, alternatively, the synthetic mesh implant will be placed. The proximal aspect is placed first, and sutures (2-0 chromic gut) are placed in the corners attaching the implant material to the tunic. Interrupted sutures are then placed on the lateral sides of the implant, stretching the implant so as to avoid crumpling of the tissue. Care is taken to not penetrate too deeply into the tunic and to avoid suture placement that impinges on the

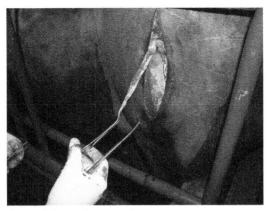

Fig. 10. Fascia lata for graft being harvested.

dorsal vasculature. The distal end of the implant is trimmed if necessary and sutured as previously described.

The edges of the apical ligament are then closed using a No. 0 chromic gut with every other or every third suture engaging the implant (**Fig. 11**). This suture will keep the apical ligament from slipping to the side, which is crucial if correcting a spiral deviation. The elastic tissues and dead space are closed with a continuous suture pattern (3-0 or 4-0 chromic gut), and the skin can be closed with a 0 chromic gut or other dissolvable suture using an interrupted pattern. The incision site is gently rinsed with a dilute Betadine solution; an antibiotic ointment (bovine intramammary infusion medication) is liberally applied; and the penis is returned to the prepuce. Systemic antibiotics are administered for 4 to 5 days, and the penis can be manually extended for examination in 7 to 10 days. Three months of sexual rest is recommended.

A vascular shunt and resultant inability to maintain an erection can follow injury (most commonly penile hematoma). It can be identified by observation of the breeding act or at VBSE when a bull loses an erection while be being electro-stimulated. A blushing of the free portion of the penis is noted as well. A fairly reliable field test is to repeat the electrostimulation following the intracavernosal injection of 40 to 60 mL of methylene blue. This test serves to make the blushing effect more evident. As there is no communication between the corpus cavernosum and the peri-penile

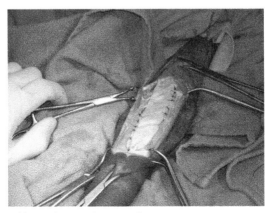

Fig. 11. Placement of fascia lata graft on penis.

vessels in a normal penis, the blue-blushing effect can occur when there is a shunt. Likewise, radiographic contrast material injected in the same manner and followed by radiography can be used.

Repair of single, readily identified and located fistula has been described. Briefly, as the specific condition alluded to results from a previous penile hematoma lesion, the surgical approach is that of the hematoma repair. The edges of the fistula must be excised (freshened) and the defect closed as described for hematoma surgery, as are the tissue layers and skin.

Denervation of the penis occurs following injury and is observed as a bull's inability to achieve intromission. Some bulls, after a period of continued unsuccessful breeding attempts, will stop seeking out and mounting cows. A caution is that attempting to confirm the diagnosis by exposing the distal penis to painful stimuli, most notably an electric cattle prod, does not always produce conclusive results, as neural pathways for pain can exist in the absence of those that allow proprioception. Observation of a breeding attempt is reasonably diagnostic for this condition. A definitive diagnosis can be achieved with electrodiagnostics[25]; however, this procedure is typically reserved for a valuable animal for whom the extra effort is deemed worthwhile. Bulls with denervation can be collected via electroejaculation and used in artificial insemination programs.

SUMMARY

Timely and correct identification of the reproductive maladies described in this article is important to increase the odds of success in treatment and in managing the costs to the producer. Likewise, if there is a poor prognosis for return to function, a decision to cull the animal before antibiotic use and loss of weight can be made. The author thinks that most large animal veterinarians have or can easily acquire the surgical skills to perform the procedures described and do so in a practical and cost-effective manner.

REFERENCES

1. Wolfe DF, Beckett SD, Carson RL. Acquired conditions of the penis and prepuce. In: Wolfe DF, Moll HD, editors. Large animal urogenital surgery. Baltimore (MD): Williams & Wilkins; 1999. p. 237–72.
2. Walker DF. Penile surgery in the bovine: part II. Mod Vet Pract 1979;60:931–4.
3. Noordsy JL. Hematoma of the bovine penis: a technique for predicting successful surgical correction. Vet Med Small Anim Clin 1981;76:1581.
4. Anderson DE. Surgery of the prepuce and penis. Vet Clin North Am Food Anim Pract 2008;24:245–51.
5. St. Jean G. Male reproductive surgery. Vet Clin North Am Food Anim Pract 1995; 11:55–93.
6. Hudson RS. Surgical correction of hematoma of the penis in bulls. In: Williams EI, editor. Proceedings of the American Association of Bovine Practitioners. San Francisco (CA). 1976. p. 67–9.
7. Hopper R, King H, Walters K, et al. Selected surgical conditions of the bovine penis and prepuce. Clin Theriogenology 2012;4(3):339–48.
8. Hudson RS. The effect of penile injuries on the breeding ability of bulls. Proceedings of the Annual Meeting of the Society for Theriogenology. Oklahoma City (OK). 1978. p. 83–6.
9. Wolfe DF. Surgical procedures of the reproductive system of the bull. In: Morrow DA, editor. Current therapy in theriogenology. 2nd edition. Philadelphia: WB Saunders Co; 1986. p. 353–79.

10. Memon MA, Dawson LJ, Usenik EA, et al. Preputial injuries in bulls: 172 cases (1982-1985). J Am Vet Med Assoc 1988;193:481.

11. Lagos F, Fitzhugh HA. Factors influencing preputial prolapse in yearling bulls. J Anim Sci 1970;30:949–52.

12. Wolfe DF. Restorative surgery of the prepuce. In: Hopper RM, editor. Bovine reproduction. Ames (IA): Wiley; 2014. p. 142–54.

13. Ross AD, Entwistle KW. The effect of scrotal insulation on spermatozoal morphology and the rates of spermatogenesis and epididymal passage of spermatozoa in the bull. Theriogenology 1979;11:111–29.

14. Kastelic JP, Cook RB, Coulter GH, et al. Insulating the scrotal neck affects semen quality and scrotal/testicular temperatures in the bull. Theriogenology 1996;45: 935–42.

15. Walters AH, Saacke RG, Pearson RE. Assessment of pronuclear formation following in vitro fertilization with bovine spermatozoa obtained after thermal insulation of the testes. Theriogenology 2006;65:1016–28.

16. Wolfe DF, Hudson RS, Carson RL, et al. Effect of unilateral orchiectomy on semen quality in bulls. J Am Vet Med Assoc 1985;186:1291–3.

17. Ivany JM, Anderson DE, Ayars WH. Diagnosis, surgical treatment, and performance after unilateral castration in breeding bulls: 21 cases (1989-1999). J Am Vet Med Assoc 2002;220:1198–202.

18. Wolfe DF. Unilateral castration for acquired conditions of the scrotum. In: Wolfe DF, Moll HD, editors. Large animal urogenital surgery. 2nd edition. Baltimore (MD): Williams and Wilkins; 1999. p. 313–20.

19. Barth AD. Vesicular adenitis. In: Hopper RM, editor. Bovine reproduction. Ames (IA): Wiley; 2014. p. 109–12.

20. Rovay A, Barth AD, Chirino-Trejo M, et al. Update on treatment of vesiculitis. Theriogenology 2008;70:495–503.

21. Waguespack RW, Schumacher J, Wolfe DF, et al. Preliminary study to evaluate the feasibility of chemical ablation of the seminal vesicles in the bull. In: Smith RA, editor. Proceedings of the 37th Annual Conference of the American Association of Bovine Practitioners. Ft. Worth (TX). 2004. p. 295–6.

22. Martínez MF, Arteaga AA, Barth AD. Intraglandular injection of antibiotics for the treatment of vesicular adenitis in bulls. Anim Reprod Sci 2008;104:201–11.

23. Walker DF. Deviations of the bovine penis. J Am Vet Med Assoc 1964;145: 677–80.

24. Walker DF, Young SL. The fascia lata implant technique for correcting bovine penile deviations. Proceedings of the Society for Theriogenology. Mobile (AL). 1979. p. 99–102.

25. Wolfe DF, Moll HD. Examination and special diagnostic procedures of the penis and prepuce: bulls, rams, and bucks. In: Wolfe DF, Moll HD, editors. Large animal urogenital surgery. Baltimore (MD): Williams and Wilkins; 1998. p. 225–7.

Management and Prevention of Dystocia

Bethany J. Funnell, DVM[a],*, W. Mark Hilton, DVM[a,b]

KEYWORDS

- Dystocia • Heifer • Utrecht method • Malpresentation • Uterine torsion
- Calving ease • Large offspring syndrome

KEY POINTS

- Dystocia is primarily an issue in primiparous females, and the most common cause of dystocia in heifers is fetal oversize.
- Assistance should be early and the delivery process should proceed in a steady and methodical manner to avoid injury to the dam and the neonate.
- Prevention of dystocia can be most effectively accomplished by breeding selection.
- Assisted reproductive technologies can present challenges for the dam during parturition and the calf during the transition to extrauterine life.

 Video content accompanies this article at http://www.vetfood.theclinics.com

INTRODUCTION

Dystocia, defined as difficult birth, is an important economic issue in the both the beef and dairy industry. Consequences of dystocia include increased calf morbidity and mortality, increased cow morbidity and mortality, reduced subsequent fertility in cows, and increased labor. Efforts to minimize dystocia will improve overall herd health and profitability.

Dystocia continues to be an important issue for the cow–calf industry despite an apparent decrease in incidence during the last 20 to 30 years.[1] The National Animal Health Monitoring System in the United States reported a decrease in hard pulls in heifers from 7.4% in 1992-1993 to 3.4% in 2007-2008.[2] During the same period, the percentage of cows requiring assistance at calving, however, did not change.

Disclosure: The authors have nothing to disclose.

[a] Veterinary Clinical Sciences, College of Veterinary Medicine, Purdue University, 625 Harrison Street, West Lafayette, IN 47907, USA; [b] Technical Services Veterinary Consultant, Elanco Animal Health, Greenfield, IN, USA
* Corresponding author.
E-mail address: bfunnell@purdue.edu

RISK FACTORS FOR DYSTOCIA
Fetal-Dam Disparity

Numerous research reports and field trials have examined the risk factors associated with dystocia. In nearly all studies, cow age, or parity, at calving and fetal-dam disparity are listed as the highest risk factors. In a 2002 study in Canada, Waldner[3] looked at 29,970 full-term births from 203 privately owned cow-calf herds with an overall dystocia risk of 8.9%. Odds ratios were calculated for cow age and dystocia (**Table 1**).

In that same study, incidence of dystocia by age was 17.3% for primiparous calving and 2.9% to 4.7% for multiparous cows (Cheryl Waldner, Saskatoon, Saskatchewan, personal communication, 2015) (**Table 2**).

The incidence of calving difficulty in first-calf beef heifers is significantly higher than in mature cows in nearly every study examined when confounding factors are eliminated.[4,5]

In dairy females the incidence of dystocia is also highest in first-calf females. In a study of 666,341 births from 1985 to 1996 in the Midwest United States, the percentage of cows in each of 3 categories (1, no assistance; 2, slight problem; and 3+, needed assistance) is annotated[6] (**Table 3**).

Abnormal Fetal Position

The incidence of malpresentation or malposture is reported to be between 0.91% and 4% of all births in beef cattle, with this factor representing 13% to 22.4% of all dystocias.[7,8] The most common abnormal presentation in beef and dairy cattle is posterior-dorsal followed by foreleg deviations, head deviations, and breech presentations.[7-9] Though fetal malposition occurs at a low incidence (<5% of all births),[4] it is the most common cause of dystocia in multiparous cows, accounting for 20% to 40% of cases.[5] Malpresented calves have a 2 times higher risk of dystocia and a 5 times higher risk of stillbirth.[4] Abnormal fetal position is most common in cases of twin pregnancies (4 times higher risk).[4] If the calf is in an abnormal presentation, position, or posture, any manipulation of the calf needs to be done when the cow is standing. To aid in manipulation of the calf, the cow should be given epidural anesthesia of lidocaine along with an intramuscular injection of 10 mL of 1:1000 epinephrine. The epidural reduces straining by the cow and the epinephrine allows relaxation of the uterus to facilitate fetal manipulations. It takes approximately 2 minutes for the epinephrine to cause relaxation of the uterus and is expected to be effective in most cases. The authors' experience is that it may not be as effective if the calf has been dead for an extended period of time.

Using obstetric lubricant is indicated on all cases of assisted delivery, especially when a malpresentation is involved. Lubricant diluted with warm water can be

Table 1			
Herd-adjusted final multivariable model of the association between cow attributes and the odds of dystocia in calving season 2002 (n = 29,970 calves and N = 270 herds)			
Cow Age Category	Odds Ratio	95% CI	P-Value
Bred replacement heifer	6.52	5.80–7.34	.00001
3 y old (2nd calf)	1.64	1.42–1.88	.00001
4 y old (3rd calf)	1.24	1.06–1.46	.01
Mature cows (5–10 y)	reference category		
Cow age ≥10 y	1.06	0.86–1.30	.61

Table 2
Incidence of dystocia by age: 29,970 full-term births

Cow Age Category	Risk	95% CI
Bred replacement heifer	17.3%	10.9–26.4
3 y old (2nd calf)	4.7%	2.8–7.9
4 y old (3rd calf)	3.7%	2.2–6.3
Mature cow (5–10 y)	2.9%	1.7–4.9
Cow age >10 y	3.2%	1.9–5.6

pumped into the uterus to not only add needed lubrication but also to expand the uterus to aid in manipulation of the calf. One word of caution is to not use a polyethylene oxide lubricant (J-Lube, Jorgensen Laboratories, Loveland, CO, USA) if there is any chance of a Caesarian section because intra-abdominal exposure has caused death in rats, horses, and cattle.[10]

If the cow is down and unable to rise, hip lifters can be used to raise the hindquarters and decrease interabdominal pressure to allow manipulation of the calf. An alternative method that will allow some manipulation of the calf is to pull both hind legs of the cow straight out behind her. This tips the pelvis forward and may allow manipulation of the calf into the correct position before delivery.

Vulval, Vaginal, or Cervical Stenosis

Incomplete dilation of the vulva and/or vagina can be a cause of dystocia in primiparous animals, whereas cervical stenosis can happen in multiparous animals. These conditions have been associated with confinement and periparturient environmental stress, premature assistance, hormonal asynchrony, and preterm calving.[4] See later discussion of techniques to dilate the vulva or vagina. Dilation of the cervix is not possible in a timely fashion and surgical intervention is likely necessary.

Uterine Torsion

Although torsion of the uterus is more common in the bovine than in other domestic species, it is still an uncommon cause of dystocia (primarily in multiparous cows) accounting for only 5% to 10% of dystocia cases.[11,12] The intermediate risk factors are excessive fetal movement during stage 1 of calving as the fetus adopts the birth posture, increased uterine instability at term, and possibly a deeper abdomen in some dairy breeds. Ultimate risk factors include fetal oversize and gender, fetal debility, and insufficient exercise.[9,11] A study from the University of Montreal and Cornell University found that uterine torsions are involved in 20% of cases of dystocia in dairy practice. It is hypothesized that this higher incidence is due, in part, to the ability of the farm staff to handle other cases of dystocia more effectively, although still requiring veterinary assistance for uterine torsions.[13]

Table 3
Percent of dairy females by parity in relation to calving assistance needed

Category	Records	Dystocia Score		
		1	2	3+
Primiparous females	167,472	71.4	9.6	19.0
Multiparous females	498,869	89.3	4.7	6.0

TREATMENT OF DYSTOCIA

Even when plans are in place to limit dystocia risk to an acceptable level (<15% for heifers, <5% for cows),[14] there are still cases of dystocia in beef and dairy herds. One of the most important fundamentals for optimum dystocia management is for the owner to know when to intervene or call for assistance. Charts are published that describe the expected duration of each stage of labor.[15] Stage 2 begins when fetal parts enter the birth canal and references give time frames of up to 4 hours. Veterinarians encounter many instances of clients waiting too long to call for assistance on a case of difficult birth and it is the authors' experience that clients who have read that stage 2 can take up to 4 hours may wait at least that long to see if the female can deliver the calf without assistance. The goal for the veterinarian is to deliver a live, healthy calf from a live, healthy female and have the dam breed back in a timely fashion. To help achieve this goal, the easy to remember rule of "progress every hour" was initiated into private practice (W. Mark Hilton, DVM, West Lafayette, IN, personal communication, 2015). If an unassisted birth is to occur, the owner should see progress every hour (ie, amniotic sac visible at 7:00 AM, feet by 8:00 AM, delivery by 9:00 AM). If not, the female should be examined or the herd health veterinarian should be called. After instituting the 1 hour recommendation, success increased dramatically. In a research study in Holstein cows and heifers, the recommendation was that intervention needed to occur within 70 minutes of the appearance of the amniotic sac.[16]

If veterinarians are surveyed to determine the best way to deliver a calf, the results will surely vary. In a natural setting, a cow lies down in lateral recumbency as she expels the calf and this is the basis of the Utrecht method of delivery. Proper execution of this technique will reduce the incidence of trauma to the calf and/or dam, and result in improved success with a low-stress delivery, a healthier calf, and a healthier dam.

The keys to the Utrecht method are:

1. Dilation of the birth canal
2. Manipulating the calf (if needed) into the correct position for delivery while the cow is standing.
3. Casting the cow in lateral recumbency
4. Applying traction only when the cow has a contraction and actively pushes.

Before dilation of the birth canal, the vulva and perineal area is thoroughly cleaned with an appropriate disinfectant (dilute iodine or chlorhexidine based solutions). In nearly all cases, it is helpful to manually dilate the vulva and vagina, especially in heifers. Dilation is accomplished 1 of 2 ways. The first method is to place both gloved, lubricated arms deep into the birth canal, clasp one's fingers together, and expand one's arms laterally. The second method is to place 1 gloved, lubricated hand on top of the calf's head and lift dorsally by extending one's ankles. In each case, progress is usually made in 2 to 3 minutes. Dilating the birth canal is time well spent because the chance of trauma to the cow and calf is now greatly reduced (Video 1).

If dilation of the birth canal and initiation of the Utrecht method of delivery is potentially dangerous due to the disposition of the female, sedation of the cow will be necessary. A reliable choice is to use a ketamine stun, in which ketamine is added to a more traditional chemical restraint combination. For a standing stun for a 500 kg (1100 lb) cow, Abrahamsen[17] suggests the 5-10-20 technique, in which the female is given 5 mg butorphanol (0.01 mg/kg), 10 mg xylazine (0.02 mg/kg), and 20 mg ketamine (0.04 mg/kg) mixed in the same syringe. This combination can be given intravenously, intramuscularly, or subcutaneously, with longest duration provided by the latter route.

It is at this point that the initial assessment of whether the calf has a reasonable chance of being delivered vaginally is done. In an anterior dorsal, frontwards delivery, if the front feet of the fetus are crossed, this is a sign of fetal-dam disparity. The feet are crossed because the shoulders are wedged into the maternal pelvis forcing the legs or feet medially. Additionally, Mortimer[18] reports, in an anterior presentation, if the fetlock can be extended 10 cm beyond the vulva, there is a reasonable chance of vaginal delivery. If it appears there is adequate room and vaginal delivery is possible, assistance should continue. If there is little or no chance of a vaginal delivery, surgical methods need to be evaluated. Although it is common to have a cow in a chute for the vaginal examination, dilation of the vulva or vagina, placement of the chains, and placement of the rope for casting, delivery should only be attempted if both sides of the chute open.

To assist a vaginal delivery, chains are placed on the legs of the calf using the double half hitch method. The proximal loop needs to be placed at the narrowest part of the metacarpus so that the chain does not slip down the leg when forced extraction ensues. The distal loop is now placed between the dewclaws and the hoof insuring that the part of the chain running parallel to the leg and between the 2 loops is taut (**Fig. 1**).

A soft lariat is now placed around the cow using the half-hitch or Burley method so the cow can be cast on her side (**Fig. 2**).

While 1 person pulls on the rope, the other should apply traction to the chains with obstetric handles. The process of applying pressure to the chains seems to stimulate the cow to contract, which makes casting her with the rope easier.

As the cow goes down she will initially lie sternal. Keep tension on the lariat or tie it off so it remains taut. Allow the cow to remain in sternal recumbency for about 30 seconds, then pull on the portion of the rope that is running horizontally down her back and ease the cow into lateral recumbency. Do not loosen the halter or the lariat because she may then jump up (Video 2).

Having the cow in lateral recumbency seems to stimulate contractions and this position has the additional advantage of allowing the pelvis to tilt slightly to aid in delivery. When initiating the delivery process, it is important to pull straight back and to apply traction only when the cow pushes. Numerous references give the recommendation of using no more force than can be applied by 2 strong people. Fetal extractors can and should be used while keeping in mind that they can exert an extreme amount of pressure. The ideal method is to alternate traction on each of the forelimbs until the shoulders have passed through the maternal pelvis, then simultaneous traction

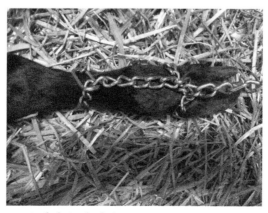

Fig. 1. Proper placement of obstetric chains.

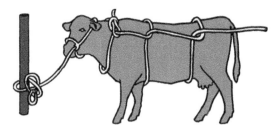

Fig. 2. The Burley method. (*Adapted from* Murray F. Restraint and handling of wild and domestic animals. 3rd edition. New York: Wiley; 2009.)

on both forelimbs is applied.[19] When the calf is in anterior presentation, the assistant should pause when the cow rests. It is very important to not rush the delivery. In nature, the cow delivers the calf lying down and will generally take a break after the shoulders of the calf have passed through the maternal pelvis. When using forced extraction, allowing the cow to rest will allow the calf to rotate slightly so that the calf does not become hip locked, and will also allow the calf to start breathing. If delivery assistance of calves in an anterior presentation is rushed, the calf does not have a chance to rotate and hip lock can be a complication (Video 3).

If the calf is in a posterior presentation, the calf needs to be delivered within 1 to 2 minutes after the calf's pelvis passes through the cow's pelvis so that the calf does not suffocate. The backwards calf does not stimulate the vagina to dilate as effectively as does the forward-presented calf due to the lack of a conical shape. Because of this, the time spent dilating the vagina is vitally important in the overall success of the deliver process.

There will be instances when a vaginal delivery is not possible and an alternative method is necessary. If the calf is alive, performing a Cesarean section is the best option and the success of the surgery is highly dependent on how quickly this decision is made after an unsuccessful attempt at vaginal delivery. If the calf is dead, performing a fetotomy is more appropriate.

Respiratory Assessment or Support for the Neonate

After delivery, the calf should be immediately placed in sternal recumbency, and if the calf is not ventilating adequately, respiratory stimulation should be initiated. This stimulation may be accomplished by inserting a slightly rigid material into the nostril and gently contacting the nasal mucosa, stimulating the calf to gasp,[20] and should be repeated until the calf is ventilating regularly. A sublingual injection of 20 mg of doxapram hydrochloride (1 mL) may also aid in initiating spontaneous respiration if a calf is struggling to take a breath. A calf resuscitator or an endotracheal tube can also be used to aid the calf in the process of inflating its lungs.

Calves that are clones (somatic cell nuclear transfer [SCNT]) are particularly challenged by respiratory issues and require a significant amount of support. This may include supplemental oxygen and even positive pressure ventilation. Blood gas analysis should be done periodically, to assess the efficacy of the intervention.[21]

Injuries to the Neonate

After respiration is completely spontaneous, the calf should be assessed for injuries. The strength of 2 strong people pulling simultaneously can cause significant bruising and potentially fracture of the bones of the calf. A fetal extractor, or calf jack, can exert much greater forces and, if used improperly, can easily cause damage to either the dam or the fetus. Fractures can be quite painful and the calf will be reluctant or unable to stand and nurse, and will require additional care. Fractures of the limbs distal to the carpus or tarsus should be splinted and closely monitored to assess adequacy of circulation to the fractured limb. The attitude of the calf (appetite, ability, or interest in standing or walking) can be a good indicator of a potential problem under a bandage or splint that may require reevaluation.[22] Fractures of other long bones can often be difficult, at best, to manage on the farm. These calves should either be referred to a specialty practice or teaching hospital for treatment or euthanized.[23]

Femoral nerve paralysis can potentially result from a hip lock or stifle lock situation, and this injury may not be readily apparent immediately after delivery. Calves that have difficulty rising should be kept in a clean, well-bedded stall, and afforded nutritional support until full examination can be accomplished.[24]

In the case of a protracted delivery, the neonate may suffer from hypoxia and may require supportive therapy. These calves will often be slow to rise, have minimal to absent suckle reflex, and will require additional assistance to make the transition to extrauterine life.[22]

Injuries to the Dam

After delivery of a calf, the astute practitioner will always palpate the dam's uterus to be certain that there are no additional calves to be delivered. This also allows the veterinarian the opportunity to assess the reproductive tract of the dam. The uterine wall, cervix, vestibule, and vulva should be thoroughly evaluated, to make certain there are no ruptures or lacerations from fetal parts. Injuries should be treated appropriately, which may include repairs, systemic therapeutics, or benign observed neglect, based on severity, labor resources on the farm, and risk for additional complications.

PREVENTION OF DYSTOCIA

Preventing dystocia, particularly in first-calf heifers, is a very important component of a successful reproductive program on any dairy or beef operation. Many factors can play a role in the incidence of dystocia and researchers have reported conflicting results associated with efforts to decrease dystocia. These topics are discussed briefly because a full discussion is beyond the realm of this article.

Sire Selection

Sire selection can have 1 of the most dramatic effects of the dystocia risk in any herd and in any breed. The sire will contribute to the growth of the fetus from a genetic standpoint but there are also reported epigenetic influences of the sire on fetal fluid weight, umbilical cord weight and length, and umbilical and placental efficiency (nutrient delivery to fetus).[25] The full extent to which the sire influences fetal birthweight are yet to be elucidated; however, there are valuable tools currently available to producers that help identify sires that will produce calves that are less likely to cause dystocia.

As previously discussed, fetal-dam disparity is the most common cause of dystocia and this type of dystocia occurs to a greater extent in first-calf heifers.[6,9] The size of the fetus, or fetal birthweight, is the single greatest influencing factor contributing to dystocia due to fetal-dam disparity.[26,27] Expected progeny differences (EPDs) have long been used as a tool to identify bulls that are likely to sire calves with low risk of dystocia. Birth weight EPDs can be used to predict the size of a sire's calves compared with other bulls and is thus an indirect measure of calving ease. Another EPD tool is calving ease direct, a figure calculated based on the percentage of a bull's calves born to first calf heifers that do not require assistance during calving and thus is a direct measure of calving ease.[28] Gestation length may influence this figure because it is highly heritable (0.61–0.64),[28] though differences in average gestation lengths between breeds are not large (279–292 days).[29,30] As gestation proceeds, the fetus continues to grow, and calves with longer gestations also have larger birth weights. By selecting cattle (male and female) for calving ease, the producer must be prepared for calves to be born early. It is not uncommon for heifers to calve up to 2 weeks before their predicted due date when bred to a calving ease sire and, in some spring calving conditions, the first calf born is often unexpected and can be at significant risk for hypothermia before it is found and given appropriate attention.

Other strategies that have been used in an attempt to decrease dystocia include crossbreeding to bulls of smaller statured breeds, or using X-sorted semen for the production of heifer calves, which typically have a shorter gestation and lighter birthweight than bull calves.[5]

Heifer Selection

Heifer selection can use the same EPD tools as bulls; however, the accuracy of EPD for females are very low because very little data is generated by each cow in her lifetime. Genetic selection for heifers can be more efficiently and effectively accomplished by the utilization or evaluation of the sire's EPDs. For instance, the calving ease maternal EPD is an estimate of the percentage of a bull's daughters that will not require assistance at their first calving. This figure can be used as an aid in the selection of a bull that would be appropriate to sire replacement heifers.[28]

Heifer Development

Proper heifer development is very important, not only for early attainment of puberty and life-long reproductive efficiency but also for the prevention of dystocia. A heifer that is not properly developed may not attain sufficient prepartum growth to successfully deliver her first calf (For a more detailed discussion on beef and dairy heifer development, please see Larson RL, White BJ, Laflin S: Beef Heifer Development and Akins MS: Dairy Heifer Development and Nutrition Management, in this issue.)

Nutrition

It is logical that producers can influence calf birth weight by manipulating dam nutrition; therefore, dystocia should be able to be decreased by the same means. However, there are many conflicting reports regarding the influence of nutrition on the incidence of dystocia. In extreme situations, both of nutrient excess and nutrient restriction during the third trimester (when the fetus is at its maximum growth rate), dystocia risk may be elevated significantly. Gunn and colleagues[31] showed an increase in calf birth weight and an increase in dystocia in heifers that were fed a nutrient dense ration (specifically excess protein) during the third trimester. In addition to a larger fetus, an excessively conditioned heifer will theoretically carry a larger amount of fat in her pelvis, which decreases the diameter of the pelvic inlet, and can cause dystocia. In some cases, the wall of the vagina may rupture and perivaginal fat will accompany the calf during delivery.

In contrast, a significantly underconditioned heifer (due to severe third trimester nutritional restriction) will lack the energy to deliver a calf in a timely fashion. In addition, the first-calf heifer has significant nutrient demands for growth, maintenance, and lactation, and late gestation nutrient restriction will delay her return to cyclicity. An anestrous 2-year old may not have an opportunity to breed back in the subsequent breeding season, thus her future fertility and longevity are at significant risk.[5,32] These conflicting findings suggest that manipulation of third trimester nutrition to decrease the incidence of dystocia may be an exercise in futility.[33,34]

Some investigators have suggested that early gestation nutrition may have greater impact on birthweight than late gestation nutrition. The theory is that the placenta is a very dynamic organ that responds to subtleties in the maternal environment in ways that compensate for inadequacies. For instance, cows fed an energy restricted diet in early gestation had a heavier placenta than those that were fed an energy adequate diet.[26] Additionally, ewes fed high levels of nonprotein nitrogen in the form of urea during early pregnancy had extended gestation lengths and delivered significantly larger lambs.[35–37]

ASSISTED REPRODUCTIVE TECHNOLOGIES

Assisted reproductive technologies (ARTs) are being incorporated in the bovine industries at a rapid rate. Specifically, in vitro production (IVP) of embryos, and cloning have gained considerable steam in the last decade.[38] These ARTs have historically been fraught with challenges. Indeed, the commercial acceptance of IVP was limited by the amount and degree of embryonic losses and fetal abnormalities that were often the result.[39] Though the culprits for the major aberrations observed in the IVP process have presumably been identified,[37,39,40] there are still challenges facing both IVP and SCNT technologies.

Large Offspring Syndrome

Large offspring syndrome has been used loosely to describe calves born as a result of IVP and SCNT that are larger than normal in birth weight. With the development of more clearly defined culture media, the incidence of abnormal offspring has decreased, with some major abnormalities nearly eliminated.[41] As a general rule, the birth weights of IVP calves born today more closely approximate those of breed averages, with a wider range of birth weights observed with IVP calves when compared with their artificial insemination cohorts.[42] Occasional exceptionally large calves can still be born as a result of IVP, but the more common abnormality with IVP calves is an enlarged umbilicus. The enlarged umbilicus presents its own set of challenges because hemorrhage must be controlled at birth. The enlarged vessels will require very close attention after delivery to prevent and manage the navel ill that IVP calves are prone to developing.[21]

Occasionally, an IVP pregnancy will progress beyond the normal gestation length, resulting in a larger birthweight calf. Interestingly, in some cases, the recipient female shows minimal signs of impending parturition (lack of colostrum deposition in the udder, minimal vulvar swelling, and relaxation). In these cases, parturition should be induced. If the pregnancy is allowed to continue, often the fetus expires before calving, whereas a live calf can often be delivered if parturition is induced by 280 days of gestation (FX Grand, St. Hyacinthe, Quebec, CA, personal communication, 2015).

Supportive therapy is often of critical importance for survival of IVP or SCNT calves. Oxygen supplementation may be warranted and certainly preventative antibiotic therapy should be used to protect the at-risk neonate from navel ill. At-risk calves may also be weak or slow to stand, and colostrum may need to be administered via esophageal tube. There is often a significant financial investment in each IVF or SCNT calf, so every effort should be made to give the calf the best opportunity to transition to extrauterine life.[21]

SUPPLEMENTARY DATA

Supplementary data related to this article can be found at http://dx.doi.org/10.1016/j.cvfa.2016.01.016.

REFERENCES

1. United States Department of Agriculture (USDA), Beef 2007-08. Part V: reference of beef cow–calf management practices in the United States 2007–08; 2010. p. 16. Available at: https://www.aphis.usda.gov/animal_health/nahms/beefcowcalf/downloads/beef0708/Beef0708_dr_PartV.pdf. Accessed September 14, 2015.
2. United States Department of Agriculture (USDA), Beef 2007–08. Part III: Changes in the U.S. beef cow–calf industry, 1993–2008; 2010. p. 63. Available at: https://www.aphis.usda.gov/animal_health/nahms/beefcowcalf/downloads/beef0708/Beef0708_dr_PartIII.pdf. Accessed September 14, 2015.
3. Waldner CL. Cow attributes, herd management and environmental factors associated with the risk of calf death at or within 1h of birth and the risk of dystocia in cow–calf herds in Western Canada. Livest Sci 2014;163:126–39.
4. Mee JF. Prevalence and risk factors for dystocia in dairy cattle: a review. Vet J 2008;176(1):93–101.
5. Meijering A. Dystocia and stillbirth in cattle – a review of causes, relations and implications. Livest Prod Sci 1984;11:143–77.
6. Meyer CL, Berger PJ, Koehler KJ, et al. Phenotypic trends in incidence of stillbirth for Holsteins in the United States. J Dairy Sci 2001;84(2):515–23.
7. Holland MD, Speer NC, LeFever DG, et al. Factors contributing to dystocia due to fetal malpresentation in beef cattle. Theriogenology 1993;39(4):899–908.
8. Nix JM, Spitzer JC, Grimes LW, et al. A retrospective analysis of factors contributing to calf mortality and dystocia in beef cattle. Theriogenology 1998;49(8):1515–23.
9. Ahmad N, Al-Eknah MM, Christie WB, et al. Dystocia and other disorders associated with parturition - general considerations. In: Noakes DE, Parkinson TJ, England GCW, et al, editors. Arthur's veterinary reproduction and obstetrics. 8th edition. Philadelphia: WB Saunders; 2001. p. 205–17.
10. Frazer GS, Beard WL, Abrahamsen E, et al. Systemic effects of peritoneal instillation of a polyethylene polymer based obstetrical lubricant in horses. In: Wolfe D, editor. Proceedings of the Annual Conference of the Society for Theriogenology. Lexington (KY): 2004. p. 93–7.
11. Frazer GS, Perkins NR, Constable PD. Bovine uterine torsion: 164 hospital referral cases. Theriogenology 1996;46:739–58.
12. Laven R, Howe M. Uterine torsion in cattle in the UK. Vet Rec 2005;157:96.
13. Aubry P, Warnick LD, DesCoteaux L, et al. A study of 55 field cases of uterine torsion in dairy cattle. Can Vet J 2008;49:366–72.
14. Spire MF. Cow/calf production records: justification, gathering and interpretation. Proc Am Assoc Bov Pract 1990;23:93–5.
15. Roberts SJ. Veterinary obstetrics and genital diseases (theriogenology). Woodstock (VT): The Author; 1971.
16. Schuenemann GM, Nieto I, Bas S, et al. Assessment of calving progress and reference times for obstetric intervention during dystocia in Holstein dairy cows. J Dairy Sci 2011;94(11):5494–501.
17. Abrahamsen EJ. Ruminant field anesthesia. Vet Clin North Am Food Anim Pract 2008;24(3):429–41.
18. Mortimer RG. Calving and handling calving difficulties. In: Calving management manual. 2009. Available at: http://www.cvmbs.colostate.edu/ilm/projects/neonatal/Calving%20and%20Handling%20Calving%20Difficulties.pdf. Accessed September 14, 2015.

19. Becker M, Tsousis G, Lüpke M, et al. Extraction forces in bovine obstetrics: an in vitro study investigating alternate and simultaneous traction modes. Theriogenology 2010;73(8):1044–50.

20. van Wagtendonk-de Leeuw AM, Mullaart E, de Roos APW, et al. Effects of different reproduction techniques: AI, MOET, or IVP on health and welfare of bovine offspring. Theriogenology 2000;53:575–97.

21. Brisville AC, Fecteau G, Boysen S, et al. Neonatal morbidity and mortality of 31 calves derived from somatic cloning. J Vet Intern Med 2013;27:1218–27.

22. Murray CF, Leslie KE. Newborn calf vitality: risk factors, characteristics, assessment, resulting outcomes, and strategies for improvement. Vet J 2013;198:322–8.

23. Ferguson JG. Surgical conditions of the proximal limb. In: Greenough PR, Weaver AD, editors. Lameness in cattle. 3rd edition. Philadelphia: WB Saunders; 1997. p. 271–2.

24. Smith-Maxie L. Diseases of the nervous system. In: Greenough PR, Weaver AD, editors. Lameness in cattle. 3rd edition. Philadelphia: WB Saunders; 1997. p. 209–10.

25. Xiang R, Estrella CAS, Fitzsimmons CJ, et al. Magnitude and specificity of effects of maternal and paternal genomes on the feto-maternal unit [abstract: 97]. In: Martin G, editor. Reproduction, Fertility, and Development: Proceedings of The International Embryo Transfer Society. Versailles (France): CSIRO Publishing; 2015. p. 141.

26. Rice LE. Dystocia related risk factors. Vet Clin North Am Food Anim Pract 1994; 10:53–68.

27. Arthur PF, Archer JA, Melville GJ. Factors influencing dystocia and prediction of dystocia in Angus heifers selected for yearling growth rate. Aust J Agric Res 2000;51:147–53.

28. American Angus Association. EPD and $Value definitions. Available at: http://www.angus.org/Nce/Definitions.aspx. Accessed August 28, 2015.

29. Crews DH Jr. Age of dam and sex of calf adjustments and genetic parameters for gestation length in Charolais cattle. J Anim Sci 2006;84:25–31.

30. Joubert DM, Hammond J. A crossbreeding experiment with cattle, with special reference to the maternal effect in South Devon-Dexter crosses. J Agr Sci 1958;51:325–41.

31. Gunn PJ, Schoonmaker JP, Lemenager RP, et al. Feeding excess crude protein to gestating and lactating beef heifers: impact on parturition, milk composition, ovarian function, reproductive efficiency and pre-weaning progeny growth. Livest Sci 2014;167:435–88.

32. Bell AW. Maternal nutrition, other factors affect birth weight. Feedstuffs 2005;77: 10–2.

33. Funston R. Nutrition and reproduction interactions. In: Proceedings, Applied Reproductive Strategies in Beef Cattle. San Antonio (TX): 2010. p. 175–91.

34. Hickson RE, Morris ST, Kenyon PR, et al. Dystocia in beef heifers: a review of genetic and nutritional influences. N Z Vet J 2006;54(6):256–64.

35. Wallace JM, Regnault TRH, Limesand SW, et al. Investigating the causes of low birth weight in contrasting ovine paradigms. J Physiol 2005;565:19–26.

36. McEvoy TG, Robinson JJ, Aitken PA, et al. Dietary excesses of urea influence the viability and metabolism of preimplantation sheep embryos and may affect fetal growth among survivors. Anim Reprod Sci 1997;47:71–90.

37. Young LE, Sinclair KD, Wilmut I. Large offspring syndrome in cattle and sheep. Rev Reprod 1998;3:155–63.

38. Perry GA. International Embryo Transfer Society Data Retrieval Committee: 2013 statistics of embryo collection and transfer in domestic farm animals. 2014

Available at: http://www.iets.org/pdf/comm_data/December2014.pdf. Accessed August 28, 2015.

39. van Wagtendonk-de Leeuw AM, Aerts BJG, den Daas JHG. Abnormal offspring following in vitro production of bovine preimplantation embryos: a field study. Theriogenology 1998;49:883–94.

40. Hill JR. Incidence of abnormal offspring from cloning and other assisted reproductive technologies. Annu Rev Anim Biosci 2014;2:307–21.

41. Constant F, Guillomot M, Heyman Y, et al. Large offspring or large placenta syndrome? Morphometric analysis of late gestation bovine placentomes from somatic nuclear transfer pregnancies complicated by hydrallantois. Biol Reprod 2006;75:122–30.

42. Bonilla L, Block J, Denicol AC, et al. Consequences of transfer of an in vitro-produced embryo for the dam and resultant calf. J Dairy Sci 2014;97:229–39.

Index

Note: Page numbers of article titles are in **boldface** type.

A

Abnormal fetal position
 dystocia related to, 512–513
Abortion
 diagnosis of, 430
Adenitis
 vesicular
  in bulls, 505–506
Advanced reproductive technologies
 in embryo transfer, 383
Age
 as factor in beef heifer puberty development, 286–290
Anestrous
 postpartum
  infertility in cattle related to, 337
Anovulation
 in dairy cows
  management of, 397–399
Antibody detection in sentinels
 in diagnosis of viral diseases of reproductive importance, 428–429
Artificial insemination
 fixed-timed
  in beef cattle
   in reducing breeding season length and its effects on subsequent calf value, 342–345
 in beef cattle, **335–347**
  economic implications of combining with estrous synchronization, 341–342
  introduction, 335–356
 in dairy herds, **349–364**
  for replacement dairy heifers, 360–362
  introduction, 349–350
  repeat service programs for lactating dairy cows, 357–359
   early not pregnancy diagnosis, 357
   presynchronization before resynchronization, 357–359
  timed programs before first services for lactating cows, 350–357
   Ovsynch, 350–351
   presynchronization five-day programs, 354–355
   presynchronization gonadotropin-releasing hormone programs, 353–354
   presynchronization prostaglandin $F_{2\alpha}$ PROGRAMS, 351–353
   programs including progesterone, 355–357

Vet Clin Food Anim 32 (2016) 523–534
http://dx.doi.org/10.1016/S0749-0720(16)30021-4
0749-0720/16/$ – see front matter

Moving?

Make sure your subscription moves with you!

To notify us of your new address, find your **Clinics Account Number** (located on your mailing label above your name), and contact customer service at:

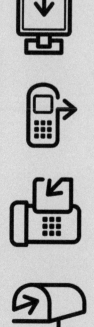

Email: journalscustomerservice-usa@elsevier.com

800-654-2452 (subscribers in the U.S. & Canada)
314-447-8871 (subscribers outside of the U.S. & Canada)

Fax number: 314-447-8029

Elsevier Health Sciences Division
Subscription Customer Service
3251 Riverport Lane
Maryland Heights, MO 63043

*To ensure uninterrupted delivery of your subscription, please notify us at least 4 weeks in advance of move.